ANIMAL WELFARE AND MEAT SCIENCE

NEVILLE G. GREGORY

AGMARDT Professor of Animal Welfare Science, Massey University, Palmerston North, New Zealand

and a chapter by

TEMPLE GRANDIN

Assistant Professor of Animal Science, Colorado State University, Fort Collins, Colorado 80523, USA

CABI *Publishing*

CABI *Publishing* – a division of CAB INTERNATIONAL

CABI *Publishing*
CAB INTERNATIONAL
Wallingford
Oxon OX10 8DE
UK

Tel: +44 (0)1491 832111
Fax: +44 (0)1491 833508
Email: cabi@cabi.org

CABI *Publishing*
10 E 40th Street
Suite 3203
New York, NY 10016
USA

Tel: +1 212 481 7018
Fax: +1 212 686 7993
Email: cabi-nao@cabi.org

A catalogue record for this book is available from the British Library, London, UK.

Library of Congress Cataloging-in-Publication Data
Gregory, Neville G.
Animal welfare and meat science / by Neville G. Gregory : with guest chapter by Temple Grandin.
p. cm.
Includes bibliographical references and index.
ISBN 0–85199–296–X (alk. paper)
1. Animal welfare. 2. Slaughtering and slaughter-houses.
I. Grandin, Temple. II. Title.
HV4731.G74 1998
636.08'32—dc 21
98–25756
CIP

ISBN 0 85199 296 X

Typeset in 10pt Garamond by Columns Design Ltd, Reading
Printed and bound in the UK at the University Press, Cambridge

Contents

Preface

The origins of an organized meat industry date back to the beginning of the 14th century. The first European public abattoirs were built at about that time and their purpose was to slaughter the large number of animals that became available in the late autumn and early winter months. Much of the meat was salted and stored in casks, whilst some was smoked or dry fermented. The animals arrived at the abattoirs on foot, and in some cases they walked long distances before reaching their destination. The traditional methods of meat production and slaughter at that time had some ugly features. For example, 400 years ago British butchers were required by law to bait bulls with dogs before slaughter. Bull baiting helped to make the meat more tender. Thankfully, that practice is now illegal. Society is now very sensitive to malpractices such as this, and there is increasing concern for those animals which are unable to protect themselves or improve their own conditions because of constraints imposed by farming, transport and abattoir conditions. There is concern about some practices which are done to improve product quality but may be considered unnecessary, such as force-feeding geese, castrating pigs and swimwashing sheep. There is also abhorrence for most forms of intentional injury to animals. The principle that underlies these concerns is one of being fair and reasonable to animals. It is held that we have a duty of care to animals that are under our control. At the other extreme some people take the view that life is not fair, and so whether they or anyone else are unfair to animals does not concern them.

The problem that faces modern society is in knowing, agreeing and deciding about what is fair and reasonable. There are widely differing views on whether it is fair to:

- remove baby chicks and calves from their mothers;
- breed animals with physical features that create problems with parturition, breathing, exercise and joint pain;
- confine animals in pens or cages;
- kill animals without any form of stunning.

It will take time before we come to agree on these issues, and there are three ways in which changes in attitude will come about. Legislation will force some changes. For example, legislators in the USA will probably soon decide that chickens should be stunned before they are killed in processing plants, and they will make the appropriate modifications to the law. Changes will also occur because people in charge of animals will modify their attitudes about what is fair and reasonable. Thirdly, changes will occur when it is recognized that there is profit in taking good care of animals. The profit motive is a particularly effective way of bringing about change. Part of the profit motive for being fair to animals rests in the assumption that good welfare is good for meat quality. This book brings together the evidence that lies behind that assumption.

Neville G. Gregory
Massey University
Palmerston North
New Zealand

List of Synonyms

The meat and livestock industry uses many jargon words, and these are apt to cause confusion. Quite often there is more than one word which means the same thing. For example, in many parts of the world a hogget would be the term used for a two-tooth sheep, but in some English-speaking regions it would be known as a teg, gimmer or chilver. The following list summarizes some of the synonyms which crop up in this book.

Auction market – saleyard
Blood splash – ecchymoses, petechial haemorrhages
Cardiac arrest stunning – stun-kill, head-to-back stunning, head-to-leg stunning
Counting-out pen – count-out pen, unloading pen, first holding pen
Electric goads – electric prods, hot shots
Electric stunner – electrolethaler
Exsanguination – sticking, neck cutting, killing, bleeding out
Forcing pens – crowding pens
Haulier – trucker, lorry driver
Humane killer – captive-bolt gun
Lairage – holding pens, stockyards
Mob – group, flock, herd
Mustering – gathering
Rig – cryptorchid, short-scrotum castrate
Slaughterhall – killing floor, slaughterboard
Slaughterhouse – abattoir, freezerworks, meatworks, processing plant
Tenderstretch – hip suspension
Truck – lorry, transporter
Weasand – oesophagus, gullet.

Chapter 1

Animal Welfare and the Meat Market

The novelist John Galsworthy once wrote:

> Butchers and slaughtermen perform a necessary task from which most of us would shrink, and it is unbecoming and nonsensical to suggest intentional cruelty on their part. I do not for a moment. But I do say that it is the business of the law so to control the methods of slaughter as to obviate, as far as possible, needless suffering, however unintentionally it may be inflicted.

Many of us would probably agree with these sentiments, and we would go further in saying that there should be effective control and prevention of needless suffering in almost all aspects of animal handling and husbandry (Rollin, 1997). This is the basic reason for studying and for being concerned about animal welfare.

WHAT IS ANIMAL WELFARE?

Animal welfare is a concern for animal suffering and for animal satisfaction. Animal welfare science is the science of animal suffering and animal satisfaction. Neither suffering nor satisfaction can be measured directly, but the consequences of different causes of suffering and satisfaction can be compared in various ways. For example, animal welfare scientists have found that it is more stressful physiologically for a lamb to have its tail docked with a knife than with a rubber ring (Lester *et al.*, 1996), and that it is more satisfying for a sow confined in a stall or farrowing crate to have snout contact with a neighbouring sow than to be in total isolation. One way of evaluating different causes of suffering is to measure the animal's stress responses. A *stress response* is a physiological reaction in an animal to threatening or harmful situations. *Distress* is the emotional state that is created by the threatening or harmful situations. For example, distress would include the fear that causes some animals to shake uncontrollably when confronted with the novel sounds and situations at an auction market or abattoir. *Suffering* is a less precise term. Humans suffer in many different ways, including sickness, anxiety, fear, emotional deprivation, and through cold, heat, physical discomfort, pain, extreme thirst or hunger. No doubt animals also experience these feelings, which in extreme situations cause suffering.

Some people adopt the view that society is largely to blame for animal suffering. 'We have stuffed it up' is a phrase I hear from students. However, not all forms of suffering are caused by humans. We have no control over the weather, although we may be in a position to try to protect animals from adverse weather. We do not have good control over all diseases, and these are a major cause of suffering in livestock. In many cases, where humans are to blame for suffering it has not been inflicted on purpose. Instead, it has occurred as a by-product of some other motive or aim. For example, it was inexperience by the broiler breeding companies that led to leg disorders and lameness in the modern broiler chicken; it was not intentional.

In practice there are four situations where humans have some responsibility for animal suffering, and these are known as the *Four I's.* They are:

- **Ignorance** – not knowing what to do.
- **Inexperience** – knowing what to do but not knowing how to do it.
- **Incompetence** – inability to do it.
- **Inconsideration** – not caring.

In cases of cruelty it is unwise to bring a cruelty charge against a first-time offender where the cause was ignorance, inexperience and incompetence. Education or guidance can help to avoid or correct ignorance and inexperience. Incompetence is more difficult to correct, and often there is a human tragedy behind the situation. For example, the person in charge of the animals may be unstable, taking drugs or misusing alcohol. If it was a repeated offence which involved ignorance, inexperience and incompetence, it is likely there is inconsideration as well, and the offender should have taken steps to avoid its recurrence. In this case it would be more appropriate to raise a charge. Inconsideration is more difficult to tolerate and prosecution is more appropriate, especially where there has been callousness.

There are three *reasons for being concerned about animal welfare*:

- respect for animals and a sense of fair play;
- poor welfare can lead to poor product quality;
- risk of loss of market share for products which acquire a poor welfare image.

The first reason is a moral one, and each of us will differ in our values and outlook. Some feel that animals are less important than themselves or other humans and so they warrant less concern. For example, a well known behaviour scientist once gave a talk on hen welfare to a group of farmers.

At the end of the presentation one perplexed farmer stood up and asked, 'Do you mean to tell me that you care about what a chicken thinks?' Others take the view that animals deserve rights and freedoms comparable to those of humans. Most of us, however, fall between these two attitudes.

Society has grown to accept that, to satisfy the world's appetite for meat, animals must be farmed intensively as well as extensively, but some hold strong views about how the animals should be kept. As a guide to moral standards many countries have adopted the *Five Freedoms.* These are a set of goals towards which animal owners and handlers should strive. They are:

- freedom from thirst, hunger and malnutrition;
- the provision of appropriate comfort and shelter;
- the prevention or rapid diagnosis and treatment of injury, disease or infestation with parasites;
- freedom from distress;
- the ability to display normal patterns of behaviour.

Some countries go so far as to include freedom from fear as a goal instead of freedom from distress. This, perhaps, overstates the goal, as fear is an everyday occurrence and one that is needed, for example, in mustering animals together. The suffering associated with disease is one of the worst animal welfare problems that exists today (Gregory, 1998), and in some countries climatic stress is a common welfare insult (Gregory, 1995b). In overall terms these two forms of suffering receive insufficient attention simply because they are not sensitive politically.

The Five Freedoms (or, more correctly, the *Five Needs*), for animals are based on our perception of what animals need. We know what it feels like when we experience hunger, thirst, fear, cold and pain and we project these feelings on to animals. We cannot claim to have a complete appreciation of what animals feel, and we can only infer feelings by interpreting the animals' behaviour and physiology. To be precise, we must apply a different set of definitions for humans from those for animals. Take thirst, for example. Thirst in a human is the sensation that accompanies dehydration. In animals, the definition that would satisfy most people would be the tendency to seek and consume water when unimpeded and whilst experiencing dehydration. Physiologists would clarify the situation by determining whether dehydration was present. This could be done by measuring the concentration of total protein in the plasma, the packed cell volume or the plasma osmolality. For humans, we refer to sensations; for animals, we are more cautious and refer to behavioural and physiological experiences.

Livestock breeders have a particular responsibility to animal welfare because their actions can lead to genetic antagonisms which can affect a sizeable proportion of the population. *Genetic antagonisms* occur when genetic selection for particular traits results in unwanted traits emerging in the progeny. This can occur either because the wanted trait is genetically correlated to the unwanted trait, or because insufficient attention is paid to removing unwanted traits that inadvertently start increasing – for example, through line breeding. Some examples of genetic antagonisms involving meat production traits and animal welfare are:

- dystocia, conformation and body size in particular cattle breeds;
- exercise stress disorders and muscularity in double-muscled cattle;
- osteochondrosis and growth rate in pigs;
- stress-induced deaths and muscularity in particular pig breeds;
- PSE meat and muscularity in particular breeds or strains of pig and turkey;
- leg disorders, lameness, conformation and growth rate in poultry;
- green muscle disease and muscularity in turkeys and chickens;
- ascites and genetic selection for breast meat yield and growth rate in chickens.

Poor welfare can lead to inferior meat quality (Gregory, 1993). In the fresh meat trade it results in loss of yield and loss of sales through rejection or downgrading of poor quality product. The links between poor welfare and downgrading apply to the following conditions in the fresh meat or carcass:

- abnormal meat colour;
- pale soft exudative (PSE) meat in pork and turkey;
- dark firm dry (DFD) meat in pork, beef and lamb;
- poor shelf life;
- dry meat;
- heat shortening in poultry;
- bruising;
- torn skin;
- broken bones.

In some situations poor welfare may also aggravate problems with:

- gaping in meat;
- boar taint.

It would be inaccurate to say that poor welfare always leads to poor meat quality. There are many instances where there is no effect at all. For example, cold stress during transport before slaughter does not usually have any detrimental effect on meat quality or yield. In some situations stress can even improve some quality features; for example, physical exhaustion before slaughter can make the meat more tender. However, animal welfare is in itself becoming a quality issue because some retailers are imposing animal welfare standards in their specifications for suppliers. The retailers want to have a *caring image* – for animals and for the company's customers. Some of the major supermarket companies are setting standards on animal welfare within the market. The specifications on welfare and product quality are taken seriously by the meatworks which supply them because they need to secure the supermarkets' business.

Market forces created by the meat processing industry can also have a bearing on animal welfare. The industry is one of the major users of meat that is downgraded because of minor blemishes created by poor handling or stress. Sometimes there is a good market for meat from animals that have been ill-treated. For example, there is a well-established market for high pH_{ult} beef as hamburgers. This type of meat is unsuitable for the fresh meat trade because of its objectionable dark colour, but it is accepted by the processing sector because of its high water-holding capacity. With poultry there may be little difference in value in using a carcass for processed meat production in comparison with selling it as a whole bird. So, if the carcass is unfit for presentation as a whole bird because of an ante-mortem tear in the skin, the value of the carcass can often be maintained by sending it for further processing.

The meat quality features that are most important depend on the way in which the meat is used. For instance, a bone fragment (arising from a broken bone) might be disregarded in a whole chicken, but if it was present in a manufactured take-away product it could lead to a consumer complaint. Bruising and abnormal meat colour are important in the fresh meat trade, but less important in the ground meat trades. Hock burn in poultry is a serious appearance defect in the whole-bird market, but it is of little concern in the boneless meat market because it is trimmed out. Some meat processors run separate standards in their processing and quality control for different customers, but not all plants are sufficiently organized to know the destination of a batch of animals at the time they are slaughtered or when the carcasses are graded. In that situation a high standard in overall quality control has to be aimed for, or the plant has to concentrate on supplying a limited number of specialized outlets.

From the meat processor's and consumer's perspective, further processing fulfils seven functions:

- **Convenience** – ready-to-eat products, fast foods.
- **Preservation** – extending the storage life of meat.
- **Providing alternative products** – bacon or ham instead of fresh pork.
- **Adding value** – coated meat products, re-formed meats.
- **Upgrading low value meats** – buffalo wings, hamburgers manufactured from dark-cutting beef.
- **Spreads seasonal glut over the year** – salted meats, dried meats.
- **Allows distribution of meat over longer distances** – low water-activity meats.

It must be emphasized that only a small proportion of the total amount of meat that goes for further processing has in fact been downgraded because of a welfare-associated product quality problem.

Animal welfare is becoming more important in the *international trading* of meat (Gregory, 1995c). Meat-exporting nations depend on agricultural produce for their livelihood. If sentiment goes against a country because it has unacceptable welfare, hygiene, environmental or sociopolitical standards, meat buyers may take their custom elsewhere. Consider the following example. Suppose that Country X exports beef to Country Y. There is a television programme broadcast in Country Y which shows hot-iron branding, and farmers in Country X are identified with this practice. The animal welfare pressure groups use the opportunity to lobby the public to stop buying beef from Country X. A sector of the public responds, but more importantly the supermarkets in Country Y decide to stop sourcing beef from Country X because of its tarnished image. The market forces that set this off originated with the animal welfare pressure group. Animal welfare pressure groups try to influence purchasing behaviour through their publicity. This may or may not have much effect on the way consumers spend their money, but it can influence the purchasing patterns of the major retail companies which try to promote the image of a reputable and caring business.

Animal welfare has not been used as an official barrier to trade between countries. This is because there are no provisions under the World Trade Organization (WTO) agreements for an animal welfare issue to become an acceptable technical barrier which one government could use as a reason for disallowing importations from another country. If a country did adopt an animal welfare issue as a technical barrier for trade, the matter could be taken before the WTO for arbitration. However, some EU meat-importing countries have argued strongly that transport duration for livestock should be limited by EU regulations to eight hours, whereas some of the meat-exporting countries have argued that there should be no limit on journey time. This is an example where an animal welfare issue could become a barrier to trade, assuming that a mutual agreement was reached. In practice, it is pressure from retailers, animal welfare pressure groups and consumers that is likely to have more influence on market positioning in animal welfare issues.

From the public's perspective the two least acceptable features of modern farming practice are close confinement of animals with limited ability to exercise, and mutilations without anaesthesia. These practices raise three recurring questions. Are they fair? Are they necessary? Are there alternatives? *Close confinement systems* which inevitably limit movement and exercise include:

- farrowing crates;
- dry sow stalls;
- sow tethers;
- battery hen cages;
- veal calf crates;
- rabbit, mink and quail cages.

Mutilations are procedures that involve removing or damaging part of an animal's body as a routine husbandry procedure. Many of them are done without anaesthetic. Working from the front of the animal and moving backwards, they include:

- nose ringing;
- beak trimming;
- teeth clipping;
- antler removal;
- disbudding;
- dehorning;
- dubbing;
- desnooding;
- ear notching;
- wing and feather clipping;
- branding;
- pizzle dropping;
- mulesing;
- tailing;
- castration;
- toe clipping.

Disbudding, dehorning, toe clipping and turkey beak trimming are done to reduce the risk of damage to the animals and hence the final product. Castration is performed in pigs to ensure that the meat does not possess undesirable taints. Other procedures are done to prevent animals escaping (wing clipping); as a means of identifying animals (dubbing, desnooding, ear notching, branding); to reduce the risk of parasitism, body damage and disease (teeth clipping, pizzle dropping, mulesing, tailing); as a way of collecting a product (antler removal); or as a way of controlling damage to pasture (nose ringing and toe clipping). In the future there will probably be more pressure on farmers to move away from methods which involve close confinement and to farm without mutilations.

CHANGING PATTERNS IN MEAT CONSUMPTION

Over the past 25 years the world consumption of meat has been rising. The largest increases have been in countries where the standard of living has been improving. However, in many industrialized countries where the standard of living and economy have been stable, the consumption of red meats has been declining, whilst that of poultry meat has been increasing. For example, in the USA, Canada, Australia, New Zealand and the UK, beef consumption per capita has reduced by 24%, sheepmeat consumption has fallen dramatically by 45% and poultry meat consumption has increased by 96%. Pigmeat consumption has not changed. In summary, the English-speaking countries in the world are in an era of reduced redmeat consumption and increased whitemeat consumption.

In order to understand the *reasons for reduced redmeat consumption* it is helpful to examine the attitudes and beliefs that vegetarians and semi-vegetarians have about meat (Gregory, 1997). Semi-vegetarians are people who eat some kind of meat but only on an occasional basis (e.g. once or twice a month), and they usually avoid red meats. Vegetarians do not eat any meat. In the UK during the1980s and 1990s, between 2 and 5% of the population were vegetarian, and about 15% of the adult population are now semi-vegetarian. In Australia, 16% of adolescents (16-year-olds) are semi-vegetarian. Vegetarians represent only a small section of the meat-reducing public, but by studying their attitudes and those of semi-vegetarians we can identify more easily the key features which lead to more generalized reduced redmeat consumption. In addition, examining the attitudes and beliefs of young vegetarians and young semi-vegetarians is helpful in deciding whether consumption of red meats is likely to carry on decreasing in the next generation.

A familiar theme throughout human history is that things which are highly prized by some individuals are thought to be highly defiling by others. This applies in the case of the different meats we eat. Red meats, and in particular beef, have the highest status for meat eaters, and yet they are the ones which are first avoided by semi-vegetarians.

If one asked a vegetarian or semi-vegetarian what images they associated with meat or meat eating, the likely answer would be:

- animality;
- animal cruelty;
- depriving animals of the right to life;
- the consumption of dead flesh.

Many vegetarians believe that humans behave like animals when they eat animal flesh. It increases animality in humans. Along with this, meat eaters are thought to be more aggressive and they acquire animality through that particular food.

The full vegetarian is a morally motivated individual whose primary concern about meat eating is cruelty in modern farming systems and ethical concerns about animal slaughter. They see the health gains of being vegetarian as a bonus. There is a sense that the health gains are a symbolic reward for moral rectitude. Modern *semi-vegetarianism* is a diluted form of vegetarianism. The semi-vegetarian is also morally charged. In fact the primary concern amongst Australian semi-vegetarian women about eating meat is animal cruelty (Table 1.1). The negative sensory features of meat are an important additional deterrent, and about one-third of teenage semi-vegetarian and vegetarian women were reduced meat eaters principally because they thought that meat was fattening. It might be thought that the present trend toward reduced meat eating reflects a desire to live a long and healthy life. However, the evidence suggests that only 19% of full and semi-vegetarian adolescent women viewed meat eating as unhealthy, and this outlook existed in only 3% of non-vegetarians.

Table 1.1. Main concerns about eating meat amongst Australian adolescent women who were either vegetarian or non-vegetarian. (From Worsley and Skrzypiec, 1997.)

	Proportion of individuals (%)	
	Full and semi-vegetarian	Non-vegetarian
Animal cruelty	61	37
Sensory (bloody, smell, etc.)	44	5
Red meat is fattening	30	13
Meat is harmful to the environment	25	13
Meat eating is unhealthy	19	3

Most modern vegetarians and semi-vegetarians share the outlook that humans, as individuals, are not innately cruel to animals or disrespectful of the environment, but cultural values have forced society towards being cruel and wasteful. To some vegetarians and semi-vegetarians, applying logic in resolving such problems is less important than feeling at peace with the world and fellow creatures. For example, by denying themselves the right to eat animals they do not stop animal slaughter but they do quell any personal anxieties about being responsible for an animal's death. The mind and conscience are eased. Perhaps many of us are closer to this outlook than we realize. For example, when a large sample of meat eaters in the United Kingdom was confronted with the hypothetical prospect of having to kill animals themselves in order to eat them, the majority said that they would cease eating meat altogether (Richardson *et al.*, 1993).

Beardsworth and Keil (1992) held detailed interviews with 76 self-defined vegetarians in the United Kingdom, and some of the comments were revealing. In connection with animal welfare, one interviewee made the following point:

> I've always been fond of animals and when you reach the age where it is blatantly obvious that meat is animals, I didn't want any more to do with it.

Another interviewee changed abruptly to vegetarianism after seeing a television programme, which:

> showed them electrocuting pigs and I sat down in the canteen at work the very next day, and everybody was saying how awful this programme was, and they were all tucking into bacon cobs. I'd bought one of these cobs as well and I took one bite of it and it tasted awful and I thought, well if that pig's gone through all that for me ... and I've never touched it since. That was five years ago.

There are pronounced cultural differences in attitudes to animals and animal welfare. Kellert (1988) classified the attitudes people have towards animals into nine categories:

1. **Naturalistic** – an interest and affection for animals and the outdoors.
2. **Ecologistic** – concern for the environment as a system, for interrelationships between species and their habitat.
3. **Humanistic** – interest and strong affection for individual animals such as pets or large wild animals, with strong anthropomorphic associations.
4. **Moralistic** – concern for the right and wrong treatment of animals, with opposition to presumed over-exploitation and/or cruelty towards animals.
5. **Scientific** – interest in the form and functioning of animals.
6. **Aesthetic** – interest in the physical attractiveness and symbolic appeal of animals.
7. **Utilitarian** – interest in the practical value of animals, or in subordination of animals for some practical benefit.
8. **Dominionistic** – interest in mastery and control of animals.
9. **Negative** – avoidance of animals due to indifference, dislike or fear.

Moral attitudes would equate most closely to concerns about livestock welfare, but animal welfare would also feature to some extent in humanistic attitudes towards companion animals. In a comparison of Japanese, Germans and US Americans it was found that the moralistic attitude was very strongly developed amongst the Germans (Fig. 1.1). The Japanese had a well-developed humanistic outlook and Americans varied according to the part of the country in which they were raised (Kellert, 1993).

In Australia, up to a third of teenage women experience difficulties in divorcing the image of the living animal and its production and slaughter from meat. Approximately half of the female interviewees said that they felt rearing animals to be killed was either 'cruel' or 'wrong'. In the same survey, it was reported that about one-third of the teenage women were in some way vegetarian, but only 21% of the women looked upon themselves as being vegetarian or semi-vegetarian. This indicates that either they did not like or wish to label themselves as vegetarian or that they took their abstention from meat consumption for granted without recognizing that it was synonymous with vegetarianism. Only 26% of all teenage females in the survey agreed with the statement: 'I think meat production is done humanely.' The majority of teenage Australian males had a different outlook: only 6% were semi-vegetarian and 65% agreed that they were not bothered that meat comes from animals. Their appreciation of eating meat was stronger than concerns about welfare. Nevertheless, fewer than half (46%) of all the teenage males agreed with the statement: 'I think meat production is done humanely' (Worsley and Skrzypiec, 1997).

The reduced meat eater would typically progress towards vegetarianism by giving up first red meats, then poultry and finally fish. The species of origin, the appearance of blood and the redness of the meat are thought to be key features which create this hierarchy (Twigg, 1979). An important issue for the pigmeat and veal industries is where their products fit within the hierarchy of meats. Are they white meats, in which case they may be

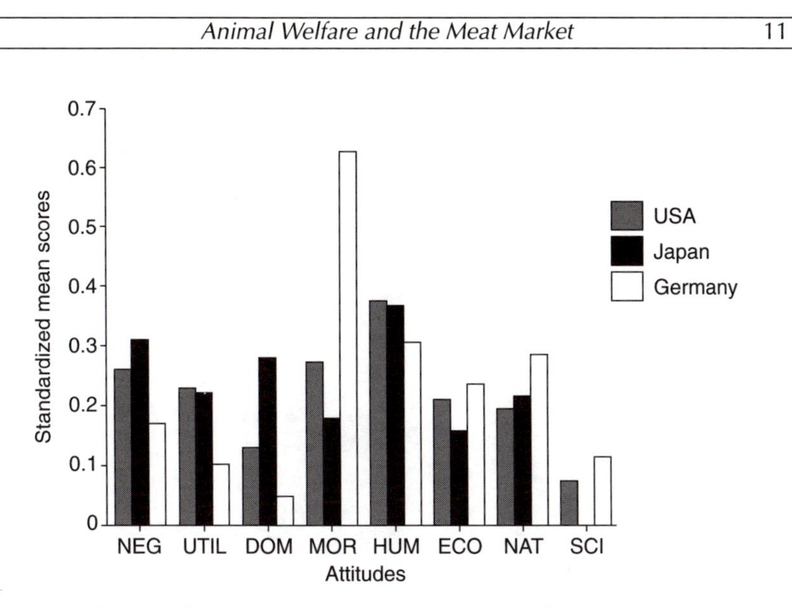

Fig. 1.1. Different cultures have different attitudes towards animals. NEG = negative; UTIL = utilitarian; DOM = dominionistic; MOR = moralistic; HUM = humanistic; ECO = ecologistic; NAT = naturalistic; SCI = scientific.

acceptable to semi-vegetarians, or are they regarded as redmeats and so are likely to be rejected? Alternatively, do they share the live-animal images of beef and lamb as distinct from chicken and fish, in which case they would be avoided along with beef and lamb? A survey of Australian adolescents conducted by Worsley and Skrzypiec (1997) indicated that pork and veal are in fact ranked along with red meats (Table 1.2).

The vegetarian's outlook about vegetarian eating conjures up a different set of symbolic images:

- purity of lifestyle;
- healthiness;
- femininism;
- crispness;
- freshness;
- light eating.

The images of crispness, freshness and light eating fit well with heightened awareness about youthfulness and one's body shape. All these images help to influence an individual's attitudes and beliefs, which in turn helps to decide whether he or she is a meat eater.

Surprisingly, some vegetarians have a nostalgia and a craving for particular meats and especially for the taste and smell of bacon. Others find most cooked meats repulsive to the extent of causing nausea. Some people find preparing and cooking meat particularly offensive. The stickiness of

Table 1.2. Hierarchy of meats amongst 16-year-old Australian semi-vegetarians. (Adapted from Worsley and Skrzypiec, 1997.)

Meat	Number of semi-vegetarians who eat the respective meat for every meat eater who consumes the same meat
Beef sausages	0.41
Pork	0.43
Crumbed veal	0.46
Lamb	0.46
Steak	0.47
Bacon	0.47
Roast beef/veal	0.51
Casserole (not chicken)	0.55
Mincemeat	0.56
Cold meats	0.65
Processed meats*	0.67
Chicken	0.82
Fish	1.05

* Sausage rolls, pies, hamburgers.

raw meat and the elasticity of meat when it is chewed can be objectionable. Notwithstanding this, the main reason people eat meat is because they enjoy it. It may be an acquired or habit-based enjoyment as other people live quite comfortably without it. For some, the taste of meat helps to reinforce that enjoyment and this is one of the main reasons why would-be vegetarians resist becoming vegetarian.

The meat and livestock industries have little to gain from trying to convert full vegetarians back to an omnivorous diet. Instead, they need to address the concerns that lead to reduced meat eating in would-be semi-vegetarians. Since animal welfare is one of the most important issues leading to semi-vegetarianism (Table 1.1), the contents of this book are pertinent to the long-term future of the industry.

It is not easy to know how the ethics of animal slaughter for meat consumption should be approached. Some take the view that in the long term it may be counterproductive to try to divorce meat from the living animal as this could create a greater reaction amongst adolescents and adults against meat eating when they realize where meat comes from. Others take the view that most meat eaters do not want to know where their meat comes from and there is a risk that frankness about animal slaughter may put them off altogether. A balance between these two would be to introduce society at an early age to the notion that we eat animals and that this is a normal activity. As such the image of meat eating needs to be promoted in a positive light, showing that it is part of the vital nutrition for normal, active, healthy people of both sexes.

It is worth asking how animal welfare problems have arisen in the first place. In some respects the meat and livestock industry has been a victim of its own efficiency. During the first 70 years of the 20th century the emphasis in farming was towards greater efficiency in terms of return for capital invested. This was achieved by increasing feed conversion efficiency, stocking density, growth rate through genetic selection, and reproductive performance. In some situations this striving for economic and biological efficiency has out-competed the welfare of the animal. Examples include:

- expansion in farm size leading to difficulties in handling stock because less time is spent familiarizing the stock with the handling procedures;
- overstocking livestock buildings, leading to respiratory disease, excessive dust and ammonia, and hockburn in poultry;
- genetic selection for growth rate, resulting in leg disorders in broiler chickens and pigs;
- confinement in dry sow stalls and stereotypic behaviours;
- insufficient space inside the abdomen, leading to diarrhoea in dairy cows, prolapses in broiler breeder hens and prolapses in twin-bearing ewes;
- inappropriate use of bulls from breeds of large mature size, and dystocia in heifers and cows.

It should not be overlooked that there have been many improvements in animal welfare standards during the 20th century. These include:

- more prescriptive legislation on animal welfare and cruelty;
- more effective prevention and control of infectious diseases;
- better understanding of how to avoid malnutrition and undernutrition;
- fewer male animals being castrated;
- better methods and standards in stunning and slaughtering in meatworks;
- in some countries, the abolition of some less humane practices and systems (e.g. sweatbox piggeries, tethered sow stalls, veal calf crates, hot-iron branding, surgical caponizing).

The methods used for slaughtering livestock species such as cattle, sheep and pigs have improved considerably in recent years. Unfortunately this does not apply to all farmed species. For example, a common method for slaughtering farmed frogs has been to chill the live animal and then cut off the hindlegs, which are the edible part, with a large pair of shears. On some frog farms, the live frogs are held in iced water containing 200 ppm chlorine before pithing with a spike in the head, and the chlorine at this concentration would undoubtedly have an irritant action before loss of consciousness.

There is a perception amongst some consumers that a product produced under natural or free-range conditions is inevitably better to eat. I was once told that 'a free-range hen is bound to produce tastier eggs because it has a happy life'. To biologists, the basis for this statement is not immediately obvious. Is there a link between happiness in hens and flavour in their eggs and, if so, why? This book gives a scientific view of the possible relationships between welfare and meat quality.

Chapter 2

Livestock Presentation and Welfare before Slaughter

MEETING THE ABATTOIR'S NEEDS

Modern meatworks operate at fast line speeds. Pig abattoirs in the USA slaughter up to 1100 pigs per hour, lamb meatworks in New Zealand kill up to 24,000 animals a day and broiler processing lines in various parts of the world put through up to 220 birds a minute. At these throughput rates the companies cannot afford to make mistakes. The hourly capital cost in running a plant is high and any stoppage or slowing of the line is likely to reduce efficiency and financial return. If there are interruptions and the line is idle, staff are being paid for doing nothing. Interruptions in the supply of livestock are minimized by ensuring that there is always a sufficient reserve of stock waiting in the holding pens in the lairage. Holding animals in pens before slaughter has an added advantage. It gives them a chance to have a drink of water if they are dehydrated, and it provides a rest period before slaughter, which in some situations can be beneficial to meat quality. Where holding-pen space is limited it is important to schedule truck arrivals precisely, and this is not always easy to control.

When animals are presented for slaughter the abattoir needs them to be:

- clean;
- healthy;
- fasted;
- free from blemishes;
- unstressed;
- easy to handle;
- well muscled and not overfat.

Making sure that there is a continuous supply of suitable stock to the killing floor has implications for line efficiency and animal welfare in four ways.

- Animal handling becomes more critical. The animals must arrive in a continuous stream at the stunning point. Uncontrolled behaviour in the stock can create interruptions in this flow.
- The animals must be healthy and free from blemishes. Diseased and bruised or blemished tissue needs to be removed, and the additional inspection and trimming this involves can slow the line or require extra staff.
- Animals must be fasted to reduce gut contents and so lower the risk of rupturing the digestive tract during evisceration, which would cause contamination of the carcass with digesta or faeces.
- Animals must be presented in a clean condition. Stock which are dirty with dung, mud or dust on their surface create a risk of spreading dirt. If dirty carcasses enter the dressing area, the veterinarian or supervising meat hygiene officer may be obliged to stop or slow the line in order to ensure either that the dirty carcasses are handled appropriately and do not contaminate equipment or other carcasses, or that further dirty stock do not enter the killing floor.

Some of these features can also affect carcass yield or value. Diseased tissues have to be trimmed and so they cause a reduction in yield. Meat which is bruised or blood-splashed or has an abnormal colour cannot be sold in the high value markets. If the blemish is severe the meat will be rejected and used as pet food. In less serious cases it may be used for making mince, burgers or lower value products which have a lower profit margin. In modern plants, carcass contamination with faeces or digesta is removed by trimming with a knife along with some underlying tissue, and this also incurs a reduction in yield. Certain preslaughter stress conditions can reduce yield by increasing the amount of drip, evaporative loss and the thawing loss from the resultant meat. Stress can also adversely affect the colour of the meat, which may be downgraded to low value product.

The greatest *hygiene* risk from processing dirty stock occurs when the skin is being removed. When the hair, wool or skin is covered with dung, mud or dust there is a risk of contaminating the carcass either if the dirty side of the hide or pelt rolls on to the carcass, or as the brisket skin is being opened or during bung (anus or anus plus vulva) dropping or bung removal. In the case of sheep that have been folded on a forage crop, the fleece is likely to be contaminated with mud and ideally they should be taken off the crop and allowed to graze pasture to provide a cleaning-up period. If there is excessive dung on the hindquarters they should be dagged (dirty wool shorn off) before slaughter. These procedures involve extra handling of the sheep, which inevitably imposes some stress, but they are important from the perspective of carcass cleanliness.

There are a number of counteracting influences which determine the optimum length of wool that sheep should carry when they are presented for slaughter. In some countries the welfare requirement is that sheep should not be presented for slaughter within 3 weeks of a complete shearing, as this period is needed for the healing of shearing scars. Consideration should also be given to any risk of chilling during long journeys if the sheep have been recently shorn, but at the other extreme shearing before despatch can help to reduce the risk of heat stress in the truck. If greasy-wool prices are depressed, farmers will be more inclined to send sheep for slaughter without shearing them. At the meatworks, longwool sheep are more difficult to dress hygienically, but there can be more profit in processing these sheep if fibre length meets the needs of the higher quality slipe wool trade (70–120 mm fibre length).

Cattle and sheep often develop diarrhoea when they graze lush spring pasture. Although the diarrhoea is not directly harmful to the animal, it is an indirect cause of a number of welfare and hygiene problems in the meat, dairy and wool industries. In some countries dirty sheep and cattle are swimwashed or spraywashed at the meatworks just before slaughter as a way of removing visible dirt. This is stressful for the animal and it has been shown to affect meat quality adversely in sheep. Springtime diarrhoea is also an important reason for the extra handling and stress involved with crutching, dagging, tailing and mulesing sheep and in some countries it is the main reason for tail docking dairy cattle.

The reasons that cattle develop diarrhoea when grazing spring pasture are not fully understood. The old adage that it is because the grass is lush is only a superficial explanation. One possiblity is that there is insufficient cross-linking of the fibre components in young grass and this leads to poor binding of the faeces. In mature herbage the cross-links between lignin and hemicellulose are through ferulic and *p*-coumaric acids, which are lacking in young pasture. In addition to this there could be volume overloading of the colon and rapid transit through the colon in cattle. The colon is responsible for absorbing water from the gut contents before evacuation as faeces. The bovine's colon is only a little longer than the sheep's colon; the transit time through the colon is faster in cattle and so it has less time to absorb water. These features lead to real practical problems with dirty stock entering meatworks.

A typical stress response in cattle is to void faeces. When animals are crowded together in a pen or a truck the faeces spread on to other stock. To help to reduce this, the animals are taken off feed before they are despatched for slaughter. No doubt this results in hunger and if feed is withheld for unnecessarily long periods it will cause loss of carcass yield as well. Stress can also promote loss of digesta when it is linked to exercise. Light exercise speeds gastric emptying, but strenuous exercise slows it. Running has been shown to increase the plasma concentration of the hormone motilin, which helps to stimulate gastric emptying and colonic motility. Running can also induce a sense of urgency and defaecation through movement of the contents of the colon. The sloshing of the digesta inside the colon stimulates the colon to contract. It is also thought that in some species the psoas muscles compress and massage the emptying of the colon and rectum during the hip flexion involved in running movements.

If an animal becomes infected with *Salmonella* or *Campylobacter*, these bacteria usually get established and multiply within the caeca. A wide variety of mental and physical stresses can cause increased emptying of the caeca into the colon and faster propulsion of the digesta through the colon. In laboratory rats, passage of digesta along the colon to the rectum takes about 1 hour during fear stress instead of 15 hours in unstressed control animals (Enck *et al.*, 1989). During fear-induced evacuation the faeces are more moist as there has been insufficient time for the colon to absorb water, and they have the stronger odour of an upper large intestine stool. When farm animals are stressed before slaughter they excrete more salmonellas in their faeces, and part of the reason for this is the greater evacuation of the caecum and large intestine. In addition, salmonella-free animals become infected and this can magnify the hygiene risk in the abattoir (Berends *et al.*, 1996).

In some countries, when lambs or sheep have been presented to a meatworks in an *overfat condition* they have been withheld from slaughter. Instead they have been put through a crash weight-reduction schedule for a week or more on a bare paddock and then slaughtered once they reached the appropriate body condition. This practice would not necessarily apply to many animals, as it is not in the best interests of either the farmers or the meatworks companies. According to anecdotal comments, the meat from these animals has been tough.

CARCASS DAMAGE, TRANSPORT STRESS AND DEATHS

Farmers usually have to bear the financial loss if an animal dies during transport to the abattoir. The farmer does not have direct control over this mortality, but the genotype that is selected can influence susceptibility to *transport deaths*. There is more than one cause for death during the stress that accompanies transport. In poultry it is often linked to congestive heart failure, in pigs to hyperthermia and in sheep to asphyxiation from smothering. Congestive heart failure is a condition which broiler chickens acquire during the growing period on the farm. The heart is unable to pump blood adequately and blood builds up in the pulmonary veins. This congestion with blood is obvious in the lungs, which at autopsy are dark in colour from stagnant blood, and in the swollen pulmonary blood vessels. In advanced cases the heart is enlarged through stretching, the lungs are oedematous and a serous fluid leaks into and accumulates within the body cavity, producing the condition of water belly or ascites. This disorder is particularly common in birds farmed at high altitudes, where there is low atmospheric oxygen. It is due to an inability of the heart to meet the blood and oxygen needs of the body, and it has been suggested that this is a feature of insufficient correction for the condition when stock have been selected genetically for a high growth rate.

Most of the pig deaths that occur during transport happen in the warmer seasons. The heat stress triggers a metabolic acidosis, and this is more common in strains of pig which have been genetically selected for muscular hams. Linked to these traits is a semi-lethal recessive gene known as the halothane gene (*n*). Pigs that are homozygous for this gene have an abnormality in their muscle metabolism which makes the muscle over-reactive to stressful stimuli such as high temperatures and to certain drugs, such as halothane. The muscle is prone to excessive metabolism, the pig develops hyperthermia and lethal blood potassium levels.

In cold seasons there are similarities in the pathology seen in pigs that die during transport with that in humans who die from over-exertion. One cause of over-exertion death in unfit humans is as follows. During exercise there is an increase in haematocrit to allow greater oxygen transport by the blood. The blood is also more viscous, partly because the haematocrit is increased and also because the red cells become more rigid and less deformable when they are exposed to adrenaline. Under these conditions (high haematocrit and viscous blood), the red cells in the artery tend to flow in the centre of the bloodstream, where they rotate and collide with one another, creating turbulence that drives platelets against the vessel wall. The higher the haematocrit, the greater is the force with which the platelets impact with the vessel wall. If a part of the artery becomes denuded of endothelium, platelets that impact with this region stick to the vessel wall and a clot forms. The higher the haematocrit, the greater is the likelihood of forming this type of clot. If clots form in the coronary arteries, the heart muscle can be starved of blood and a cardiac arrest will result. Cardiac arrest from occlusion of the coronary arteries can be recognized post-mortem from pale necrotic patches in the heart muscle. These lesions have been found to be common in pigs that died during transport during cold seasons in Canada (Clark, 1979).

Being physically unfit increases the risk of developing a thrombosis during exercise or stress. Physical fitness helps to reduce the viscosity of the blood and it helps to promote fibrinolysis, which is the body's main clot-dissolving mechanism. During exercise the fibrinolytic agent, tissue plasminogen activator (TPA), is released from blood vessels. TPA binds to plasminogen, which is present in a clot, and converts plasminogen to plasmin, which dissolves the clot.

Causes of *smothering* and death from suffocation include poultry panicking during catching and the birds piling on top of one another at one end of the shed, overstocking of poultry transport crates so that weaker birds are being trampled and smothered by others, and sheep going down during yarding or transport and being trampled by other sheep. The general signs of asphyxia in the dead animal are relatively non-specific. They can include blood splash, cyanosis and pulmonary oedema, but these can occur in non-asphyxial deaths as well. If an animal takes a long time to die during the smothering, it tries hard to breathe in and this creates sub-atmospheric pressures within the lungs which disrupt the alveolar–capillary barrier, leading to the release of a frothy blood into the trachea and mouth. Other situations can cause frothy blood to appear at the mouth, so here again this is not diagnostic; it is only indicative. The circumstances in which the dead animals are found are likely to be more informative in deciding whether death was due to suffocation.

The longer the journey before slaughter, the greater is the likelihood that there will be some deaths during the transport period. Particularly long journeys occur when livestock are sold between nations. At the end of the 19th century and the beginning of the 20th century there was a sizeable international trade in live cattle for slaughter. Cattle were shipped from North America to northwest Europe, and large numbers travelled long distances within Europe. Modern transport has reduced the journey times associated with the international trade in fatstock, but even so some journeys can take up to 3–4 weeks. This is the case during the export of live sheep from Australia or New Zealand to the Middle East. These sheep are sent to the Middle East for the *haj*, a religious pilgrimage and festival during which Muslims arrange for and witness the slaughter of an animal, part of which is distributed as meat to the poor. Large numbers of sheep are needed at this time to satisfy demand. The concerns from the welfare perspective are in the conditions during transport and unloading, and in the method of slaughter. On the vessels that leave New Zealand the mortalities are usually low (less than 1%) and there is a veterinarian on board who is responsible for the sheep's health and welfare. Occasionally things go wrong and there are heavy mortalities. In 1996, a ship from Australia caught fire and all the sheep were lost. A more common risk is with the condition of the manure underfoot. Normally the manure is not cleared out during the journey; instead, it is allowed to accumulate and dry out. If the weather turns foul it does not dry out and can turn into a faecal mud, which by the end of the journey is about 20 cm deep. Heavy losses from smothering in the faecal mud have occurred when sheep have been trodden down during competition for feed at the troughs, or from competition for fresh air at the ventilation hatches if it has become hot and humid. About eight million sheep are sent from Australasia to the Middle East every year, and the vessels typically hold about 60,000 sheep. At present, the biggest oceanic trade in live cattle is between Australia and countries on the Pacific rim.

Mortality from *heat stress* during road transport occurs in chickens and pigs, but it rarely happens in sheep and cattle. A truck may hold 4000 to 5000 closely confined chickens, which together produce sizeable amounts of heat. Normally, the birds would be kept cool by wind passing through and between the crates, but if the truck breaks down or gets stuck in a traffic jam, the temperature in the vehicle can quickly rise and some birds will die. The hottest spots are usually immediately behind the headboards, especially if these are solid and do not allow much airflow (Kettlewell *et al.*, 1993). In the future, temperature needs to be monitored at this point and relayed to the dashboard in front of the driver, who can then take corrective action when appropriate.

Heat exchange between an animal and its environment occurs in four ways:

- conduction;
- convection;
- radiation;
- evaporation.

The high risk situations that occur during transport are failure in forced convection (wind), high humidities which compromise evaporative cooling from panting, and exposure to solar radiation. During transport the animals are not able to express all the behaviours that normally allow them to keep cool. Depending on the species, animals seek shade, wallow, lick their fur (to promote evaporative cooling) and stretch their wings or legs (to increase surface area and convective heat loss). They are able to sweat and pant, and these are the principal methods of increasing evaporative heat loss for most meat-producing species (Table 2.1). Physiologically, pigs are at greatest risk from heat stress because they do not pant or sweat.

There are two simple ways of assessing whether or not an animal is heat-stressed. The first is to look for the signs shown in Table 2.1. However, these do not always give an unequivocal diagnosis. Panting could be due to exercise (especially in sheep) or to high levels of CO_2 in the atmosphere, but these can usually be discounted by the time stock on a truck arrive at the abattoir. Paradoxically, prolonged exposure to intense heat can sometimes be associated with no apparent panting. For example, chickens will start to pant (more than 60 breaths per minute) if their body temperature reaches 42.6°C, but beyond 45°C they stop panting in order to conserve body water (Fig. 2.1). The second method is to measure rectal temperature. The normal ranges are shown in Table 2.2, and any temperatures which exceed the normal range indicate hyperthermia. Lethal body temperatures are usually stated in terms of the temperature at which 50% of the animals can be expected to die. In chickens it is 47.2°C, but it will be lower than this if there is a slow rise in body temperature.

Table 2.1. Main evaporative heat loss mechanisms used by the livestock species.

Species	Main evaporative method
Cattle	Panting – nose
Sheep	Panting – mouth
Deer	Panting – nose
Pig	Wallowing and evaporation
Chicken	Panting – mouth

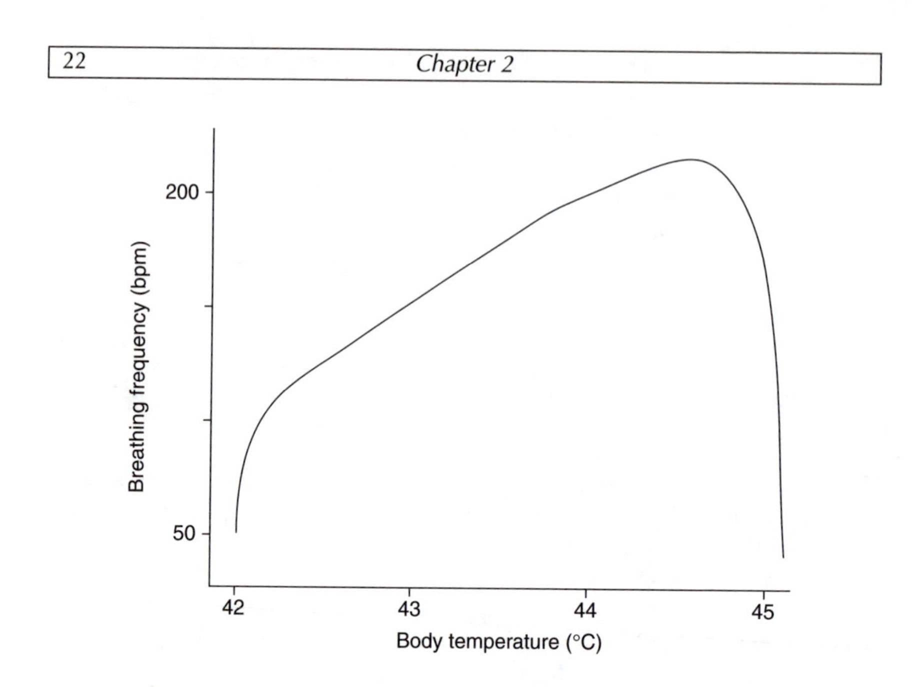

Fig. 2.1. Relationship between body temperature and panting in the chicken.

Table 2.2. Body temperatures in livestock species.

Species	Average rectal temperature (°C)	Normal range (°C)
Beef cow	38.3	36.7–39.1
Dairy cow	38.6	38.0–39.3
Deer	39.0	38.5–39.5
Ostrich	39.0	37.9–40.7
Sheep	39.1	38.3–39.9
Goat	39.1	38.5–39.7
Pig	39.2	38.7–39.8
Rabbit	39.5	38.6–40.1
Chicken	41.7	40.6–43.0

Ways of minimizing the risk of hyperthermia include the following.

- Park in the shade.
- If there is no shade, do not park; keep the vehicle moving to allow cooling with an airflow.
- Transport stock during the cooler times in the day.
- Reduce load density during hot weather.
- Insulate the roof of the truck to reduce radiant heat gain.

Dehydration is an added complication in heat-stressed stock on transport vehicles. The effects of severe dehydration include severe thirst, nausea, a dry tongue, loss of coordination, and concentrated urine of small volume. The ability to cope with dehydration varies between species. Under hot, dry (tropical) conditions, sheep can survive whilst losing up to 7% of their body weight daily when they are without water. Over a 10-day period, losses of 31–33% of body weight have been recorded. Some sheep breeds adapt by increasing their packed cell volume. Other species do not usually increase their packed cell volume and they are unable to withstand reductions in blood volume associated with dehydration without going into circulatory shock. Instead, they depend on peripheral vasoconstriction for maintaining adequate blood pressure. This has important consequences for their ability to survive during heat stress. Normally, when an animal is heat stressed it dilates the blood vessels in its skin to dissipate excess heat, but if it is dehydrated and its blood volume drops it has the conflicting need to vasoconstrict in its skin to maintain blood pressure, and to vasodilate to dissipate heat. Vasodilation in the skin whilst dehydrated is a key feature which causes collapse from heatstroke.

In temperate climates, preslaughter dehydration is most common in animals that are transported long distances. Water is never provided during road journeys, except when stock are off-loaded at a market or rest area, or when they reach the holding pens at the meatworks. The rate of dehydration is likely to be high during dry hot weather and when airflow through the moving truck is high. Bobby calves are particularly susceptible to dehydration because they have not learnt how to drink from a trough and so they fail to drink the water provided at the abattoir. The effect of dehydration can be aggravated by other stresses. For example, in one study where 6-month-old calves were severely stressed during loading and transport, the time taken for the plasma protein levels to rise, which would indicate dehydration, was as short as four hours (Kent and Ewbank, 1983). Normally, dehydration takes longer than this to set in. In these animals there were unusually large amounts of fluid loss from stress-induced salivation and voiding of faeces and urine.

When animals become dehydrated, the skin loses its pliability. A tough, unpliable skin is a useful indicator of dehydration in both the live animal and freshly killed carcass. In the live animal the decreased pliability is obvious from the skin's resistance to tenting; it is more difficult to lift a fold of the skin with a finger and thumb, the skin feels thicker and it does not fall back quickly to its original position when released. In meatworks, dehydration is a hindrance to slaughterfloor staff because the toughness makes it more difficult to remove the skin from the carcass. This is due to strengthening of the matrix of collagen fibres within the skin and between the skin and the carcass as water is lost. Normally, the water content of the skin is regulated by colloidal osmotic pressure. The collagen matrix acts as a colloid with the osmotic pressure controlled by glycosaminoglycans associated with the collagen. As water is lost the collagen fibrils compact and it is more difficult to tear them apart. During dehydration, the skin becomes substantially drier; in a 380 kg liveweight steer the total amount of water held in the skin falls by up to 1.8 litres as the animal becomes dehydrated (Bianca, 1968). During rehydration, the water content in the skin and subcutaneous tissues returns to normal in response to their raised osmotic pressure (Heir and Wiig, 1988).

Dehydration also results in a drier, sticky meat which has a higher water-holding capacity. The meat may also be slightly darker and have a slightly higher pH_{ult} (Joseph *et al.*, 1994). Eye muscle area can be reduced in severely dehydrated pigs, and the yield of offal and chymozin from calf vells (abomasums) is reduced.

Stock usually rehydrate by drinking water whilst they are held in the lairage. In many countries it is a requirement that water should always be available in the holding pens. If sheep become excessively thirsty during transport, they may over-drink when they get access to water at the meatworks. This leads to a condition known as wet carcass syndrome. The carcass has a wet, shiny appearance due to the accumulation of water in the subcutaneous tissues (Joubert *et al.*, 1985). Affected carcasses have poor keeping qualities and an unacceptable sloppy appearance and handling properties. Providing salt blocks in the holding pens makes the condition worse, as they cause further water intake.

In tropical countries it is common to see emaciated animals submitted for slaughter when there is a drought. There are nine signs of *emaciation* in live cattle (Fig. 2.2):

- visible ribs;
- concave longissimus dorsi muscle;
- thin dewlap;
- hollowness in gut fill, between the ribs and pelvis;
- concave rump;
- protruding pin bones;
- protruding hip bones;
- concave plate muscles, between hip bones and tail head;
- raised tail head.

Poor muscling and underdeveloped subcutaneous fat can also be seen in the carcass. In addition, the fat depots in the offal may be unusually red or grey. Redness is due to a high ratio of blood to fat; when the lipid in the fat is depleted, the blood vessels become more apparent. The fat can look grey because the whiteness of the fat is masked by the greyness of the connective tissue. A grey fat may also appear to be wetter because of its lower lipid and higher water contents.

In live sheep, emaciation is judged by palpating the top of the loin with the palm of the hand. The dorsal processes of the vertebrae are clearly felt against the palm of the hand and the lateral processes are felt with the

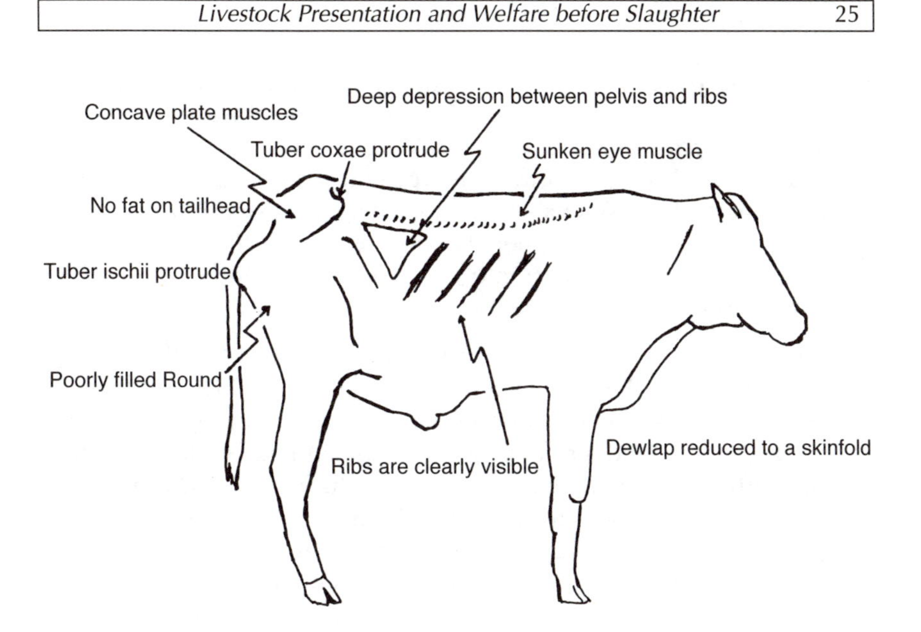

Fig. 2.2. Signs of emaciation in live cattle.

fingertips. These bony protruberances feel like knuckles if there is only a limited covering of muscle over the bone. In live deer, emaciation is usually gauged from the cover of flesh over the ribs, and in birds the breast is palpated with the palm of the hand to judge the plumpness of the breast muscles and protrusion of the ridge of the keel bone.

Motion sickness is associated with a variety of unpleasant sensations in humans which are linked to activation of the autonomic nervous system. These include dizziness, nausea, cold sweating, anorexia, malaise, epigastric awareness, retching and vomiting. Salivation, headache, increased intestinal peristalsis, fatigue and mental depression may also occur. Humans and dogs are thought to be particularly susceptible species, but some features of motion sickness are also thought to occur in cats, horses, cows, monkeys, poultry and songbirds. Not all species vomit when they develop motion sickness. Pigs can vomit, whereas sheep do not.

In those species that do vomit, the vomiting can be divided into three phases:

- **Anticipatory phase.** This can include nausea, salivation, sweating, facial pallor, tachycardia, weak pulse, feeling of faintness, headache and diarrhoea. These are largely attributable to parasympathetic and sympathetic nervous activity. They do not necessarily involve higher-centre activity, as they have been observed in a decorticate man subjected to a rough airplane journey, and in a midbrain-transected dog.

- **Retching phase.** This is a pre-expulsion phase in which there is a series of large negative pressure pulses in the thorax at the same time as positive pressure pulses in the abdomen. This causes the gastric contents to rock back and forward between the stomach and oesophagus.
- **Expulsion phase.** After a period of retching, the diaphragm is flattened and a quick jerk of the abdominal muscles expels the contents of the upper part of the stomach into the oesophagus and out through the mouth/nose.

In a study on pigs, one or more pigs vomited during 24% of the journeys (Riches *et al.*, 1996). Overall, 1% of the pigs vomited. Besides vomiting, the signs of travel sickness in pigs may include repetitive chewing, slight foaming at the mouth and prolonged bouts of sniffing at the air whilst intermittently standing and lying down (Bradshaw *et al.*, 1996). Between bouts of vomiting, stomach motility in humans is reduced and this is brought about by reduced vagal nerve activity and the release of vasoactive intestinal peptide (VIP) and lysine vasopressin. VIP inhibits gastrointestinal motility and its concentration in plasma has served as a useful physiological indicator of motion sickness.

Motion sickness results from stimulation of the vestibular apparatus in the inner ear, particularly when there are discrepancies between the signals coming from the vestibular apparatus and visual sensations. The vestibular system has two components: the vestibular sacs and the semicircular canals. The vestibular sacs respond to the force of gravity and inform the brain about the head's orientation. The semicircular canals respond to angular acceleration (i.e. changes in rotation of the head). Low-frequency stimulation of the vestibular sacs can produce nausea, and stimulation of the semicircular canals can produce dizziness and rhythmic eye movements (nystagmus). Changes sensed by the vestibular apparatus send nervous impulses to the reticular formation of the medulla oblongata in the brain. This region of the brain controls expulsive activity during vomiting, and a region which is dorsolateral to this structure controls retching activity. Projections from the medulla are responsible for the autonomic and sensory effects that occur during motion sickness.

Vibration of the truck during transport can create discomfort and it may lead to motion sickness. Vibration arises from acceleration, deceleration and uneven road surfaces. Chickens find 1.0 Hz vibration in the horizontal axis particularly aversive, and for humans vertical motion at about 8 Hz produces pronounced physical discomfort. Frequencies around 0.2 Hz can lead to motion sickness. A comparison of four pig trucks showed that the twin-axle trailer which farmers often use to transport up to about ten pigs are likely to produce the worst types of vibration pattern. The large fixed-body transporters with air suspension provide the smoothest journeys, and small or medium-sized fixed-body transporters are intermediate (Randall *et al.*, 1996).

Bruising is evidence of poor animal handling. A bruise is painful for two reasons. Firstly, the insult which leads to the bruise could have been painful itself; and secondly, the subsequent swelling and inflammation at the site of the injury leads to a longer-lasting pain and sensitivity to pressure.

Two mechanisms operate in bruise formation which limit the size of a bruise. The first is platelet aggregation. Platelets from the bloodstream adhere to collagen in the damaged surfaces of the blood vessels and surrounding connective tissue. This response is very rapid, and is capable of stopping a haemorrhage within 2 minutes. A longer-lasting, stronger clot is produced by fibrin deposition. This involves a series of reactions which take time, but the end result is the conversion of soluble plasma fibrinogen to insoluble fibrin which enmeshes and strengthens the platelet clot. A platelet clot is white, but when fibrin is added it traps red blood cells, giving a bruise its blood-red appearance.

As a bruise ages it changes colour, from red to yellow. The changes in colour are due to different pigments which are formed as haemoglobin in the bruise is broken down (Fig. 2.3). The rate of the changes is accelerated by exposure to sunlight, and the green and yellow pigments fade in carcasses which are stored in the presence of UV light.

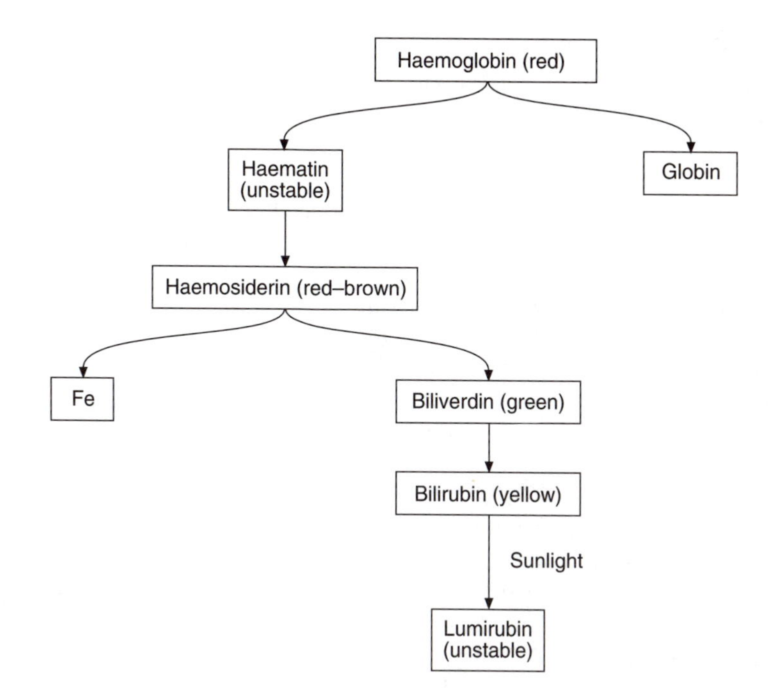

Fig. 2.3. Chemical pathway involved in the colour changes occuring as a bruise ages.

Table 2.3. Ageing bruises in chicken.

Age of bruise	Colour of bruise
2 min	Red
12 h	Dark red–purple
24 h	Light green–purple
36 h	Yellow–green–purple
48 h	Yellow–green (orange)
72 h	Yellow–orange
96 h	Slight yellow
120 h	Normal

In chickens the changes in colour can be used to determine the age of a bruise (Table 2.3), but this may be less reliable for redmeat species.

In redmeat species bruises can be aged by looking for macrophages at the bruised site histologically. After the fibrin has been deposited, leucocytes, neutrophils and macrophages are recruited to the wound as part of the defence against infection. The recruitment of macrophages starts at a later stage than that of the other white blood cells. They are only present in bruises that are at least 4 hours old, and this can be used in diagnosing the age of a bruise. The macrophages engulf the spent red blood cells at the bruise, and they break down the haemoglobin to haemosiderin. This takes time, and the absence of haemosiderin within the macrophages at a bruise indicates that the bruise is less than 24 hours old (Gregory, 1996b). Clearly these methods would not be used routinely, but they may have use in legal prosecutions and defences.

The prevalence of bruised carcasses which require trimming in New Zealand meatworks is shown in Table 2.4. This bruising was sufficiently severe to warrant trimming by the Meat Inspection Service, and it does not include light forms of bruising. The main sites of bruising in a carcass vary between handling systems, but commonly in beef carcasses the hips, round and the top of the back are most affected. The main sites in lamb carcasses are the hindleg and the leading margin of the foreleg (Table 2.5) (Thornton, 1983). Bruising tends to be less serious in pig carcasses, but it can be found around the femur and in the leading margin of the hindleg. In poultry it is particularly common in the wings if the birds have been flapping their wings violently before slaughter.

At saleyards and meatworks, bruising occurs when stock are unloaded, drafted and weighed. The animals strike against fences, gates and sharp corners, often bumping their hindquarters against the obstacle. Bruising no doubt occurs when stock fall over, and this happens when animals push into each other as they are being moved, when they are forced too quickly by the stock handler and when they pass over ground that is covered with wet, slippery manure. Once an animal goes down, it is prone to being trampled by the others and so picks up more bruising. The risk is greatest

Table 2.4. Prevalence of wounds and bruises in carcasses in New Zealand meat-works that required trimming by meat inspection staff.

	%	Source
Cattle	6.0	Selwyn and Hathaway, 1990
Deer	4.3	Selwyn and Hathaway, 1990
Calves	3.5	Biss and Hathaway, 1994
Lambs	0.8	Thornton, 1983

Table 2.5. Common sites for bruising in lamb carcasses.

Position of bruise	Percentage of all carcasses with bruising
Lateral hindleg	33
Medial hindleg	27
Rump	7
Back	6
Shoulder and thorax	9
Brisket	0
Distal foreleg	13
Generalized	4

during transport and it is often said that animals need to be stocked reasonably tightly in the truck, otherwise they are more prone to going down. Eldridge and Winfield (1988) provided support for this when they monitored 400 kg cattle stocked at 0.9, 1.2 and 1.4 m^2 per animal. It was only at the low density that some cattle went down during transport. Owing to this, bruising was worst at the lowest density in this particular study.

Bruising occurs during unloading from the truck if the stock panic or rush at the entrance, if they crush each other against the doorway, and as they manoeuvre to face the right direction. In some countries each deck of a cattle truck is divided into sections with three to five animals in each section. The section nearest the door on the upper deck should be lightly stocked, otherwise there is a risk that the first animal to be unloaded will come down the ramp backwards or bruising will be incurred as it manoeuvres to face the right direction. In trucks fitted with a sliding door there is usually a set of metal or rubber flaps which fold from the ramp and act as a bridge to the truck. It is important that the flaps are not displaced by the stock as they move off the truck, otherwise a hindleg is liable to slip between the ramp and the truck, and the animal goes down and gets wedged in the gap. Guillotine gates in races at the meatworks are an important cause of back bruising, and they should be padded to reduce any insults.

Other less common forms of bruising and trauma include:

- dislocated hips in broilers;
- ruptured livers in poultry;
- dislocated wings in poultry;
- bleeding noses in sheep;
- broken backs in pigs;
- chest perforation from antlers in deer;
- broken metacarpal or neck in deer;
- old bruises which have formed scar tissue.

In many of these situations, if the animal died it would be from hypovolaemic shock (loss of blood). Damage to internal organs, such as rupture of the liver or aorta, often leads to massive bleeding, collapse and death. The extent of blood loss around a broken bone depends on the pressure and space available around the leaking blood vessel. Often there can be significant blood loss following a broken pelvis, hip or shoulder, but there is less loss of blood with fractures of the long bones.

Haemorrhaging from the liver into the abdominal cavity can also be fatal. Although the liver is in a well protected position in the upper abdomen, it is prone to three types of damage: lacerations, subcapsular haematomas and rupture. Lacerations occur, for example, when a hard-antlered deer pushes its antler through the chest wall of another animal. Subcapsular haemorrhages can take the appearance of tiger stripes at the surface of the liver and may occur when an animal is thrown or when it experiences some other form of abrupt blunt impact. Rupturing of the liver is the most common form of liver damage, especially in species with large, soft or fatty livers.

Bruising tends to be more common in the following.

- Stock sold through saleyards (auction markets) in comparison with stock sent straight from the farm to the meatworks. In Britain, carcasses from cattle that were put through saleyards were found to be more stick-marked than those sent direct to meatworks (McNally and Warriss, 1996).
- Unshorn sheep in comparison with shorn sheep. Unshorn sheep acquire more wool-pull bruising. Wool-pull bruises often appear as a shadow under the fascia of the hot carcass when the surface is moved with the hand. They are less obvious in chilled carcasses.
- Entire male pigs that are allowed to fight.
- Stock with less fat and poor conformation.
- Sheep that are swimwashed at the meatworks.
- Cattle that have been showing a lot of mounting behaviour before slaughter.
- Horned cattle in comparison with hornless cattle.
- Cattle that are tightly or too loosely stocked on trucks. At high stocking densities, this is probably linked to damage occuring at unloading. At

very low loading densities, the animals are able to mill around in the truck and this can also result in more bruising and some cattle going down.

- Long journeys. In Australia, where the interval between leaving the farm and slaughter can be as much as 10 days, longer transit times have been linked with more bruising.

Not all bruising occurs before the animal is slaughtered. Some types of bruising occur post-mortem. In poultry, if the carcass is poorly bled or if there is blood left in a wing vein, the plucking operation can damage the vein and massage blood out of the vein, causing a post-mortem bruise (Gregory and Wilkins, 1989). A similar effect sometimes occurs in the skin of the hindleg during flail dehairing in pigs. There are no known situations where bruising has occurred post-mortem in sheep and cattle. In sheep, as soon as the animal has lost 50% of the blood that is due to leave the carcass, bruising will no longer occur (Gregory and Wilkins, 1984). Bleeding an animal promptly after stunning can reduce the severity of a bruise that occurs at or just before stunning. Inducing a cardiac arrest at stunning causes a prompt reduction in arterial pressure, and if the carcass acquires an insult between stunning and sticking, the fall in blood pressure from the cardiac arrest makes it unlikely that a bruise will form.

Bruising can lead to downgrading of carcasses and, at best, trimmed bruises will only find a market in the ground meat trade. Besides being unattractive, bruised meat is often considered unfit for human consumption on hygiene grounds, and in the case of poultry meats there is some justification for this view. Bruised chicken has higher burdens of *Staphylococcus aureus* (Hamdy and Barton, 1965). It is thought that proteolytic enzymes in bruised tissue increase the permeability of chicken skin and tissue at the site of the bruise, and this allows bacteria to penetrate the injured tissue. The situation is less clear in the redmeat species. Bruised tissue from redmeat species normally has a low bacterial count and, contrary to popular opinion, the additional blood does not affect the rate of bacterial proliferation if the meat becomes contaminated (Gill and Harrison, 1982). Blood in the bruise contains sodium and this imparts a salty flavour if the bruised tissue is incorporated into minced meat. Bruised meat has a higher pH than unbruised meat, and bruised carcasses are more likely to have generalized high pH_{ult} meat than unbruised carcasses.

Incidental measurements of meat quality in trauma cases which survived the insult and were subsequently slaughtered have shown that they can have exceptionally high ultimate pH (pH_{ult}) values. This may be linked to the release of large amounts of adrenaline into the bloodstream.

When old wounds are examined in carcasses it is often found that damaged muscles have been replaced by scar tissue, some regenerated muscle and adipose tissue. The damaged area may not have filled to the same extent as the corresponding position on the opposite side of the carcass.

After wounding, muscle regeneration starts with myoblast proliferation and is most active 2–3 days after the injury. Subsequent differentiation of the myoblasts into muscle cells requires an intact nerve supply. If a muscle has been denervated by an injury, the myofibres degenerate and they are instead replaced by connective tissue. Applying the normal tension to a regenerating muscle helps that muscle to take up its normal morphology. From the eating quality point of view, old wounds are unacceptable because the scar tissue makes them tough and because they are abnormal in appearance or unsightly.

Preslaughter accidents resulting in trauma to the animal sometimes involve *bone damage*. Pain is a common feature of bone, joint and ligament injury. It is caused by activation of pain receptors through tearing and displacement of periosteum and muscle fascia. The pain is generally less severe if there is little diplacement of the fractured bone within or through the surrounding muscle. However, where there is a displaced or comminuted fracture, moving or even touching the injured area creates small pressures which will trigger pain. The two most important principles in managing slaughter stock that have damaged bones, joints and ligaments are to limit the animal's movement and to despatch the animal promptly. This means that slaughter equipment must be taken to the animal instead of taking the conscious animal to the slaughterline.

Bone and joint trauma can occur during live animal handling, during stunning and after stunning when the carcass is convulsing. Table 2.6 classifies some of the injuries that are seen in slaughter stock and their carcasses.

Injection site blemishes are due either to an infection developing at the injection site, or to a reaction developing because the material injected was an irritant (Dexter *et al.*, 1994). Infections occur when dirty needles are used for vaccinating or treating livestock. The risk of infection is greater if the stock are wet when they are injected. When the injection itself acts as an irritant, the responses in the animal can include discomfort (e.g. limping), soreness to touch, heat and swelling. Injected materials may act as irritants because of the solvent that is used, and when the irritation is severe it may lead to muscle fibre necrosis and fibrosis. The scar tissue tends to persist and it will make the area of meat inedible when the animal has been slaughtered.

During mustering, yarding, loading and transport, *torn skin* occurs in the following ways:

- contact with barbed-wire, nails, metal stanchions and hinges (cattle, sheep and pigs);
- dog bites (sheep);
- horn damage (cattle);
- fighting (pigs);
- claw damage to the back during catching and transport (ducks, turkeys sometimes);

- contact with cages (farmed salmon);
- rubbing against nets (marine fish).

All these faults decrease the value of the skin and the value of products that are eaten with the skin on (e.g chicken breasts and flat fish). Skin damage

Table 2.6. Types of bone fracture and dislocation.

Classification	Description	Example
Direct bone fractures		
Tapping fracture	Transverse fractures resulting from deceleration applied to a small area. Little soft tissue damage.	Damage to keel and ischium as hens are pulled out of their cages.
Crush fracture	Comminuted or transverse fractures with soft tissue damage. Bone fragments may be displaced and float in the soft tissue. Blood vessels and nerves are often damaged.	Crushed skulls in broilers when drawers of transport modules are closed.
Penetrating fracture	Bone broken by a missile. Bone usually fragments and the smaller pieces can act as secondary missiles.	Damage to cranium by captive-bolt gun.
Indirect bone fractures		
Traction fracture	Bone or joint pulled apart.	Hip dislocation in carcasses that are convulsing whilst suspended from the bleeding line by one leg (rare).
Compression fracture	Compression resulting in buckling and eventually cracking of a bone.	Broken shoulder blade at stunning in pigs.
Joint injuries		
Joint dislocation	Disruption and separation of bones at a joint.	Hip dislocation in broiler chickens during catching.
Chondral fracture	Cartilage fragment shears off the articular surface and floats freely within the joint.	Lameness due to osteochondrosis in pigs.
Ligament injuries		
Ligament avulsion	Complete separation of a ligament from its point of attachment.	Green leg condition in poultry.

is responsible for substantial downgrading of carcasses in the poultry industry. Damage to the skin also allows entry of bacteria into the meat. From the welfare perspective the main concern is with pain produced by the injury. Torn skin is painful because of activation of pain receptors in the skin which occurs, for example, when the cut ends of the skin are rubbed. The pain receptors are free nerve endings and they activate type III and type IV nerve fibres, which provoke an initial sharp pain and a dull burning pain, respectively.

In 1994, a vertically integrated turkey company experienced serious problems with skin damage in the form of back scratching which occurred during the catching procedure before slaughter. The problem arose because the company employed inexperienced staff to do the catching for the Christmas kill. In subsequent years the company controlled this problem by amputating the last joint of each toe of the turkeys when they were poults. More recently, the company has stopped amputating the toes and has introduced a staff training programme instead.

Torn or scuffed skin in pigs occurs when unfamiliar pigs are mixed either before they are transported or when they are held in pens at the abattoir. The pigs fight each other using their lower incisors to gash the opponent along the flank, side, shoulder, neck and ears. This produces bright red weals in the skin, which do not usually penetrate deeply into the fat or muscle. These marks, which are known in the pigmeat industry as rindside damage, do not disappear with scalding, dehairing or chilling of the carcass, and they are often associated with a high pH_{ult} in the meat because of the muscle exercise during fighting. The condition is more common in entire males than in castrates (barrows) or gilts, and it is sometimes found in pigs that are held overnight and squabble because the pens are stocked too heavily.

Problems with barbed-wire scratches in cattle have decreased in those countries where farmers have changed from barbed-wire to electric fencing. Shearing scars in sheep are still a considerable problem in the leather trade. These are usually old scars which have healed, and they form obvious blemishes which downgrade the value of the skin. In New Zealand, it is estimated that 23% of lamb pelts and 74% of sheep pelts carry identifiable shearing scars. The typical regions that are affected are the sternum, the leading margin of the hindleg, the neck, the flank and belly. This damage has obvious welfare implications.

PRESLAUGHTER HANDLING

There are two approaches to trucking animals to meatworks. Small stock can be containerized on the farm and then the container is loaded on to the truck. This approach is used for broiler chickens, end-of-lay hens, ducks, rabbits and most turkeys. The other approach is to walk the stock on to the truck and drive off. This is the usual procedure for cattle, sheep, pigs and deer. Attempts have been made to containerize pigs but they proved too costly.

The modern system for poultry is to load them into crates which are stacked as drawers in a module. A fork-lift truck unloads the empty modules individually from the transport vehicle and carries a module into the grower shed on the farm. The modules are filled with birds by a team of catchers, and then the fork-lift truck returns the full module to the transporter, which is standing outside the shed. Feeders and drinkers inside the shed have to be cleared away beforehand, otherwise they will be damaged by the fork-lift truck. The catchers drive the birds away from the shed entrance, but it is important not to overcrowd the birds otherwise there is a risk of smothering and death from suffocation. The catchers usually grasp the birds by one leg and carry up to seven birds at a time to the module. This procedure can cause damage, especially if the birds become aroused and start wing-flapping whilst they are held. When the birds are being caught the catcher should bend down at the knees to floor level and the birds should be accumulated in one hand with their bodies resting on the floor. Once the correct number has been accumulated they can be lifted. A wrong way is to accumulate birds by one leg in the hand with the birds' other leg standing on the floor. This causes the birds to 'do the splits' and it can lead to hip damage.

Large turkeys are often caught and carried by holding a wing at the shoulder with one hand and the opposite leg with the other hand. Geese and ducks have short legs and so they are often caught by the wings or the neck. When birds are caught and held by the wings it is important to grasp the wings at the shoulder and not to cause too much pressure on the shoulder joint if it struggles. There is a risk of dislocating the humerus from the shoulder joint in young birds. If the bird actively struggles, pause briefly to try to arrest the movement. Birds should not be held by the neck if it creates a risk of compressing the trachea. Ostriches are sometimes handled by holding the lower beak with a thumb in the mouth and leading the bird forwards, with one or more people behind pressing into the bird and directing it. Alternatively a very effective method is to confine the bird and stand alongside its shoulder. Then with a cut-off sleeve covering the right arm, quickly draw the neck of the animal down by grasping the back of the neck with the left hand. Hold the beak with the right hand and evert the cut-off sleeve over the bird's head to cover its eyes. The hooded bird can then be guided to the truck, stunning pen or wherever it has to be taken. Some hooded birds move better in reverse, whereas others are better at moving forwards. Emus should not be hooded. They are best moved individually to the stunner by standing alongside and slightly to the rear of the bird and guiding it with the arms around its girth.

Moving pigs on the farm requires patience. Points worth noting are as follows.

- Some animals, especially fat lop-eared pigs, can be slow to move. They have poor vision and may lack incentive to move fast.
- If the handler tries to rush the pigs they get stressed and once this happens they form a scrum and stick together. They may become less predictable. Often they will turn and try to get back to where they came from. Or they may push into each other and this stresses the other pigs and so the chaos becomes contagious.
- Pigs do not always move as a group. If a gap is available one or more pigs will find it and break away. Good gates, corridors, raceways and ramps are essential.
- When pigs are moved in large groups, the ones at the front will turn back. Handlers often resort to exerting pressure on the pig at the back in order to control the behaviour and direction of the pigs at the front. This can lead to stress. Pigs should be handled in small groups. The level of noise from the pigs is a good indicator of how bad the handling system is. It is possible to move pigs without them screaming.

Cattle handling is discussed in Chapter 3. It is also worth noting how mustering and driving animals on the farm influences foot damage. Young cattle have relatively soft feet which are prone to bruising when walking on rough tracks. Observations made on dairy cows as they are being brought to the milking shed have shown that they normally walk with the head down, carefully placing each front foot to avoid damaging the sole. The hind feet are placed close to the front feet and so they are usually safe from bruising by angular stones in the track provided the cow can focus on positioning its front feet. If the cows are rushed, they are not able to assess the track and place their feet safely. The risk of foot damage is also increased whenever the cattle are crowded. For example, at gateways the cows make unplanned foot placement as they jostle and push each other for position. There are three important lessons from this:

- On rough uneven surfaces, the handler should be patient and allow cattle to move at their own pace.
- Points of congestion pose a higher risk of foot injury.
- Taking cattle over soft ground avoids foot damage, but where tracks are needed to prevent poaching (pugging) of the ground, they should be well maintained. The aim in track maintenance should be to provide an even, well-drained surface with few loose angular stones.

Loading and unloading stock can be very stressful for the animals. Some of the best loading and unloading facilities have no *ramps*. Instead, single-deck trucks, of a standard size and height, back on to a level unloading platform; they have sliding doors instead of tailboards, and bridging flaps span the small gap between the unloading platform and the truck floor. Where multi-deck trucks are used, the unloading platform acts as an adjustable ramp. This is preferable to having ramps fitted inside the truck, as the slope will be less. Alternatively, for multi-deck pig trucks there can be a tailgate lift. The pigs walk on to the lift, which is then raised vertically by a hydraulic pump to the level of the truck floor. Where inclined ramps or tailboards are used, they must be stable; it is generally recommended that the incline does not exceed 20° for cattle, and it should be level for pigs and calves. In the case of pigs, if the incline is steeper than 20° it takes longer for the pigs to pass over the ramp (Fig. 2.4) (Warriss *et al*., 1991). Difficulties are often experienced in ascending and descending ramps inside the trucks, because of their steepness. With pigs, one approach is to get them to slide down the internal ramp, but this causes damage to the small claws on the heel of the hindlegs.

The lighting inside and immediately outside the truck can influence the ease of loading and unloading. Providing a non-glaring light inside the vehicle can encourage cattle on to the truck. Similarly a well lit unloading platform or counting-out pen will make unloading that much easier. Electric goads are commonly used for unloading pigs and cattle, and there are two types: ones that operate off the mains electricity supply and deliver a current at mains voltage; and ones that are battery powered and deliver a current by capacitance discharge. When electric goads have to be used it is recommended that they should only be applied to the rump of the animal, but many modern meatworks companies have now stopped using them, for welfare reasons. The need to use them is sometimes a reflection of some inadequacy in the facilities, such as poor lighting.

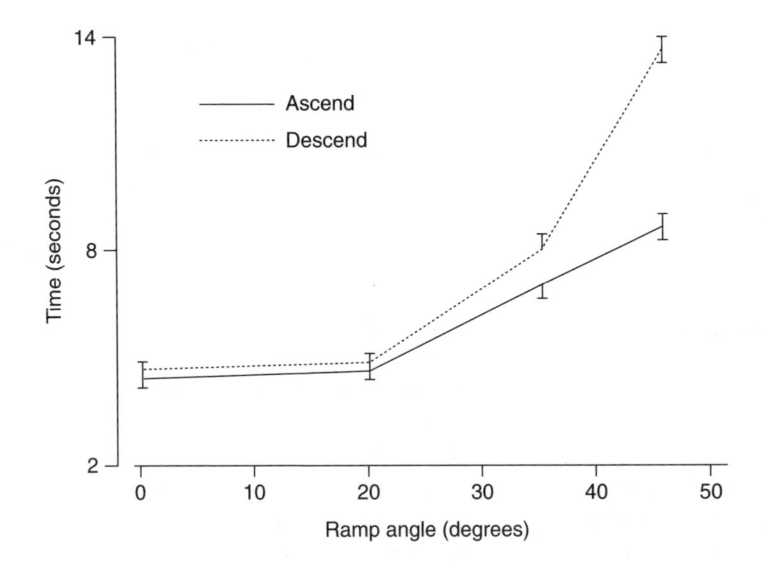

Fig. 2.4. Time taken by pigs to ascend and descend ramps of different slope.

Another difficult situation during preslaughter handling is driving the animal up to the stunning position. In some countries it is a legal requirement to restrain an animal at stunning. This helps to ensure accurate application of the stunning gun or tongs, but it inevitably leads to stress for those animals that do not want to enter the restrainer or that object to being restrained. The usual method of restraint is with a restraining conveyor. Loading the restraining conveyor can pose a problem. The animals first have to be reduced to a single file at the entrance of the conveyor. This is done with either a funnel race, a stepped race or a crowding pen (Fig. 2.5). Each system has its strengths and weaknesses (Warriss, 1994).

Once the animals are in a single file race they are usually loaded into a semi-automatic conveyor which takes them to the stunning position. Figure 2.6 shows the layout for the stunning area for a pig abattoir which has a restraining conveyor. The conveyor grips the pig between two moving walls and conveys it automatically to the stunner, who controls the conveyor with a foot-operated switch. When the pig arrives at the end of the conveyor, the conveyor is stopped and the pig is electrically stunned. When the stunning current flow is completed the conveyor is started again and the stunned pig slides down a chute to a slatted table or platform where it is bled, shackled and hoisted to an overhead rail. There are variations on this arrangement. In beef meatworks the race may lead to a stunning box where the animal is shot with a captive bolt. Another system is to drive a batch of sheep or pigs into a room, then electrically stun them individually, followed by hoisting and conveying out of the room to a bleeding area where they are stuck.

Some animals can be very difficult to handle, and in particular those that are unfamiliar with humans. The handling of pigs and calves early in life helps to familiarize them with humans, makes them less fearful and makes subsequent handling easier (Tanida *et al.*, 1995; Le Neindre *et al.*, 1996). There is also a genetic component to ease of handling (Le Neindre *et al.*, 1996). These are features which the meatworks cannot control. All it can do is design facilities that are appropriate for all types of stock – from the almost wild animals which come from extensive properties, to the pet animal which was reared in someone's back paddock.

In terms of smooth animal handling during the lead-up to stunning, the following difficulties can arise:

- Cattle refuse to enter the stunning box, because they recognize that there is no exit.
- Pigs back in the reverse direction down the lead-in race. This is sometimes reduced by installing heelbars, which the pigs have to walk over when proceeding forwards but which stop them if they go into reverse. One-way push-through gates are sometimes used instead.
- Pigs and sheep show reluctance to enter the restraining conveyor because of a visual cliff effect at the entrance.
- Pigs crowd each other in the race, and do not respond well to the stop–start routine of the restraining conveyor.

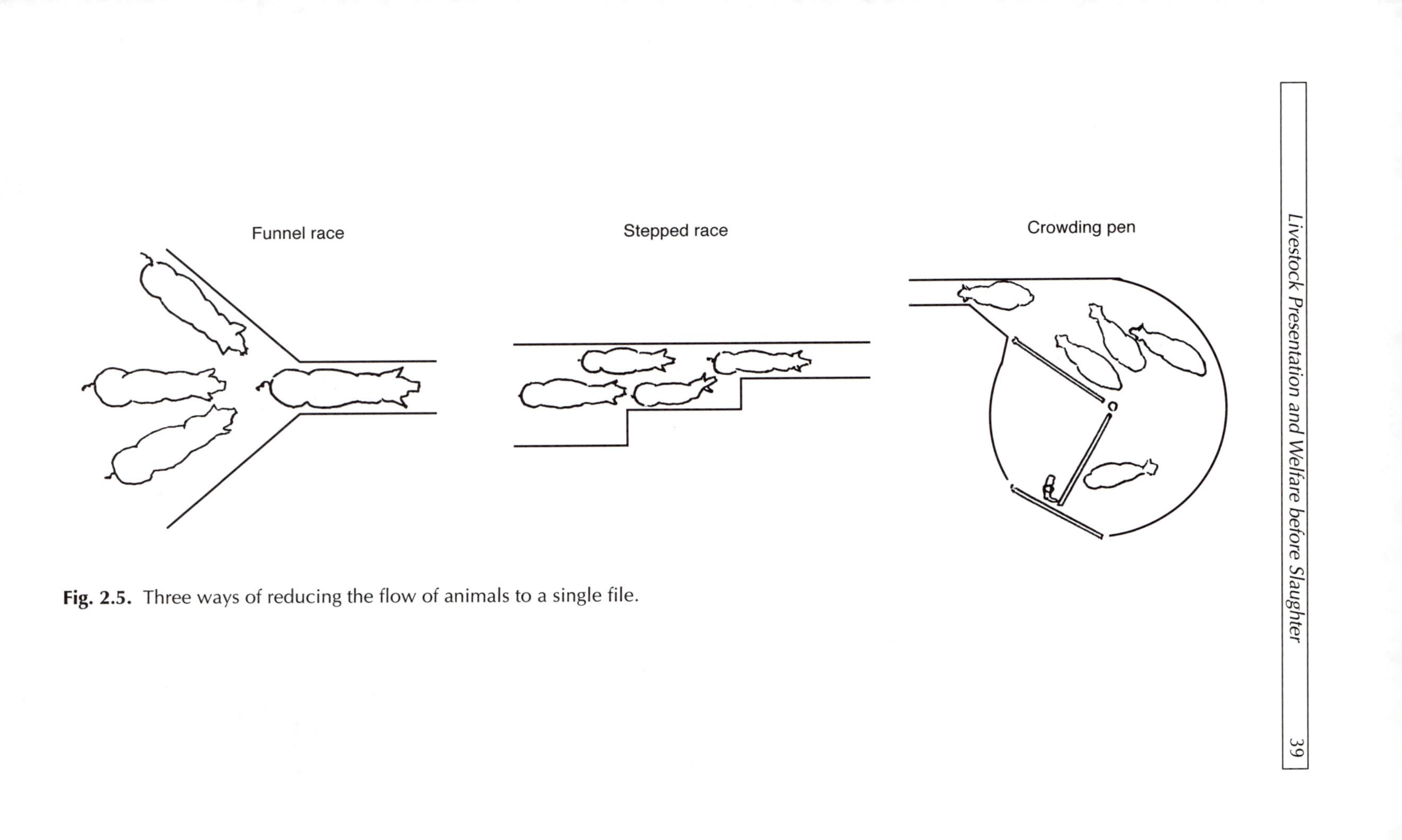

Fig. 2.5. Three ways of reducing the flow of animals to a single file.

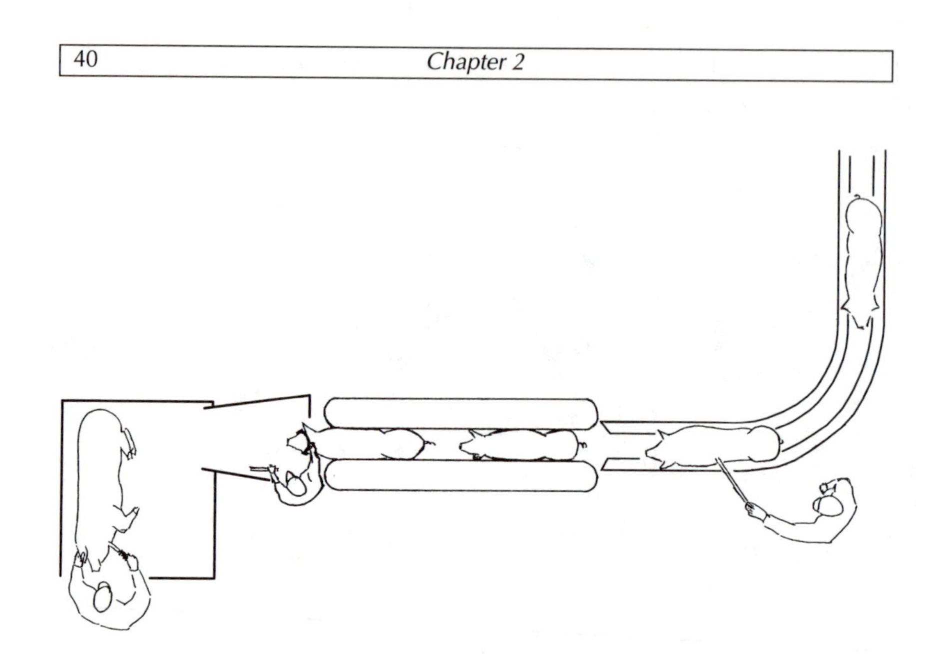

Fig. 2.6. Lead-in race, restraining conveyor, stunning and sticking at a pig abattoir.

Many meatworks try to reduce the problem of difficult handling by conveying the animals. There are two other types of conveyor besides the restraining conveyor. The straddle conveyor supports the animal under the sternum and belly. The walls of this conveyor are static and the moving part of the conveyor is the support on which the animal rests. In the oval tunnel gas-stunning system (see Fig. 13.8), pigs travel on a moving floor conveyor through a gas unit which is filled with carbon dioxide.

Abattoirs do not appreciate receiving *diseased animals*. Extra work is involved in trimming the diseased tissues and if there are a lot of diseased animals the line speed will need to be reduced. There is the risk that microorganisms from the infected tissues will contaminate edible parts of the carcass. In addition the extra trimming reduces meat yield. Practical experience shows that when there is an economic downturn in agriculture the number of diseased stock submitted for slaughter rises. Farmers reduce their veterinary costs and they are more likely to send in sick animals rather than treat them.

Theoretically one might expect that for some infectious diseases the edible meat that comes from the trimmed carcasses could be more tender than normal meat. During the inflammatory response in diseased animals, muscle catabolism is increased. The proteins are hydrolysed to produce amino acids which are used in the liver as part of the body's defence against the infection. If the enhanced proteolytic activity in muscle persists post-mortem, the meat from diseased animals might tenderize more rapidly.

Periodically livestock farmers are faced with a problem of deciding whether an animal is *fit for transport* to the abattoir from the welfare perspective. There are three general rules which can be used as guidelines:

- Can the animal bear weight on all four legs? If it cannot, there is a risk that it will lose balance during the journey and go down. If it goes down it could injure itself or get trampled by other stock.
- Is it likely to suffer unduly during the journey? An example might be a heifer which has severe skin sores from facial eczema. The skin would inevitably be rubbed during the journey. In this case it would be better to allow the skin to heal before transporting the animal.
- Will the animal be in a worse condition as a result of the journey? An example would be animals which are weak and emaciated. The journey would sap their strength, and if they are weak some might collapse, get trampled and be unable to walk off the truck.

Some examples of diseases and disorders which pre-empt submission for slaughter for welfare and hygienic quality reasons include:

- active arthritis;
- acute fractures and dislocations;
- ascites;
- bloat stabs;
- metritis;
- necrotic cancer eye;
- gangrenous mastitis;
- skin conditions such as subacute photosensitivity and suppurative epitheliomas.

If a *casualty animal* is identified on the truck or in a holding pen and it is likely that it is in pain, it should be slaughtered immediately. This might disrupt the routine of the slaughterline, in which case provision should be made for separate staff and equipment to be available for deployment to do this job. There should be convenient access to the slaughterline for carcasses from casualty stock.

It is sometimes suggested that one way of pre-empting the stress of transport and preslaughter handling is to slaughter the animals on the farm of origin. This, in fact, occurs at some feedlots where the meatworks is within walking distance of the feedlot pens. Several *mobile slaughterlines* have been designed which tour farms and provide a slaughtering and dressing service for farmers. Their throughput, however, is very low (about ten EC cattle units per day). It is feasible to slaughter and dress an animal in a mobile slaughterline and comply with EU hygiene regulations at the same time (Gregory, 1992a).

Chapter 3

Solving Livestock Handling Problems in Slaughter Plants

Temple Grandin

INTRODUCTION

Animals should move quietly at a walk through pens and races with a minimum of visible excitement or agitation. Most animals should walk calmly into a stunning pen or a restrainer without the use of an electric goad. If animals balk and refuse to move through a facility, it is important to determine the cause of the problem. Are handling difficulties caused by an equipment problem, or are they due to a lack of employee training and supervision? This chapter provides a practical guide for monitoring livestock handling procedures and for solving problems, and contains step-by-step information for locating and correcting handler and equipment problems. The information contained in this chapter is based on experience in handling animals in over 100 slaughter plants. The author has designed handling facilities and restraint equipment in slaughter plants in the United States, Canada, Australia, New Zealand and other countries.

The importance of reducing stress during slaughter is clear. In pigs, reducing excitement and agitation during handling in the stunning race will improve welfare and help to preserve meat quality (Sayre, 1963; Barton-Gade, 1984; Grandin, 1994). A study by Warriss *et al.* (1994) indicated that the sound level of vocalizing pigs in a slaughter plant was correlated with reduced pork quality. Furthermore, Voisinet *et al.* (1997) found that cattle which become agitated during handling and restraint had tougher meat, and more borderline dark cutters. In many different pork slaughter plants, the author has observed that reducing the use of electric goads and preventing pig pile-ups in the stunning race resulted in a reduction of PSE (pale soft exudative meat) by approximately 10%. Pork slaughter-plant managers have reported that when handling practices were improved, 10% more pork was accepted for export to Japan.

NEED FOR OBJECTIVE SCORING OF WELFARE

There is a need for objective scoring methods for assessing animal welfare during handling and stunning. Objective scoring could be used to monitor the performance of both people and equipment. When animals are handled quietly at slaughter plants, cortisol levels are similar to those during on-farm handling and restraint (Mitchell *et al.*, 1988; Ewbank *et al.*, 1992; Tume and Shaw, 1992; Zavy *et al.*, 1992; Grandin, 1993, 1997a). Scoring methods must be objective and simple enough to use under commercial conditions. The author was commissioned in 1995 and 1996 by both Agricultural Canada and the US Department of Agriculture (USDA), to conduct surveys of large and small slaughter plants. Information was used from these surveys to develop objective scoring methods for assessing animal welfare during handling and restraint. The following objective measures are recommended:

- percentage of cattle stunned with one captive bolt shot;
- percentage of animals where electric stunning electrodes are placed in the correct position to insure that the electric current flows through the brain;
- percentage of animals slipping or falling during handling and stunning;
- percentage of cattle vocalizing during handling, restraint and stunning;
- sound level measurements of pig squealing;
- percentage of pigs which squeal either during stunning or while they are in the restrainer;
- percentage of animals prodded with an electric goad;
- percentage of possibly sensible animals on the bleed rail.

Measurements should be done at both the beginning and the end of a shift, because performance declines when people get fatigued.

VOCALIZATION SCORING FOR WELFARE ASSESSMENT

Vocalization scoring during handling or restraint for stunning is a simple and practical way to identify objectively problems which would be detrimental to good animal welfare. Monitoring the percentage of cattle or pigs that vocalize during restraint can help plant management to determine if a restraint method to hold animals for stunning is aversive. Increased levels of vocalizations such as bellowing and squealing are an indicator of animal distress. Dunn (1990) reported that restraining beef animals in an apparatus which turned them on to their backs resulted in a significantly greater percentage of cattle vocalizing compared with restraint in a device which held them in an upright position. Inverting the animal also increased the number of vocalizations per animal and its cortisol levels. Studies in pigs indicate that the sound level and pitch of squealing are associated with pain and distress (White *et al.*, 1995). Warriss *et al.* (1994) found that the intensity of pig squeals during handling in a commercial slaughter plant was correlated with physiological indicators of stress. The intensity of pig squealing was measured by recordings from a sound meter.

Survey results indicated that plants with good equipment and well trained employees in the stunning area attained low cattle vocalization percentages of 3% or less (Grandin, 1997b). In a plant with careful quiet handling, and a state-of-the-art restraining conveyor system, over 300 feedlot heifers were scored for vocalization. Only 1.3% vocalized while riding on or entering the restrainer. No attempt was made to quantify the intensity or number of cattle vocalizations per animal. Each animal was scored as being either a vocalizer or a non-vocalizer. Vocalization scoring should only be done in the stunning area, which consists of the stunning pen, restraining conveyor, the single-file race and the crowding pen which leads to it. There is little point in vocalization scoring in the lairage area or holding pens, as cattle standing undisturbed in the lairage will often vocalize to each other. Cattle vocalizations were scored in six different plants during the USDA survey. In four plants, the cattle were handled carefully and electric goads were only used on animals that refused to move; the percentage of cattle which vocalized in the stunning area was 1.1%, 2.6%. 6.6% and 7.5%. In two plants with rough handling and excessive goad use, 12% of the cattle vocalized in the first plant, and 32% vocalized in the second plant. When excessive use of electric goads was stopped, the percentage of cattle that vocalized dropped from 12% to 3% in the first plant, and from 32% to 13% in the second plant.

Unless something obviously aversive happens to cattle, they usually do not vocalize when they are being driven through a race or into a stunning pen or restrainer. In the USDA survey, a total of 1125 cattle were scored for vocalization in six slaughter plants; of these, 112 cattle (10%) vocalized in the stunning area during handling. With the exception of two cattle, all of the animals vocalized in response to an observable aversive event such as prodding with an electric goad, slipping on the stunning pen floor, missed captive-bolt stuns, pinching by moving parts of a restrainer apparatus, or excessive pressure exerted by a restraint device powered by either pneumatic or hydraulic cylinders. The effects of excessive pressure were easily observable. The animal remained calm as the apparatus slowly squeezed it, and then it bellowed as the steadily increasing pressure caused discomfort. In one plant, excessive pressure caused 35% of the cattle to vocalize. This would be a serious animal welfare problem.

Vocalization scoring will not work for sheep. Sheep quietly walking up the stunning race often vocalize to each other, whereas cattle seldom vocalize during handling unless an obvious aversive event occurs. However, vocalization scoring can be used to evaluate restraint equipment for pigs. In one plant that was surveyed, 14% of the pigs vocalized in a restraining conveyor where a missing part caused the pigs to be pinched. In several plants none of the pigs squealed in the restrainer. Since counting individual pig squeals in a large group of pigs is impossible, a sound meter could be used to quantify squealing during handling.

Vocalization scoring is not possible if an animal is immobilized by being paralysed with an electric current. This procedure prevents the animal from vocalizing. Several meatworks have considered introducing electroimmobilization to restrain cattle before stunning. Studies conducted in a number of laboratories indicate that this procedure is very aversive (Lambooy, 1985; Grandin *et al.*, 1986; Pascoe, 1986; Rushen, 1986). It is the author's opinion that the use of electricity to restrain conscious animals should be banned. Electrical immobilization, which must not be confused with proper electrical stunning, does not make an animal insensible (Lambooy, 1985). Electrical stunning uses high amperages which are passed through the brain, inducing instantaneous insensibility. The low amperages and voltages used in electrical immobilization are sufficient to paralyse the muscles but the animal will still be conscious.

TRAINING HANDLERS

People who handle livestock need to understand the basic behavioural principles of moving animals. The expertise of the people handling the animals will affect stress levels (Weeding *et al.*, 1993). In pork and beef plants, the most common handling mistake is overloading the crowding pen leading up to the single-file race (Grandin, 1996). Cattle and pigs need room in which to turn. Handlers should be instructed to fill the crowding pen no more than three-quarters full; half full is best. Figure 3.1 shows the proper operation of the crowding pen. Note that the crowding gate is not pushed up against the animals. Cattle and pigs should enter the race easily when they are moved in small groups as shown in Fig. 3.1. If they balk and refuse to enter the race, either there is something wrong with the facility, or they can see a moving person up ahead. In the figure, the man in the dark shirt is standing back so that the approaching cattle do not see him.

In many plants, over-use of crowding gates is often a problem, especially if they are powered gates. Handlers must not attempt to push animals forcibly with a crowding gate. When pigs and cattle are handled, they should be moved towards the stunning area in small groups, and handlers should also avoid overfilling the corridor that leads up to the crowding pen – it should be only half full. Handlers also need to learn how to time movements of each group of animals between the yards and the

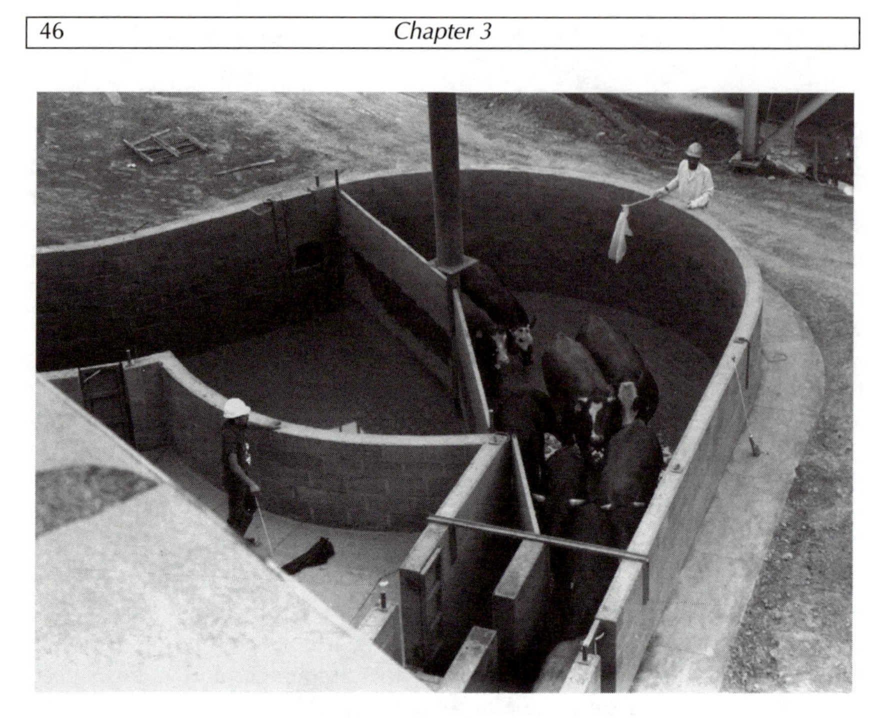

Fig. 3.1. A small group of cattle moved quickly into a single-file race from a forcing pen.

crowding pen: the pen should not be filled with the next group of animals until there is space in the single-file race. Filling the crowding pen when the race is full will often cause cattle and pigs to turn round.

Whereas cattle and pigs should be moved in small bunches, this principle does not apply to sheep. Due to their strong following behaviour, it is important never to break the flow. Sheep can be moved in large groups and should be moved through the crowding pen in a steady stream. The crowding pen may be completely filled but the sheep must not be squeezed tightly with the crowding gate. A good way to visualize how sheep move through a race is siphoning water: the animals are 'sucked through' by their intense following behaviour.

FLIGHT ZONE PRINCIPLES AND POINT OF BALANCE

Figures 3.2, 3.3 and 3.4 illustrate the animal-handling principles of flight zone and point of balance. These principles work for all livestock. To make an animal go forward, the handler must be behind the point of balance at the shoulder (Fig. 3.2). A common mistake made by many handlers is to stand in front of the animal's shoulder and attempt to move it forward by prodding it on the rear. An animal will not move forward until the handler is behind the point of balance at the shoulders.

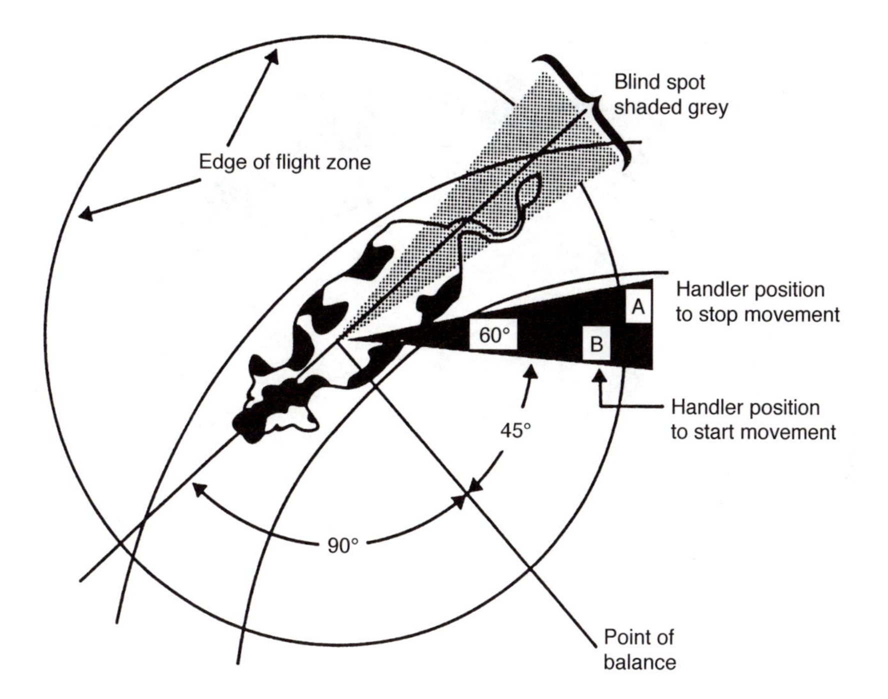

Fig. 3.2. Basic flight zone diagram showing the point of balance and the blind spot.

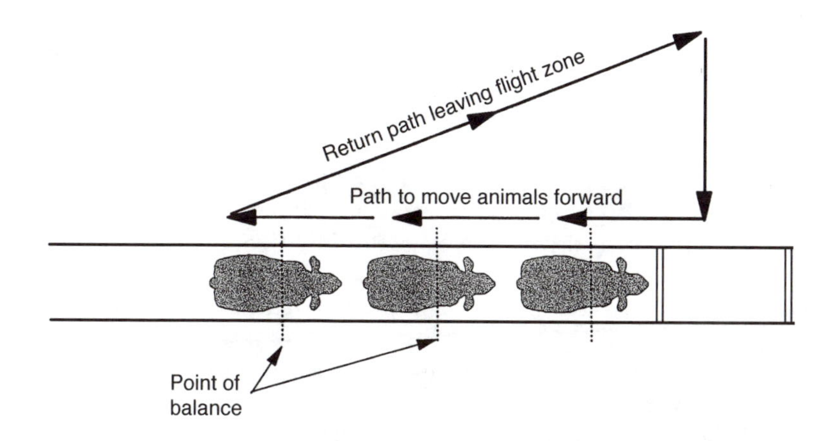

Fig. 3.3. Handler movement patterns for inducing animals to move forward in a straight race. Cattle will move forwards when the handler passes the point of balance at the shoulder of each animal. The handler walks in the opposite direction alongside the single file race.

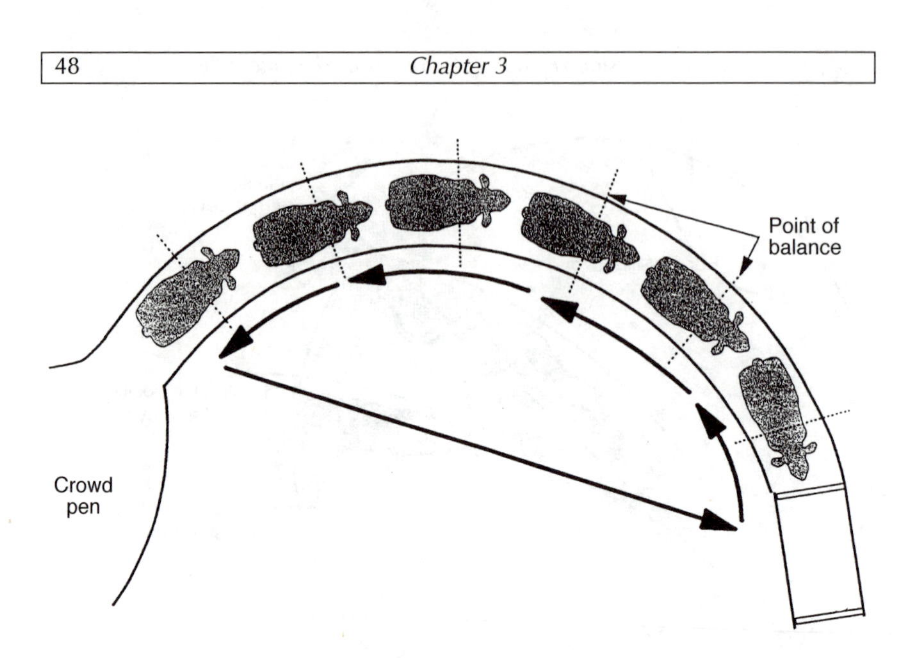

Fig. 3.4. Handler movement patterns for inducing animals to move forward in a curved race. Cattle will move forward when handler crosses the point of balance of each animal.

Animals that are not completely tame have a bigger flight zone, which is the animal's safety zone. If the animal is in a large pen, it will move away when a person enters the pen. When a person is outside of the flight zone, the animal will turn round and look at them, but when the handler enters the flight zone, the animal will turn away. A wild animal may panic if it cannot escape from a confined area when its flight zone is invaded. Extensively raised cattle with a large flight zone may rear up in a race in an attempt to get away from a person. In this situation the handler should back up and get out of the animal's flight zone. Tame animals which are accustomed to people and handling are less likely to attempt to escape by rearing or turning back on a handler. A completely tame animal has no flight zone and is sometimes difficult to drive. However, the flight zone becomes smaller when there is a solid barrier such as a fence covered with steel sheeting between the animal and a person. The solid barrier makes the animal feel safe.

Animals can be moved quietly, and are less likely to become agitated, if the handler works on the edge of the flight zone. Figure 3.5 illustrates the collective flight zone of a group of sheep. Figures 3.3 and 3.4 show the handler positions for inducing animals to move forward in a race. Animals will usually move forward when the handler penetrates the flight zone and walks in the opposite direction of desired animal movement. The animal goes forward when the handler crosses the point of balance at the shoulder. The handler should remain inside the animal's flight zone when walking in

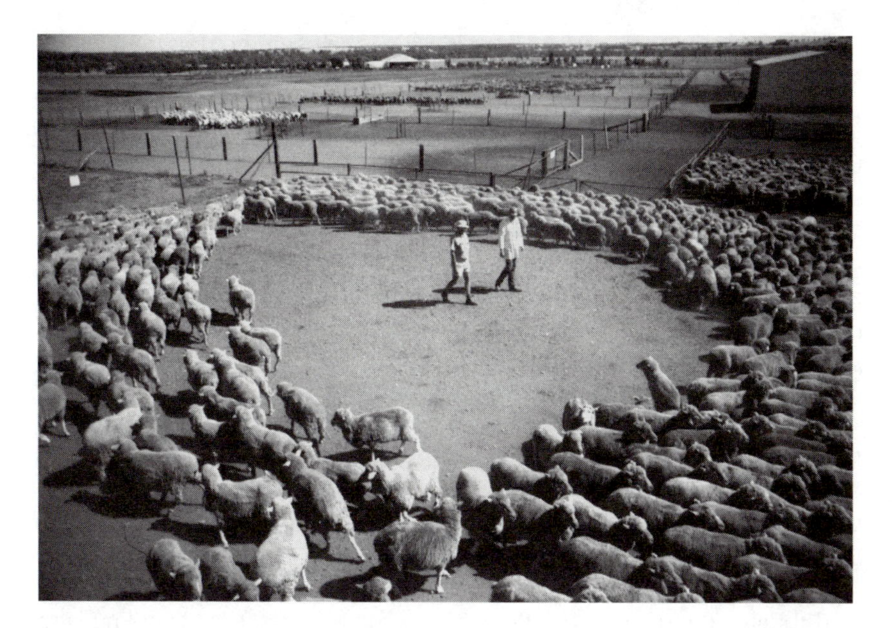

Fig. 3.5. Collective flight zone of a large flock of sheep. Note that the sheep move in the opposite direction to the handler.

the direction opposite to desired movement. A handler walking in the same direction as the desired movement should be outside the flight zone. The movement pattern in Fig. 3.3 can be used to induce an animal to enter a stunning pen or restrainer. Handlers should stand outside the flight zone until they want the animal to move.

Continuous pressure caused by standing deep in the animal's flight zone is counter-productive. The handler should not apply pressure to the animal's flight zone until movement is desired. To move only one animal, the handler should stop moving back in the opposite direction to the desired movement after the point of balance of the first animal is crossed. For further information on flight zone principles, refer to Grandin (1993a, 1998), and Kilgour and Dalton (1984).

Cattle, pigs and sheep can become highly stressed if they are isolated from other animals. In sheep and cattle, confinement and isolation cause an elevation in cortisol concentration which is much higher than with restraint (Parrott *et al.*, 1994; Boissy and Boissou, 1995). A lone isolated cow can be very dangerous to handle. Isolation makes the animal fearful and it may charge handlers in an attempt to rejoin its herdmates. A lone agitated cow or steer is a common cause of handling accidents, and handlers should be instructed never to enter a crowding pen containing an agitated lone bovine. If the animal refuses to enter the race, it is often best to let it go or put it in with another group of cattle. A single animal must never be left alone in a restrainer or stunning pen during coffee breaks or lunch.

If a cow or steer escapes and is loose on the plant grounds, employees should not chase it. If it is left alone it will usually return to the cattle pens. Employees should be instructed to stay out of its flight zone until it has calmed down. When it calms down, it can be carefully directed back to the lairage by working on the edge of its flight zone.

Cattle will sometimes rear up in a race or stunning pen. The animal rears because the handler is deep in its flight zone and it is attempting to get away. It will often settle down again if the handler steps back and removes himself from the animal's flight zone. Handlers should not forcibly attempt to push a rearing animal back down: this will often increase the animal's agitation because the handler is penetrating even deeper into its flight zone.

REDUCING OR ELIMINATING ELECTRIC GOADS

When an animal becomes agitated and fearful, many people do not realize that it can take a long time for it to calm down. In cattle, it can take up to 30 minutes for the heart rate to return to normal if the animal has been handled roughly (Stermer *et al.*, 1981). The secret to quiet, easy handling is to avoid getting the animal excited. Good stockmen have known for years that 'slow is faster' (Bud Williams, Canada, and Burt Smith, University of Hawaii, personal communication, 1997). Calm animals are easier to move and are less likely to balk. To keep animals calm, handlers should use slow, deliberate movements. Sudden jerky movements cause animals to become excited: in the wild, sudden movements are associated with predators and danger. Handlers should also refrain from yelling and making loud noises.

Electric goads should be replaced as much as possible with other driving aids, such as a stick with a flag or plastic streamers on the end. The flag should be used to direct the animals gently and should not be shaken vigorously (Fig. 3.6). An animal will often move forward if the flag is moved across the point of balance in the direction opposite to the desired movement. Brooms or small solid boards can be used to move pigs quietly into the races (Fig. 3.7).

Teaching handlers the behavioural principles of handling can greatly reduce the use of electric goads in large slaughter plants. For example, this was examined at three large slaughter plants with chain speeds ranging from 100 to over 200 cattle per hour. After the employees had been instructed in the use of behavioural principles for moving cattle in the yards, crowding pen and race, it was possible to move 90% to 95% of the cattle through the entire system without electric goads. In four beef and pork plants, rough handling and excessive use of electric goads was reduced after only 5 minutes of instruction. Plant employees were simply instructed to fill the crowding pen only half to three-quarters full, and to attempt to move each animal by tapping it on the rear before resorting to an electric goad. Electric goad usage in the stunning race decreased from 64% of the animals

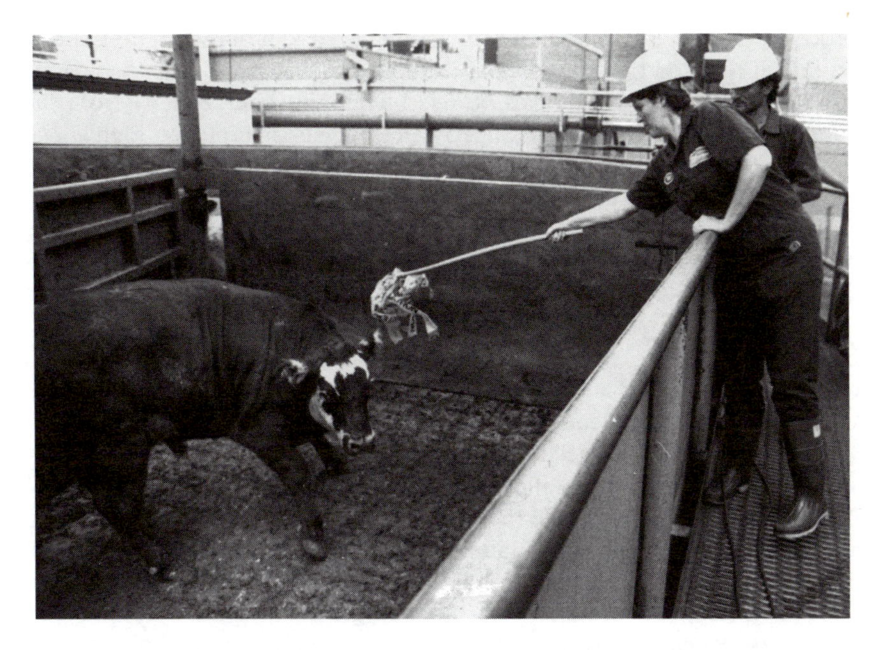

Fig. 3.6. Temple Grandin demonstrates the use of a stick with plastic streamers on the end for turning a steer in the forcing pen.

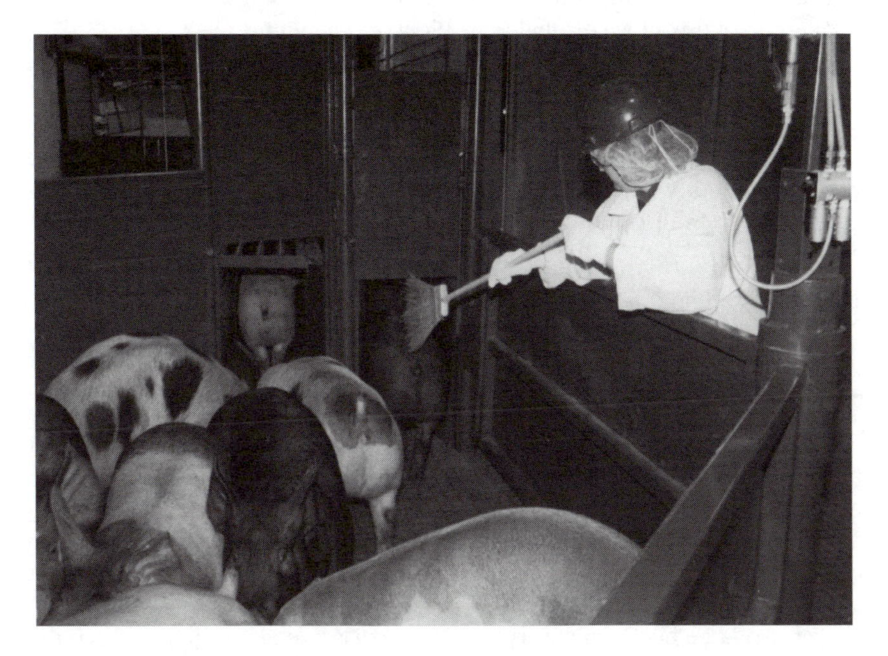

Fig. 3.7. A broom is used to move pigs into races.

prodded to only 16%. The handlers were able to keep up with the slaughter line at reduced prodding rates (Grandin, 1997b).

In sheep plants, goats can be used to move sheep quietly from the lairage into the crowding pen. Sheep will flow easily through a high speed sheep line and electric goads should never be used. It is the author's opinion that the use of dogs in a slaughter plant should be banned.

DISTRACTIONS CAUSING BALKING

In some plants, it is extremely difficult to reduce the use of electric goads because animals balk and refuse to move through a race or corridor. Even with well trained handlers, cattle and pigs will still balk at distractions such as shadows and shiny reflections. In eight pork and beef plants in the USDA survey, two plants had very high electric goading scores due to distractions. It was not possible to reduce the use of electric goads and still be able to keep the slaughter line filled. Handlers had to use electric goads on 64% of the cattle and 80% of the pigs in these two plants (Grandin, 1997b). Both plants had easily correctable distractions. In the beef plant, the cattle could see a person's hand moving under the stunning pen exit door. In the pork plant, the pigs refused to move from a crowding pen illuminated with sunlight into a darker stunning race. The problem in the beef plant was corrected by installing a piece of conveyor belting to block the gap at the bottom of the stunning pen door. In the pork plant, pigs moved more easily after a solid wall was installed to block the sunlight.

Problems caused by distractions usually fall into one of five categories: (i) lighting problems; (ii) seeing moving equipment or people up ahead; (iii) seeing contrasts; (iv) excessive noise; and (v) air drafts blowing in the faces of approaching animals. Distractions that make animals balk can ruin the performance of well designed equipment. The following sections discuss how to correct these problems.

Lighting problems

Animals tend to move best from a darker place to a more illuminated place (van Putten and Elshof, 1978; Grandin, 1982). Animals will not enter a race, stunning pen or restrainer if the entrance is too dark. Lamps aimed at the entrance of a race or restrainer will often facilitate entry (Fig. 3.8). The light must not shine directly into the eyes of approaching animals – animals will not approach blinding light. Lamps can also be used to induce animals to put their head into a head restraint device. A portable lamp can be used to experiment with lighting and to determine the best position for a permanent lamp.

In two large beef plants surveyed, there was adequate lighting when the systems were new, but balking increased as the sodium lamps dimmed with

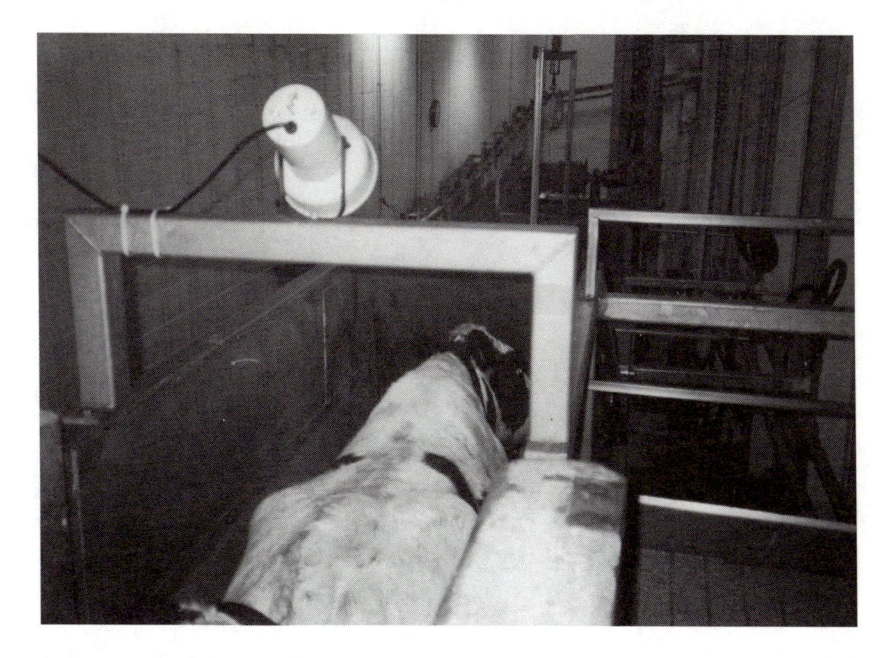

Fig. 3.8. A spotlight aimed at a restrainer entrance will help to induce all species of livestock to enter.

age (Grandin, 1996). There can also be time-of-day effects in facilities with natural lighting. The sun may make a shadow in the morning, but not in the afternoon. The author has observed several plants where animals moved easily on cloudy days, but balking increased on sunny days due to shadows and harsh contrasts of light and dark (Fig. 3.9).

Sparkling reflections on shiny metal, dripping water or a wet floor will also make animals stop. To see the reflections or shadows, get down to the animal's eye level. In indoor facilities, problems with reflections can often be eliminated by moving a lamp slightly. Lamps installed directly over the centre line of a race or restrainer sometimes create greater reflection on wet floors. This can be corrected by installing lamps slightly off the centre line. Reflections can sometimes be eliminated by covering the top of the race. To solve lighting problems, one has to experiment.

Seeing motion or people ahead

All livestock may balk and refuse to move if they see people or equipment moving rapidly up ahead. Races and crowding pens should have solid sides to block the animals' vision. Installing a shield for a person to stand behind can also prevent balking. Cattle and sheep are prey species animals with visual systems tuned to detect slight movement in the environment.

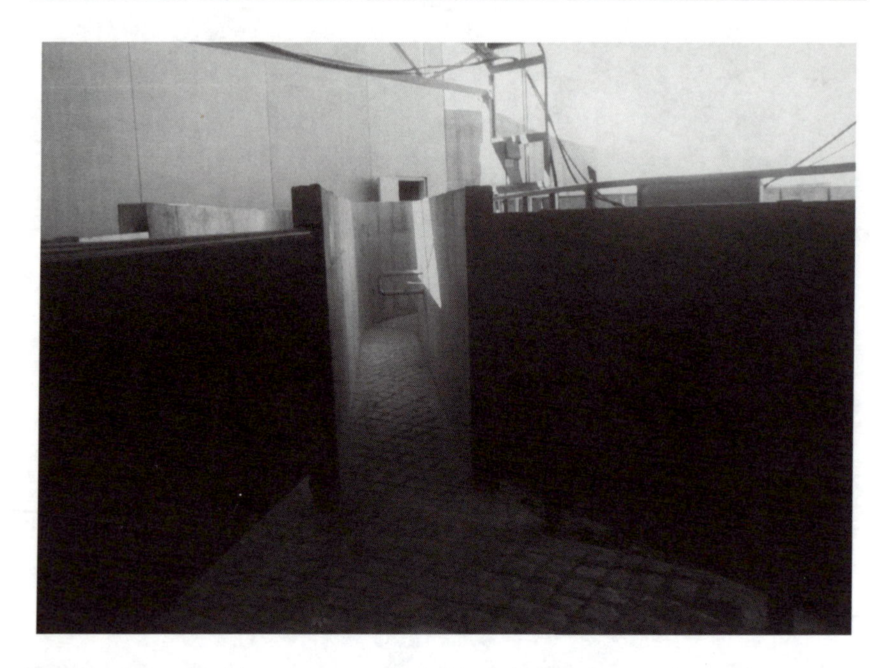

Fig. 3.9. Animals will tend to move from this darker forcing pen into a more brightly illuminated race, but they may balk at the sharply contrasting bright patch of sunlight on the inside of the race.

Livestock are very aware of slight intermittent movements of gates or other equipment as they move into crowding pens and races. They may stop if they see a piece of chain moving over a race, or a metal panel that rattles and moves. In one surveyed plant, pigs refused to move through a race because of a loose gate in the side of the race. The pigs moved more easily when the gate was tied shut with wire. Moving fan blades can also make animals balk. Figure 3.10 illustrates a facility where cattle balked at plastic strips which were moved by either people passing through them or the wind.

When animals are calm and walking through a facility, it is easy to observe distractions that cause balking. Lead animals will often stop and look straight at a small moving chain or other distraction. However, when the animals are excited, they no longer look at the distraction.

Seeing contrasts

Animals are often reluctant to approach areas of high contrast between light and dark. Facilities should be painted the same colour; light and dark contrasts should be avoided. Lighting should also be adjusted so that harsh shadows are eliminated. In a corridor, animals often avoid walking on a shadow running down one side.

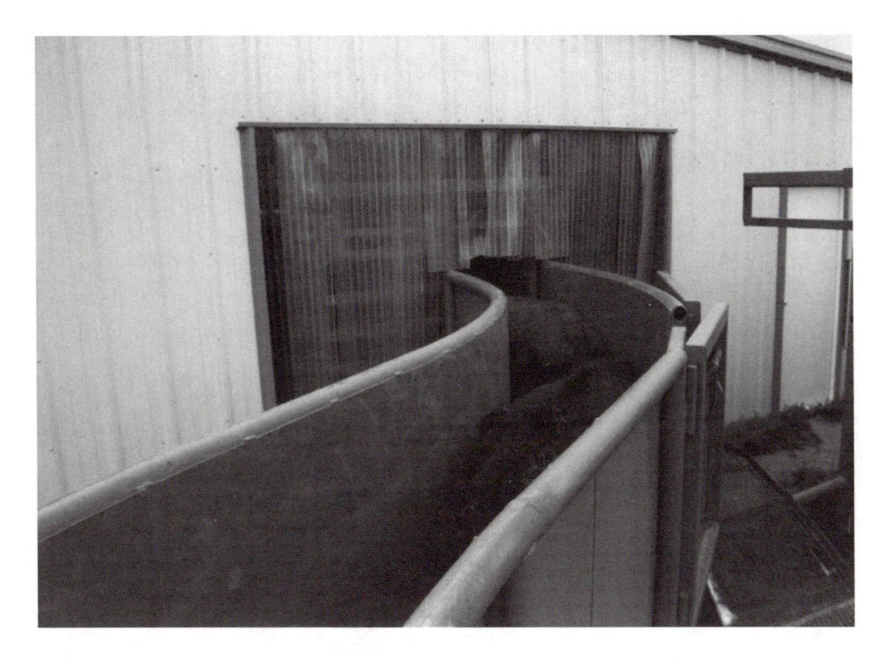

Fig. 3.10. Cattle balked when the plastic strips moved.

A drain grate located near a race entrance can also make animals balk. When new facilities are built, drains should be installed outside areas where animals walk. In an existing facility, changes in lighting may help to reduce balking at a drain grate.

Something as simple as a coat flung over a race fence may cause the animals to stop. Anything that makes a visual contrast attracts their attention. In one beef plant, an employee dropped a white plastic water bottle near the race entrance, which caused many cattle to turn back. Almost any contrasting feature of a crowding pen or race can make animals balk. In another plant, the handlers used sticks with flags on them to move cattle quietly and effectively. However, when one of the sticks was carelessly left lying on top of the race, the animals balked and refused to move past it.

Animal movement can be improved by covering the gates along the main corridor in the lairage with metal sheeting. This prevents animals that are moving through the corridor from being distracted by animals in the holding pens.

Excessive noise

Cattle and sheep have very sensitive hearing. They are more sensitive to high frequency noise than people and are especially sensitive to high frequency sound around 7000 to 8000 Hz (Ames, 1974). Humans are more sensitive to 1000–3000 Hz (Ames, 1974). Cattle can easily hear up to 21,000 Hz (Algers, 1984) and there is also evidence that cattle have a lower hearing threshold than people (Heffner and Heffner, 1983). This could mean that sounds that may not bother people may hurt the animals' ears.

Reducing noise will improve animal movement. High-pitched noise is worse than low-pitched noise. Employees should not yell, whistle or make loud noises; clanging and banging equipment should be silenced by installing rubber stops and noisy air exhausts should be piped outside or silenced with inexpensive mufflers (muffling devices wear out and should be replaced every 6 months to keep noise levels low). Hissing air is one of the worst noises, but it is also the easiest to eliminate.

A high-pitched whine from a hydraulic pump or undersized plumbing is disturbing to animals and can make them balk. At one plant, installing larger-diameter plumbing to eliminate a high-pitched whine from a hydraulic system resulted in calmer, easier to move animals. In another plant, excessive noise from ventilation fans made pigs balk. Noise from the fans increased as the pigs approached the restrainer.

When new systems are built, there needs to be more emphasis on noise reduction. Recently, the author visited an up-to-date pork slaughter plant. Over 800 pigs per hour were quietly moved through the plant with very little balking. The race system, overhead conveyors and restrainer system were engineered to reduce noise greatly. Gates on the race had rubber pads to prevent clanging and banging; motors and conveyors were designed to reduce high-pitched noise. Well trained handlers quietly moved the pigs up the race with very little squealing.

Air drafts

Quiet handling can also be difficult if air drafts are blowing down the race into the faces of the approaching animals. At the entrance to a stunning pen or restrainer, air should move in the same direction as the animals. This is often a problem because air drafts can change at different times of day, and during different seasons. A plant may have quiet handling in the morning, but handling may deteriorate when more fans are turned on inside the plant. The prevailing wind direction will also affect handling. A wind that blows smells towards approaching animals will impede movement. Some handlers have observed that livestock become agitated and are more difficult to drive when the barometric pressure drops due to an approaching storm.

A common misconception is that animals balk in slaughter plants due to fear of blood smells. It is more likely that the novelty of the smell is what makes them stop. For example, both pigs and cattle will often refuse to enter freshly painted equipment – it is the novel smell of the paint that stops them.

Animals as diverse as cattle, pigs and rodents can smell stress pheromones secreted in saliva, urine and blood (Stevens and Gerzog-Thomas, 1977; Vieville-Thomas and Signoret, 1992; Grandin, 1994). These substances appear to be secreted in pigs and cattle after approximately 10 minutes of severe stress. When animals are moving through the races quickly and quietly, stress pheromones cause few problems. Presumably most animals are slaughtered before the substances are secreted.

FLOORING AND EQUIPMENT MAINTENANCE

Non-slip flooring is essential for quiet, calm handling. Stress levels increase when animals are slipping and falling. Cockram and Corley (1991) found that cortisol levels were high in a plant where cattle constantly slipped. Out of 29 Canadian slaughter plants surveyed by the author, six (21%) had slick floors which interfered with quiet handling (Grandin, 1996). In the USDA survey, most large pork plants had non-slip flooring, but three out of ten beef plants had serious problems with slipping in the stunning pen (Grandin, 1997b). Slipping in the beef stunning pen can be easily fixed by installing a floor grating of 2.5 cm × 2.5 cm rods spaced 30 cm apart. Rod gratings can also be used in other high traffic areas, such as scales and unloading areas.

In existing facilities with slick floors, a grooving machine rented from a concrete supply company can be used to roughen the floor. New concrete floors should be grooved in a 20 cm × 20 cm diamond pattern with 3 cm deep grooves for cattle. For pork slaughter plants, a good floor can be made by printing the pattern of expanded metal mesh into the wet concrete.

Welfare of livestock in slaughter plants can also be compromised by poor maintenance of gates, stunners and other equipment. Out of 11 US beef plants surveyed, four plants had poorly maintained captive-bolt stunners. This caused 9% or more of the cattle to be mis-stunned on the first shot. Poor maintenance is a major cause of poor captive-bolt stunning. Another problem is ergonomics of heavy, bulky pneumatic guns, which are more difficult to position than small, hand-held cartridge-fired guns. In two of the surveyed plants with bulky pneumatic guns, 12–15% of the animals were mis-stunned on the first shot due to aiming problems.

EQUIPMENT DESIGN

Detailed information on facility designs can be obtained in Grandin (1990, 1991a, 1993b). There are three major design mistakes which can make quiet, calm handling extremely difficult: a single-file race that is too wide; a race which appears as a dead end; and a crowding pen on a ramp.

Single-file races and stunning boxes must be narrow enough to prevent animals from turning round or becoming wedged beside each other. A cattle race should be 76 cm wide and races for pigs should have only 3 cm of clearance on each side of the largest pigs. For cattle, a curved race is more efficient (Grandin, 1993); and Grigor *et al.* (1997) reported that deer also enter a curved race more quickly. Curved races work well because animals entering the race cannot see people or other activity up ahead (Fig. 3.11). However, a curved race must be laid out correctly. If it is bent too sharply at the junction between the single-file race and the crowding pen, the animals may refuse to enter because the race entrance appears to be a dead end. Curved races must be laid out so that animals standing in the crowding pen can see a minimum of three body lengths up the race before it turns. Grandin (1984, 1990, 1991a) illustrated correctly curved race layouts. Weeding *et al.* (1993) illustrated a pig race that is laid out wrongly: the race looks like a dead end to the pigs and this system increased stress. Straight races will work well for pigs (Grandin, 1982).

Another serious design mistake is to build a crowding pen on a ramp. In facilities where a ramp is required to reach the stunning box or restrainer, it should be located in the single-file race. Groups of animals in a crowding pen will tend to pile up on the back gate if the crowding pen is located on a ramp. Cattle and sheep will readily move up a ramp but pigs will move easier in a level system with no ramps. New pig handling facilities should be level.

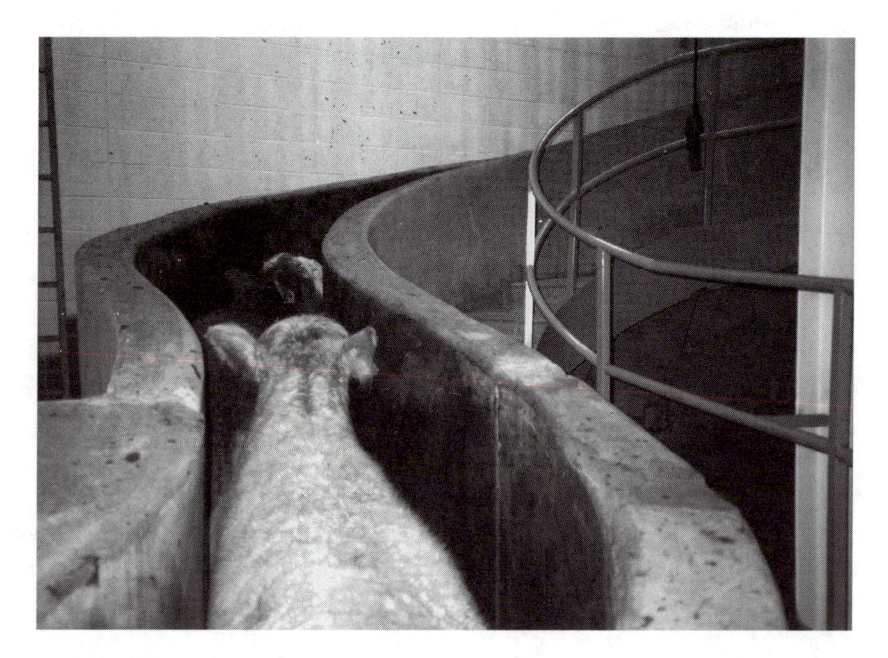

Fig. 3.11. This curved race works efficiently for cattle. Curved races must be laid out correctly.

RESTRAINT PRINCIPLES

In small plants, stress in pigs can be reduced by electrically stunning small groups of pigs while they are standing on the floor (Warriss *et al.*, 1994). When pigs or sheep are stunned while standing loose on the floor, a tong-type stunner must be used. It is clamped on the head like headphones and prevents the animal from falling away from the electrodes before the stun is completed. In plants with chain speeds of over 240 pigs per hour, electric stunning of pigs that are free-standing on the floor tends to become rough and haphazard. In large plants that use electric stunning, pigs have to be lined up in a single-file race and held in a restrainer for stunning. In the future, gas stunning systems where pigs are stunned in small groups of five or six may have the potential to reduce handling stress greatly.

Easy entrance

Design information on different restraint systems is available in Grandin (1988, 1991a,b, 1995, 1997b). To minimize stress during restraint, it is essential that animals enter a restraining device easily. When a well designed restraint device is properly installed and operated, over 90% of the animals should enter without the use of an electric goad. It must be free of the distractions discussed previously. Balking and refusing to enter a restrainer or stunning pen can often be corrected by changing the lighting. In this section, the basic behaviour principles that apply to all restraint devices such as restrainers, conveyors, head restraint devices and restrainers for religious slaughter will be considered.

Pigs, cattle and sheep will enter a restraining conveyor more easily if they do not see a visual cliff effect. Animals will often balk when they can see that the restrainer is high off the plant floor. There are several ways to solve this problem. In an elevated restraining conveyor, illumination should be bright above the restrainer, and dark underneath it. In plants where the restraining conveyor is elevated, installing a false floor will often facilitate entry: the false floor prevents the animals from seeing a steep drop-off under the conveyor and it provides the illusion that there is a floor for the animal to walk on. The animal is picked up by the moving conveyor before its feet touch the false floor. In addition, the entrance to the conveyor should have non-slip footing so that animals can walk in without slipping. If an animal slips, it is more likely to panic and back up. The entrance ramp should never be removed from a restraining conveyor, as this would force the animals to jump off a 'cliff' into the conveyor, which will result in agitation and excitement. The entrance ramp should be long enough for the animals to walk in and be gradually picked up by the moving conveyor.

Blocked vision

Extensively raised cattle which have had little contact with people on the farm of origin should not be able to see people or a pathway of escape until they are completely held in a restraint device. If the animal can see an escape route before it is completely restrained, it is more likely to struggle because it thinks it can get away. A curtain made from conveyor belting installed at the exit of the conveyor often works well. Both pigs and cattle will ride calmly in a restraining conveyor if their vision is blocked by a solid metal hold-down rack. The animal should not be able to see out from under the rack until it has settled down in the conveyor, and its rear feet are off the entrance ramp. In many plants, extending the length of the rack will induce animals to ride more quietly in the conveyor.

In stunning pens where head restraint is used, the animals should not be able to see into the plant or see people until they are completely restrained. Shields should be installed (Fig. 3.12). To reduce stress and prevent struggling, the animal should never be left restrained in a head restraint. Head restraint devices can increase stress if the animal balks and refuses to enter them. Ewbank *et al.* (1992) reported that cortisol levels became elevated in a poorly designed head restraint where over 30 seconds

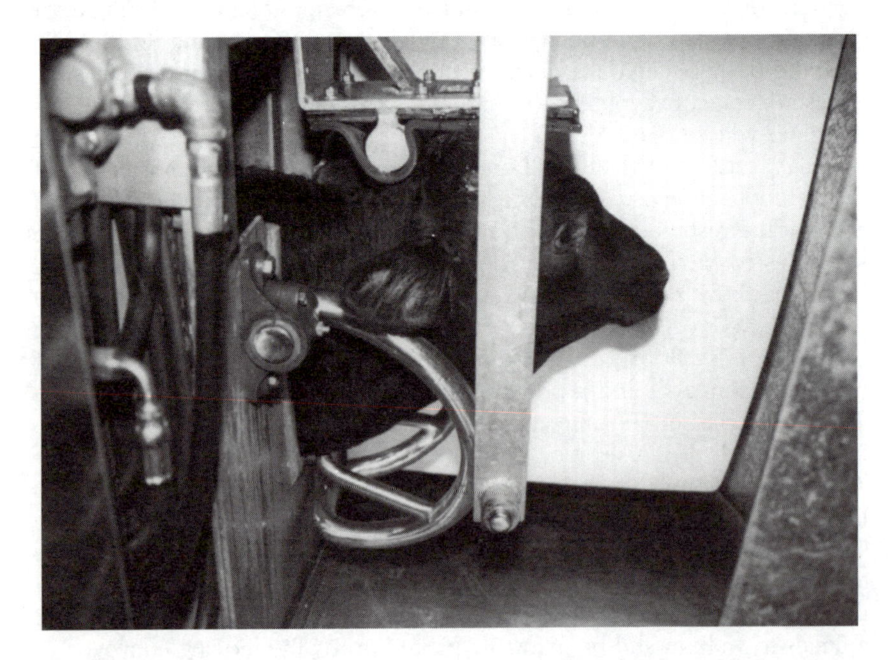

Fig. 3.12. A solid box around the animal's head will help to keep it quieter when a head restraint device is used. The box must be lit to induce the animal to place its head through the head opening.

was required to induce the animal to enter. However, Frank Shaw (1994, CSIRO, Brisbane, Australia, personal communication) stated that very low cortisol levels reported in his paper (Tume and Shaw, 1992) were obtained in a well designed head restraint device.

In some plants a passive head restraint is used to position a bovine's head for captive-bolt stunning. It is a simple shelf installed in the stunning pen which prevents the animal from lowering its head to the floor. A rear pusher gate can be used to keep the animal pushed forward so that it cannot back away from the shelf.

Smooth steady movements

Sudden jerky movement of a restraint device may cause animals to struggle or become excited. Gates and other parts of the restraint device which press against the animal should move steadily (Grandin, 1992). Devices powered by air or pneumatic cylinders should be equipped with flow controls to prevent jerky movement or sudden bumping of the animal. Parts of a restraint device that press against the animal will operate more smoothly if they are controlled by high quality, manually operated control valves which enable the operator to control the flow of fluid or air. On pneumatic systems, return-to-centre valves enabling the operator to stop an air cylinder in mid stroke should be used. Solenoid-controlled valves often create jerky movement unless they are very carefully designed.

Optimum pressure

Many people make the mistake of squeezing animals too hard with a restraint device. Pigs and cattle will struggle when they are held too tightly and many people make the mistake of applying more pressure. It is also important to determine the cause of struggling. Is it due to too much pressure, or is it due to another problem such as slipping on the floor or seeing a person who is in their flight zone? For example, in one beef plant the author was able to prevent cattle from struggling in a restraining conveyor system by blocking their vision with a piece of cardboard. Handlers and engineers must strive to restrain animals using behavioural principles, and not force.

There is an optimum pressure for holding an animal (Grandin, 1995). A restraint device needs sufficient pressure to give the animal a feeling of being restrained, but excessive pressure which causes pain must be avoided. If an animal struggles, pressure should be gradually reduced. However, if the pressure is reduced suddenly, the animal feels the sudden movement and may continue to struggle.

Animals vocalize in restraint devices when excessive pressure or a pinch point causes pain or discomfort. In seven pork plants, pigs vocalized in the V restraining conveyor in four plants, and in one of these plants 14% vocalized due to pinching caused by a missing part (Grandin, 1997b). In three of the plants, none of the pigs vocalized and this was because the restraining conveyor fully supported their bodies. The author observed that very muscular pigs with large hams often vocalize vigorously in a V restraining conveyor, because it pinches their hams. These animals would probably be more comfortable on a centre-track conveyor that supports them under the belly. Pigs will often vocalize and struggle if one side of a V restraining conveyor runs faster than the other. Even a slight difference in conveyor speeds will cause struggling.

In two plants, excessive pressure applied by an upright pen fitted with restrainers for kosher slaughter caused 6% to 12% of the cattle to vocalize. When a kosher head-restraint device was operated correctly, the percentage of cattle that vocalized was 0% in one plant and 3.7% in another. The shape and size of the animal can also cause problems. In one plant, 35% of the large Holsteins vocalized because they were too long to fit in the apparatus. If the animal vocalizes when its body first contacts the restraint device, it is likely that it is being pinched by a moving part. If it stands quietly when the device initially starts to apply pressure, and then vocalizes as the pressure increases, it is responding to excessive pressure.

It is also essential that the device fully supports the animal. An animal will struggle if it feels off balance or as if it is going to fall. A common cause of struggling in stunning pens is slipping on the floor. Slipping can be prevented by installing a grating on the floor: steel bars 2 cm in diameter spaced in a 20 cm square pattern.

ANIMALS DIFFICULT TO DRIVE

Genetic selection for certain types of very lean, rapidly growing pigs has caused welfare problems at the slaughter plant (Grandin, 1998). Some of these animals are very excitable, and difficult to handle in the stunning race. Lean, fine-boned hybrid pigs are more easily startled compared with pigs of a fatter type. Pigs that have been selected for both leanness and heavy muscling are often less excitable than lean, slender-bodied pigs. Handling problems with lean, excitable pigs can be reduced by either genetic selection, or training the excitable animals to being driven. This can be accomplished by briefly walking through the pens every day during fattening. The person walking the pens should teach the animals to get up quietly and flow around them as they pass through the pen. Only 5–15 seconds per pen per day is required. It is important that the person walking the pens should not stand in one corner and allow the pigs to chew on their boots – this teaches the pigs to chew on boots instead of being driven. The person should also walk carefully through the pen and never hit, kick or slap the pigs. Walking through the fattening pens will not affect weight gains and pen walking should be done throughout the fattening period. Walking the pens periodically in the alleys during fattening will also produce animals that are easier to drive at the slaughter plant (Jane Guise, 1997, Cambac Research, UK, personal communication). Overcrowding during fattening on the farm can also increase handling problems.

Lean pigs with a nervous temperament are more likely to balk at the distractions previously discussed. The author has also observed some problems with very excitable cattle. These problems are more likely to occur in lean, fine-boned feedlot heifers, which are more likely to balk at distractions and become agitated compared with fatter or more muscular types of cattle. In both pigs and cattle, the author has observed that animals which have been genetically selected for a lean, slender body and fine bones have less tolerance for sudden new experiences (Grandin, 1998). They are more likely to panic when subjected to noise and activity in a slaughter plant.

IMPORTANCE OF MANAGEMENT

One of the surprising results of the surveys was that handling of animals and employee behaviour were superior in the lairage pens compared with the stunning race area. In the USA, employees in the lairage area are supervised by the livestock buying department, and the stunning race is supervised by the slaughter department. People in the slaughter area such as the slaughter supervisor can become numb and desensitized; they need a strong manager to enforce good welfare standards. The single most important factor that determines the quality of animal handling is the attitude of management. Over the years the author has observed that handling practices in a plant improve when upper management makes a committment to improve handling.

ACKNOWLEDGEMENT

The author thanks Mark Deesing for assisting in the preparation and editing of this chapter.

Chapter 4

Physiology of Stress, Distress, Stunning and Slaughter

This chapter considers the physiology of fear, aggression, pain, stress, distress, hunger, thirst, stunning and slaughter.

FEAR AND DISTRESS

Fear is a common stress during preslaughter handling. In moderation it is not a bad thing. It allows stockhandlers to drive animals; without it the animals would be more reluctant to move. In excess, fear can make animals difficult to handle. They may become aggressive, or they may freeze; they become erratic and charge fences, or over-react to the presence of the handler and push each other unnecessarily when trying to distance themselves from the handler. The jostling between animals can result in bruising. Once stressed, pigs become progressively more difficult to handle: they crowd each other and their flow into and out of pens and races becomes disorganized. The cardinal rule is to try not to stress them early on; it makes subsequent handling easier.

Fear produces characteristic patterns of behaviour and physiological responses which can be correlated with each other. In cattle, fear can be seen from involuntary defaecation, increases in heart rate, blood pressure and plasma cortisol, refusal to move, head lowered with chin extended, head shaking and bellowing. In extreme cases of fear and where the animal is confined in a race or stunning pen, it may submit and drop to its knees. In this situation it can be difficult to get it to move on. The temptation is to strike the animal to make it rise, but this is often counter-productive as it makes the animal more submissive. Instead it is best to give it a minute or more to regain its confidence. Encourage it to stand by clearing the race ahead so that it can see a way on and is less likely to feel trapped.

Balking is a common fault in stockhandling systems at meatworks, and it is often linked to fear. It is a problem if it interrupts the flow of animals, and in some situations it can lead to bullying by the stockhandler. Some typical causes of balking at abattoirs are:

- floor drain gratings;
- contrasts of shadows and sunlight on the floor;
- distractions such as handtools or hosepipes at the side of a race or on the floor;
- change in floor material, or an obvious join between two floor sections produced when the floor was laid;
- discontinuity between ramp and floor materials;
- open gaps in solid-sided partitions;
- visual cliff effects produced by slats with light reflecting from a shiny surface below, raised floors with light coming from below, and at the entrance of restraining conveyors.

Normally, a horse will balk by moving diagonally, or sideways, as it shies from the intimidating object. Pigs stop; they may turn round and try to head back whence they came, before returning to investigate the potential danger. Alternatively, they may stop and then sniff at the object or intimidating shadow, and work it with their snouts before passing by. Individual sheep behaviour is strongly influenced by group behaviour: if the first sheep to confront the intimidating object stop and look at the object, or if they take a wide berth, or if they jump the object to clear it, the other sheep behind will probably do the same. Their cue is the behaviour of the sheep in front. Balking behaviour in cattle is reasonably similar to that in pigs; they stop, sniff and stare, shy away if they are uncertain or pass by either cautiously or in a rush if half-confident or if there is a group of cattle beyond the potential threat.

A number of tests can be used to assess fearfulness experimentally (Burrow, 1997). The strength of the regrouping behaviour can be evaluated with the *arena test*, which also provides a measure of fearfulness. It is performed by isolating a sheep or steer from its group. A potentially intimidating object or person is placed between the animal and its group. The animal has to overcome its distrust or fear of the intimidation to pass it by, and the time to joining up with its group is a measure of fear or intimidation. This can be used to assess fear of a novel object, or it can be used to test learned aversion if it is a familiar object.

The *open field test* is another one that has relevance in this context. An animal is placed in a large featureless area on its own. The usual immediate response is to stop, stand still, listen and look around. Then the animal usually moves around vocalizing. The time to onset of the movement phase, or the time to vocalizing, or the amount of walking or running and the number of escape jumps are all used as measures of fear. This test is almost identical to the livestock auction market. The animal is driven into a sale-ring, and it adopts a predation response (stops and assesses the situation), followed by a social reinstatement response (vocalizing to call to its group, searching for its group or an exit in the sale-ring). The skill of auction markets is to put the animal through before it has time to start the period of social reinstatement and adopt unpredictable panic behaviour. This will depend on how long and competitive the bidding is.

The *visual cliff test* can also be used to assess how quickly an animal adapts to an intimidating situation. The intimidating situation is an open height. Species vary considerably in their behaviour when suddenly confronted with an open height. Mountain species and species which live in trees stop and look, whereas plains-dwelling species usually back off. This fear response also varies according to age; as humans get older, they become more scared by heights. In animals the time to resumption of a particular normal behaviour pattern can be used as a measure of overcoming this fear, and sometimes it is used as a measure of an individual's innate fearfulness.

Fear of a particular procedure can be assessed by repeating it on a group of animals and seeing whether they acquire learned aversion. The aversion, which could include fear, can be assessed either from a physiological indicator or from the animal's behaviour. A truck driver once mentioned that when he had transported the same animals on repeated occasions, they did not become more difficult to load. If anything, with experience they became easier to load. This suggested to him that transport was not such an unpleasant experience for the animals as some people seemed to believe. Similar conclusions can be drawn from studies which have examined the plasma cortisol response to road transport in pigs and cattle, where the animals were transported on repeated occasions (Bradshaw *et al.*, 1996; Lay *et al.*, 1996). The plasma cortisol responses decreased once the animals became experienced travellers. This, however, does not demonstrate that the first and, for most animals, the only experience of transport is not frightening.

Some general signs of distress and discomfort in livestock include:

- vigorous tail flicking (not to be confused with tail wagging);
- head shaking;
- incontinence;
- nostril flaring;
- spasmodic body shivering;
- eyelid flickering;
- head retraction and eye closure.

However, these are not indicators of distress that can be used on their own. For example, head retraction and eye closure in a bird also occurs when it is asleep, and shivering can be due to cold as well as fear. The signs have to be recognized in the context of particular situations. They may be used as practical indicators, but they are not incontestable indicators.

When an animal experiences a surprise such as a sudden loud noise, it gives a startle response. The startle response varies with species. Rodents jump into the air, horses bolt, sheep lift their heads, cattle turn to face the threat, pigs freeze and poultry rise by leaping with their legs and flapping their wings. With sudden surprises these responses are subconscious. However, they can be affected by conscious activity and in particular by fear (Davis, 1992). If an animal is frightened by something and then it experiences a sudden loud noise, its startle response is exaggerated. In the case of the rodent, it is more 'jumpy'. A bird is more 'flighty'. The part of the brain which causes the animal to have an exaggerated startle response is the amygdala, an important centre which mediates fear, and in particular learned fears and the fear that is present in wild, untrained animals. If the amygdala is damaged by lesioning, otherwise fearful animals show reduced fear.

The ways in which fear is expressed vary between species and according to the age of the animal. Chicks start to show startle responses within 2 days of hatching and fear-linked avoidance behaviour by 7 days. Typically, when young animals such as chicks, calves, lambs and piglets are frightened they freeze and keep quiet. If the threat passes and the young animal is on its own, there follows a period of vocalizing as a call to its mother. In this situation, vocalizing is linked to fear but it is not a direct measure of fear; it is a measure of the way in which the animal is trying to attract the attention of the mother. If, on the other hand, the young animal has been caught and restrained, it is highly likely that it would vocalize from fear as well as calling for its mother.

In birds, the structure in the brain which is equivalent to the amygdala is called the archistriatum. Stimulation of the archistriatum with a small electric current elicits fear or escape behaviour, and damage to the archistriatum reduces the bird's ability to learn and memorize fear-provoking situations.

The amygdala and archistriatum can initiate many of the physiological stress responses in the body that are linked to fear (Fig. 4.1). These include stimulation of the hypothalamic–pituitary–adrenal axis (HPA), resulting in elevated plasma cortisol or corticosterone concentrations (Gabr *et al.*, 1995). Damage to the amygdala or archistriatum not only reduces startle responses, but also reduces or abolishes a wide range of other emotional behaviours and physiological responses. The amygdala integrates conditioned as well as unconditioned fear stimuli. A conditioned response is one that is consistently paired with a particular cue. For example, the sight of an electric fence in a field is a conditioned stimulus for an unpleasant shock which the animal has learned it will receive if it gets too close.

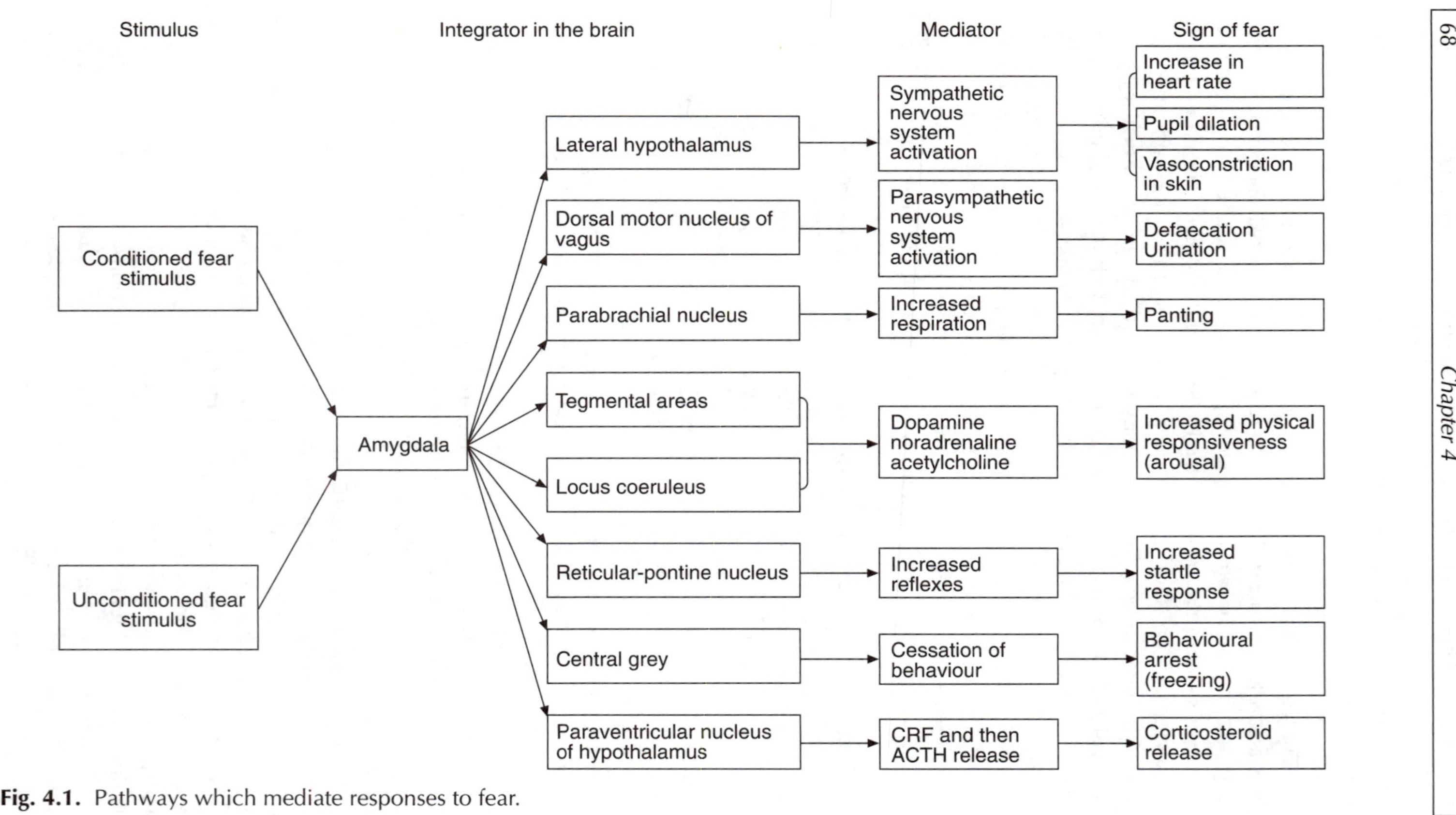

Fig. 4.1. Pathways which mediate responses to fear.

STRESS

Stress responses to fear that emanate from the amygdala are mediated largely through the sympathetic nervous system, adrenal medulla, parasympathetic nervous system and adrenal cortex. The sympathetic nervous system and adrenal medulla provoke very rapid responses, such as an increase in heart rate or blood pressure, through the release of adrenaline and noradrenaline. Adrenaline is released from the medulla of the adrenal gland, and noradrenaline is released from the adrenal medulla and from nerve endings of the sympathetic nervous system. The adrenaline and noradrenaline that are released from the adrenal gland enter the bloodstream and are distributed throughout the body. The noradrenaline that is released from sympathetic nerve endings acts on the tissue where it is released, rather than entering the bloodstream to reach its target tissue.

Adrenaline and noradrenaline are not as useful as corticosteroids as stress indicators, because they have a short half-life in the circulation (Lister *et al.*, 1982). The half-life is the time that elapses after a pulse of the hormone enters the bloodstream before half the amount of the hormone is extracted from the blood. Noradrenaline has a half-life of about 2 minutes, whereas for cortisol it is nearer 20 minutes. The short half-life of noradrenaline means that a blood sample needs to be taken immediately after a stress when measuring a stress-induced noradrenaline response, and this is not always possible. In spite of this, some of the metabolic and physiological effects of adrenaline and noradrenaline can be measured. For instance, the heart rate responses and packed cell volume responses to stresses which involve these hormones can be very useful.

The adrenal cortex releases corticosteroids (cortisol or corticosterone), which have more delayed effects. The corticosteroid response has been particularly helpful in comparing the effect of different stresses in animals. When this response is caused by fear it is mediated by the amygdala, which activates the paraventricular nucleus of the hypothalamus to release corticotropic releasing factor (CRF). This neurotransmitter passes to the pituitary via the hypophyseal–portal vessel, and it induces adrenocorticotropic hormone (ACTH) release into the general circulation. The ACTH is carried in the blood to the adrenal cortex, where it stimulates corticosteroid hormone release. In cattle, sheep and pigs the main corticosteroid hormone is cortisol. The corticosteroid hormones modulate the release of CRF and ACTH by negative feedback. The pathways are summarized in Fig. 4.2.

The main functions of the corticosteroid hormones are:

- to stimulate proteolysis;
- to stimulate gluconeogenesis;
- to bring about anti-inflammatory effects.

A common sign of fear in cattle is defaecation, and this is due to activation of the vagus nerve in the parasympathetic nervous system.

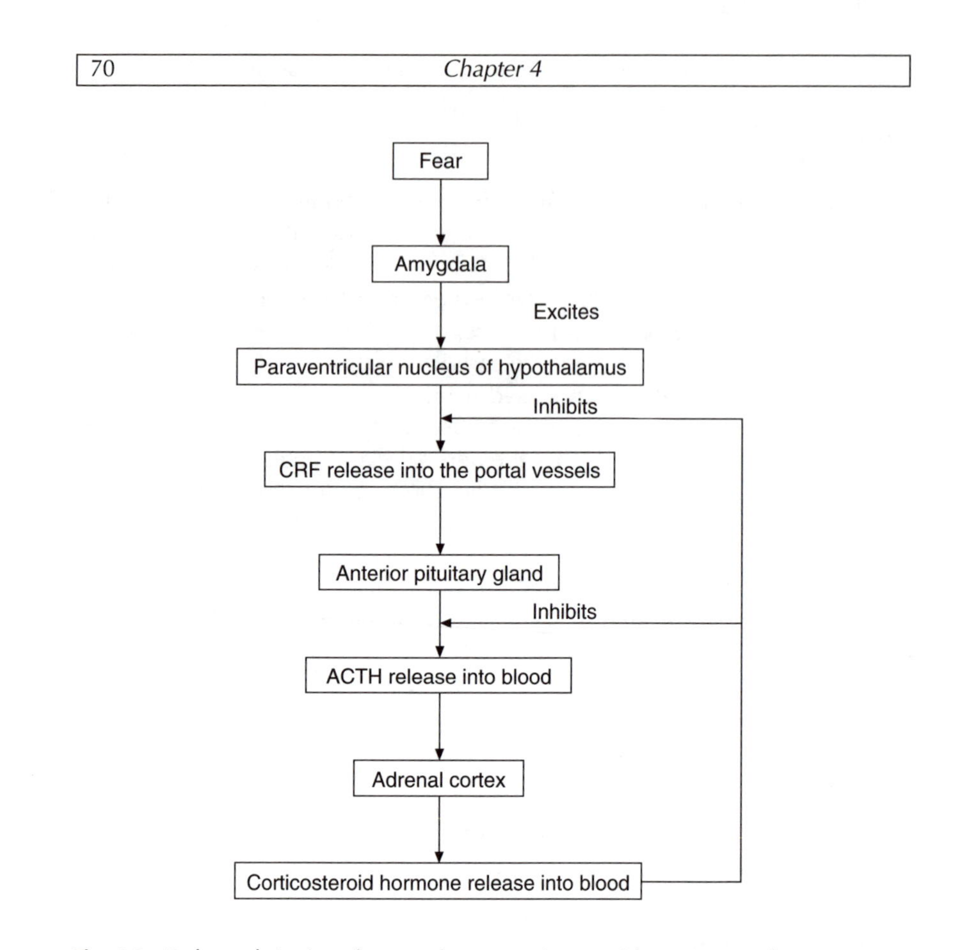

Fig. 4.2. Pathway bringing about a plasma corticosteroid response to fear.

Table 4.1 summarizes some of the potentially useful stress indicators in plasma. There are no specific plasma indicators for pain, but if pain causes muscle activity or fear, some of the plasma indicators of those reactions can be monitored instead. The value of measuring stress is in deciding which procedures are more or less stressful; from this, recommendations can be made on how to minimize or control stress. For example, in one study on pigs which were mixed when they were loaded on to a truck at a farm, the aim was to find out whether it was better to slaughter the pigs as soon as they arrived at the abattoir or to hold them in the lairage for 3 hours before slaughter (Warriss *et al.*, 1995). Holding them in the pens could either give them a rest period following the journey, or it might give the mixed pigs an opportunity to fight and the unfamiliar environment might add to their stress. The outcome is shown in Table 4.2. The cortisol and lactate levels were significantly higher when pigs were slaughtered on arrival at the abattoir. Cortisol would have indicated generalized stress, and lactate indicated

Table 4.1. Potentially useful stress indicators in plasma.

Stressor	Plasma indicators
Fasting	↓ glucose, ↑ FFA, ↑ glycerol, ↑ urea, ↑ GLDH, ↓ acetate (ruminants)
Dehydration	
without feed	↑ protein
with feed	↑ protein, ↑osmolality, ↑ PCV
Exercise	↑ PCV, ↑ adrenaline, ↑ noradrenaline, ↑ K^+, ↑ β endorphin, ↑ lactate (if anaerobic), ↑ CPK
Motion sickness	↑ cortisol, ↑ VIP
Fear/alarm	↑ adrenaline, ↑ noradrenaline, ↑ ACTH, ↑ cortisol, ↑ glucagon, ↑ prolactin, ↑ β endorphin
Heat	↑ ACTH, ↑ cortisol, ↑ adrenaline, ↑ β endorphin
Cold	↑ noradrenaline, ↑ cortisol, ↑ PCV

ACTH, Adrenocorticotrophic hormone; CK, creatine phosphokinase; GLDH, glutamate dehydrogenase; PCV, packed cell volume; VIP, vasoactive intestinal peptide.

Table 4.2. Effect of mixing before transport and holding in the lairage on two plasma stress indicators in boars and gilts.

	Pigs not mixed	Pigs mixed		
Plasma indicator	Slaughtered after 3 hours in lairage	Slaughtered after 3 hours in lairage	Slaughtered on arrival at abattoir	Standard error of deviation (s.e.d.)
Cortisol (μg per 100 ml)	5.5	5.8	14.3	0.7
Lactate (mg per 100 ml)	54	65	98	7

anaerobic muscle exercise. It was concluded that holding pigs for 3 hours in the lairage provided a rest before slaughter during which the stress levels returned to those that would be seen in pigs that were not mixed.

In pigs, a decrease in plasma glucose concentration can indicate that less glucose is being absorbed from the gut and that the pig is entering the fasted state. This can be confirmed by also measuring the plasma free fatty acid (FFA) levels. When glucose becomes less available, triglycerides in adipose tissue are broken down to FFAs and glycerol which are released into the bloodstream. Fasting may also induce protein breakdown in muscle. Amino acids enter the circulation; and when they are deaminated, ammonia is released. Ammonia is potentially toxic and it is converted into a safer form by the enzyme, glutamate dehydrogenase (GLDH). The end-product of ammonia capture is urea. Both plasma GLDH activity and blood urea concentration can be useful indicators of enhanced proteolysis.

Free fatty acids can be released from adipose tissue as a result of psychological stressors and fasting or exercise. Any stress which provokes a release of adrenaline or noradrenaline is likely to cause a rise in plasma FFA, as both these hormones stimulate lipolysis.

Different types of stress provoke different physiological and physical responses. For example, a cold stress causes vasoconstriction in the skin whereas heat stress results in skin vasodilation. Both responses are mediated by the sympathoadrenomedullary nervous system but there are selective differences in the way in which that system produces its responses:

- preferential activation of the adrenal medulla, instead of the sympathetic nerve endings;
- preferential release of adrenaline or noradrenaline from the adrenal medulla;
- differences in adrenergic receptor type in different tissues;
- selective activation of sympathetic efferent nerves which innervate particular organs, glands or regions of the body;
- selective reflex inhibition through the parasympathetic nervous system.

Some examples help to show when and how these differences occur.

1. During heat stress there is release of catecholamines from the adrenal medulla, but more adrenaline is released than noradrenaline. In skin blood vessels, adrenaline has a vasodilatory effect whereas noradrenaline has a vasoconstrictor action. The end result is adrenaline-mediated vasodilation.
2. When a particular stress causes release of noradrenaline there is an increase in heart rate and there is peripheral vasoconstriction, which causes a rise in blood pressure. The rise in blood pressure causes a parasympathetic reflex decrease in heart rate which is mediated through the vagus nerve. So, during a noradrenaline-mediated stress response, the heart rate response is brief and often inconsequential. If, on the other hand, the stress causes a release of adrenaline, the adrenaline causes a rise in heart rate and peripheral vasodilation, which can result in a fall in blood pressure. During an adrenaline-mediated stress response, the heart rate response is longer-lasting and more pronounced than for a noradrenaline-mediated stress response.
3. The adrenergic receptors which are activated by adrenaline and noradrenaline fall into two main types: α-adrenoreceptors and β-adrenoreceptors. Some tissues have predominantly α-receptors whereas in others they may be mixed or mainly β. In addition, some physiological responses are mediated by α-receptors, whereas other responses depend on activation of β-receptors (Table 4.3). Adrenaline stimulates both α and β-receptors, whereas noradrenaline has a slightly greater selectivity for α-receptors.

4. The brain is able to activate different sympathetic efferent nerves, thus producing specific responses. For example, a nociceptive (painful) stimulus applied as a pinch to the foot results in activation of nerves which cause vasoconstriction in skeletal muscle, whereas it inhibits the nerves causing vasoconstriction in the skin (Table 4.4). Inhalation of carbon dioxide has a similar effect (Janig, 1979).
5. Some stimuli result in activation of the sympathetic nervous system whereas others cause activation of the adrenal medulla. Fasting, hypoglycaemia, acute hypoxia and the immediate response to trauma, cause an adrenomedullary response, whereas sympathetic nerve endings are activated during chronic overfeeding and chronic hypoxia (Young *et al.*, 1984). During restraint stress and during bleeding out, most of the noradrenaline that is released into the circulation comes from sympathetic nerve endings, rather than the adrenal medulla.

An important difference between noradrenaline and adrenaline is their effect on glycogenolysis. Noradrenaline does not stimulate glycogenolysis in muscle, whereas adrenaline does. This implies that stresses which stimulate the release of adrenaline are more likely to cause muscle glycogen depletion than stresses which provoke a noradrenaline release.

Table 4.3. Adrenergic effects (α and β).

α-Adrenergic effects	β-Adrenergic effects
Pupil dilation	Increase in heart rate
Arteriole constriction	Arteriole dilation
Contraction of gut sphincters	Bronchodilation
Reduced intestinal motility	Reduced intestinal motility
Contraction of bladder sphincter	Trembling
Piloerection and feather erection	Muscle glycogenolysis
Splenic contraction	Lipolysis
Liver glycogenolysis	
Salivary and lacrimal gland secretion	

Table 4.4. Organization of sympathetic efferent activation during different physiologically stressful situations.

	Sympathetic nerve activation		
	Vasoconstrictor nerves in		
Stimulus	Muscle	Skin	Sweat gland nerves in skin
Nociception	↑	↓	↑
CO_2	↑	↓	↑

The response of fish to stressful situations can be assessed in similar ways to that of livestock species. When fish are stressed they can show changes in heart rate, increased release of adrenaline, noradrenaline and cortisol into the circulation and vigorous muscle activity in their attempt to escape a situation. Tissue damage such as cuts and bruises results in activation of nerves that are connected to pain receptors. Fish show avoidance behaviours in circumstances that would be expected to cause *pain*, and they learn to avoid places where they received tissue damage that probably involved pain. There seems to be little doubt that fish can experience some aspects of pain.

PAIN

The following are some examples of how pain can occur in livestock during the last 24 hours before slaughter:

- torn or grazed skin as stock are mustered and yarded;
- broken or dislocated bones in poultry during handling and loading into crates;
- periosteal pain (for example, when a bone in the leg is struck against a partition, or when the legs of birds are compressed in shackles on the killing line);
- inflammatory pain, occurring when the tissue at a wound swells during the inflammatory response;
- torn ligaments or muscle during handling injuries, especially during falls;
- bruising, resulting in swelling and activation of pain receptors through compression or swelling of tissues;
- electric shocks, delivered from electric goads, or when an animal is poorly presented for stunning and it experiences a shock from the stunning equipment before it is stunned;
- toe amputation in poultry, when transport crates with perforated floors are drawn out of the modules;
- nerve compression; for example, when a pig injures its back – this results in pain from direct stimulation of the spinal cord, and it may cause projected pain in areas served by the afferent nerves.

There are other situations where there is less certainty about whether pain occurs. For example:

- if head-to-body electrical stunning is misapplied and the animal has a cardiac arrest before it is stunned, it may experience cardiac pain;
- during transport deaths in stress-susceptible pigs, it is suspected that there is muscle pain which could be either an ischaemic pain or pain associated with cramping of the muscle;
- over-exertion during mustering resulting in muscle pain.

Animals or body parts which are unduly sensitive to painful stimuli are in a state of *hyperalgesia*. An example of this is when an animal has a wound which occurred 2 days ago, and which has become inflamed as part of the normal repair mechanism. The region is very sensitive to pressure and movement. There are two types of hyperalgesia. Primary hyperalgesia is increased pain sensitivity at the site of the wound, and secondary hyperalgesia is increased pain sensitivity at a site which is away from the wound, but the nerves from both sites converge on the same section of the spinal cord. When animals experience primary hyperalgesia, they may display various forms of *guarding behaviour* when trying to protect the painful region. They may also lick the wound, no doubt from concern and curiosity with the pain. *Analgesics* can be given to relieve pain and hyperalgesia. Analgesia is a form of insensitivity to pain whilst, at the same time, most or all other conscious mental faculties are present. During *general anaesthesia* there is absence of all conscious mental activity, including the perception of pain.

Sensitivity to pain can be influenced by the emotional state of the animal. A potential mechanism for this during preslaughter handling is the effect of stress in promoting analgesia. This mechanism is referred to as *stress-induced analgesia*, and in evolutionary terms it has given animals an advantage in allowing them to defend themselves without undue concern for the wounds gained during the fight. If the animal was preoccupied by the pain of a wound, it would be distracted from defending itself.

At least three mechanisms mediate stress-induced analgesia (Harris, 1996). All three operate through the rostral ventromedial medulla (RVM) in the brainstem, which activates descending projections on to opioid receptors in the dorsal horn of the spinal cord. The opioid receptors disrupt the transmission of pain signals passing to the brain and the site of this pain inhibition is within the dorsal horn. The three mechanisms differ in the route that they take within the brain as follows. If the stress involves a learned danger or learned fear, the amygdala is involved. It activates the periaqueductal grey (PAG) in the midbrain, which in turn activates the RVM. If the pain or stress is novel and is inescapable, the animal adopts a behavioural response called *learned helplessness*. A learning process is necessary which involves forebrain structures that are separate from the amygdala. This type of analgesia is also mediated through the PAG and RVM, and it depends in part on a corticosteroid response from the adrenal cortex. The third mechanism is probably subconscious as it is restricted to the RVM and the spinal cord, or, in unusual circumstances, to the spinal cord only.

Pain is almost inevitable when surgery is performed without an anaesthetic or analgesic. A number of mutilations are performed on livestock without any analgesics as part of routine management procedures on farms (Chapter 1). With some of these mutilations, the pain is brief; in others the pain can last for days. In general, chronic pain which is due to injury can take one of the following forms.

- **Causalgia** – prolonged, intense, spontaneous and sometimes debilitating pain which feels hot.
- **Neuroma** – distorted, sometimes enlarged parts of an injured nerve which are tender to pressure.
- **Neuritis** – spreading pain involving inflammation of a nerve.
- **Somatic pain** – pain linked to the injury of a nerve trunk emerging from the spinal column.
- **Phantom pain** – painful sensations in the stump or missing part of an amputated limb.

Neuromas have been identified in the stumps of amputated beaks, claws and tails. They develop in the following way. When a nerve is cut, the cut ends sprout and try to join up with other cut nerves. This would be the normal way in which a severed nerve would heal. The sprouts from the cut nerve grow a short length. They need to meet a Schwann cell (which normally supplies energy to the nerves) in order to continue sprouting and growing. In an amputation stump the only Schwann cells are alongside the proximal part of the nerve, and so those sprouted nerves that double back on themselves and meet up with these Schwann cells sprout again and eventually build up to form knots and bulbous swellings of nervous tissue. These swollen knots of nerves are called neuromas and they can be very sensitive to pressure. From a practical perspective, it is relevant that neuromas can form in both cut and crushed nerve endings. This suggests that whether a tail is amputated by severing or by crushing, a neuroma could still form.

It is not known whether any sheep, pigs and cattle which have their tails docked experience phantom limb sensations or phantom limb pain. In humans, phantom limb pain is more common with increasing age, and it would be uncommon in infants less than 2 years old. It is also more common if the limb was causing pain before it was amputated. These points could be used to argue that phantom limb pain would be unlikely in tail-docked stock, provided the docking was done at an early age.

There are two types of *muscle pain* or muscle soreness associated with over-exertion. Acute muscle soreness occurs during or immediately following the exercise and is due to inadequate blood flow to the active muscles (ischaemia). It is thought that this type of pain is provoked by the accumulation of H^+, lactate, potassium, phosphate or substance P in the muscle, all of which can stimulate pain receptors. In some parts of the body the nerves that convey the signals to the brain take the route of the sympathetic nervous system instead of the spinal cord. Delayed muscle soreness can be due to tearing of the muscle fibres or connective tissue or to sustained ischaemia. It occurs, for example, when active muscle is stretched or when a muscle lengthens during actomyosin formation (eccentric contraction). Tearing of muscle fibres also causes fluid to leak from the sarcoplasm and enter the bloodstream. The fluid contains proteins, including creatine phosphokinase and lactate dehydrogenase, and these enzymes have been used as indicators of muscle damage when measured in serum. Breakdown products of collagen have been used as markers of connective tissue damage, and these include urinary hydroxyproline, hydroxylysine and pyridinoline. These breakdown products are formed by enzymes which act on the collagen. In unfit individuals, heavy exercise can cause activation of cathepsin and acid hydrolase enzymes in muscle, and they can also lead to muscle cell necrosis (Salminen *et al.*, 1984).

Recognizing pain in an animal is not always easy. The most convincing way is to palpate the region which is presumed to be painful and watch for a physical reaction. This is often the approach used by veterinarians when diagnosing or assessing pain. Indicators of pain from spontaneous behaviour depend on where the pain is situated. Foot and limb pain are obvious from posture and gait. Back or hip pain in pigs can be seen when they are unable to stand on their hindlegs and they scream when attempts are made to help them up. Neck pain can be recognized from the position of the neck and head and from tension in the neck muscles. When humans have abdominal pain we often show guarding behaviour by bending over slightly with the arms across the abdomen. This protects the area when we are threatened or when we are trying to recruit sympathy, and the bent posture helps to relieve pressure inside. The equivalent posture for cattle which relieves internal pressure is standing with the four feet positioned close together and with the back arched. Abdominal pain can also be indicated by: shallow breathing with occasional groaning; grunting during expiration or walking; groaning when the abdomen is pressed; kicking at the flank with a hindleg; intermittent head-turning towards the flank; tension in the neck muscles, often with the neck outstretched; treading with the hindfeet; repeatedly getting up and lying down; reluctance to walk; trembling; and groaning when the animal rises to its feet. These are just some examples of the behaviours associated with one type of pain and comparable lists can be prepared for pain in other parts of the body.

Electric currents applied through electric goads are used for driving cattle and pigs in meatworks yards. They are intentionally unpleasant or painful to animals. The purpose of the electric shock is to make the animal move. If the shock was not unpleasant, the animal would not move. One argument that is sometimes put forward in favour of electric goads is that the discomfort they create is brief, whereas being hit with a stick causes lasting pain and damages the carcass. Electric shocks are often thought to be painful. From personal experience, perhaps a more accurate description is that they are 'shocking'. The shock may be regarded as a type of pain, but it is not typical of other forms of pain we commonly experience.

AGGRESSION

There are five causes of aggression in livestock:

- maternal instinct
- dominance
- pain
- territorial protection
- fear.

Dominance aggression and fear-induced aggression can occur during preslaughter handling. Dominance aggression occurs when bulls or pigs are mixed in the lairage. They mount, chase, butt and, in the case of pigs, bite each other during the fights for dominance. Fear-induced aggression can occur when a steer is on its own in a pen and cannot see the exit. It may turn on the stockhandler and either head-butt or charge.

HUNGER

During the preslaughter period it is necessary to fast animals to reduce their gut contents. Hunger is inevitable in this situation. When humans go without food, they experience different phases of hunger. Initially there is an enthusiasm for food, but with progressive fasting this changes to a gnawing emptiness whilst feeling weak, lethargic and sensitive to cold. No doubt these phases exist in other monogastric species.

In monogastrics, hunger is in part initiated by a drop in glucose utilization rate in specific cells in the liver and the brain. From research with fasted rats, this drop is thought to correspond to a fall of at least 5% in the resting blood glucose level. If the animal is unable to feed, the lower blood glucose fails to stimulate insulin secretion; instead, the sympathoadrenomedullary system is activated and this stimulates the fasting phase of metabolism. If the animal is able to feed and it is anticipating a meal, it has an added impetus which reinforces its hunger. This occurs through the release of acetylcholine at the pancreas just before the start of feeding, which causes the secretion of a pulse of insulin. The insulin lowers blood glucose abruptly, and this helps to intensify and sustain the hunger for a short period once it starts feeding.

In the absence of feeding, adrenaline from the adrenal medulla stimulates lipolysis, and the triglycerides stored in fat are released into the bloodstream as free fatty acids (FFA). In the pig, fat mobilization starts after about 16 hours starvation (Gregory *et al.*, 1980). The FFAs act as an alternative to glucose as a fuel for muscle metabolism, and they also have an anorexigenic effect (hunger suppression) through signals which are transmitted to the brain via the vagus nerve. With the change towards utilizing FFAs in the place of glucose, blood glucose levels start to recover and this may help to change the perception of hunger. Reduced stretching of the gut also contributes to the sensation of hunger.

The normal hunger stimuli in ruminants are not known, but the satiety signals have been identified (Baile and Forbes, 1974). Some of the products of carbohydrate digestion in the rumen are partly responsible for satisfying the animal's hunger. In the rumen, plant cellulose is broken down by microorganisms to the volatile fatty acids (VFAs) acetate, butyrate and propionate. Once these have been absorbed by the rumen wall, nearly all the propionate is converted to glucose by the liver, the butyrate is metabolized within the rumen wall to hydroxybutyrate, and acetate passes to adipose tissue (where it is used for producing long-chain fatty acids) and to muscle (where it is used in the TCA cycle for producing ATP from ADP + P_i). During fasting, glucose and acetate are replaced by FFAs as the main blood-borne sources of energy for muscle. The FFAs are derived from adipose tissue. The satiety signals in ruminants include acetate, propionate, amino acids and formate. Rumen distension following feeding also provokes satiety, and lack of rumen distension is probably important in stimulating hunger.

Absence of feed may not be an abnormal stress in fish. In temperate and cold climates it is common for fish in the wild to experience and survive long periods of feed deprivation, particularly during the winter.

THIRST

Thirst is a common occurrence during preslaughter transport. It is usually corrected by allowing the animals to drink as soon as they arrive at their destination. In physiological terms, there are two types of physiological factors which stimulate thirst: volumetric and osmotic stimuli. Thirst occurs either when there is a fall in blood volume or when the tonicity of the interstitial fluid increases. An example where both occur together is when animals are unable to drink during hot weather; thirst develops from evaporative heat loss and reduced total body water. In most species the blood volume would be reduced and it would be hypertonic. Causes of acute volumetric thirst without hypertonicity include fluid loss through haemorrhaging, vomiting and diarrhoea. One of the best physiological monitors of dehydration is the concentration of total protein in the plasma.

PHYSIOLOGY OF STUNNING AND SLAUGHTER

The purpose of stunning from the welfare perspective is to render the animal insensible. The purpose in slaughtering the animal is to kill it before it can recover from the stun and regain sensibility. This section describes the key physiological aspects of the main stunning and slaughtering methods.

Stunning

Concussion is used for stunning cattle, deer, heavy pigs and some sheep. It is one of the most effective ways of disrupting brain function and stunning an animal. It is instantaneous and it can be permanent. This has been demonstrated using evoked potentials, which are electrical potentials in the brain that occur in response to an external stimulus, such as a flash of light. When animals are correctly stunned with a captive bolt, the evoked potentials are lost immediately and they do not return.

There are four stages (or depths) of concussion. In Stage 1 the subject is slightly disorientated and the memory is affected. In Stage 2 the subject has poor coordination and impaired memory. In Stage 3 the subject is on the ground and breathing is maintained. In Stage 4 the subject is prostrate on the ground and there is no breathing. Stage 4 concussion is very dangerous for humans. If respiration is not reinstated, the blood will become progressively deoxygenated and brain function will eventually fail altogether. From the point of view of stunning animals, the aim should be to induce Stage 4 concussion every time, and absence of breathing should be used as the measure of success.

The heart is not immediately stopped during concussion. This has two important consequences. Firstly, if the animal is breathing or resumes breathing, the continued beating of the heart will enable the animal to recover once the concussion wears off. Secondly, since the heart is beating, blood will pass from the captive-bolt wound to the carcass. Any bacteria attached to the bolt could be washed off by the blood and end up in the carcass, and so it is important to have a clean bolt. Also, from the hygiene point of view, it should be noted that captive-bolt stunning has been linked to shedding of epithelial cells from the mucosa of the first part of the small intestine (Badawy *et al.*, 1957). The consequences of this have not been fully investigated, but it is usually thought that bacteria do not invade the carcass from the gut in freshly killed animals (Gill *et al.*, 1978).

Concussion is thought to work in the following ways:

- Torsion at the brainstem. When the head is accelerated by the shot, the brain oscillates within the skull and shear forces are set up at the brainstem which can disrupt brainstem function, including breathing.
- Impact of the midbrain against the tentorium. When the head is accelerated by the shot, there is localized pressure at the midbrain as it jars against the rigid edge of the tentorium. This would disrupt nervous function associated with midbrain structures.
- Disruption of synaptic transmission. Pressure gradients within the brain could be responsible for inhibiting neurotransmission at nerve synapses.
- Nerve transection. The bolt from the captive-bolt gun cuts through nerve pathways as it penetrates the brain and disrupts the functions that those pathways serve.
- Coup injuries. These occur when the brain strikes the inside of the skull as it oscillates following the shot. Localized brain haemorrhaging can develop at the point of contact, and at regions where the brain surface rubs along the inner surface of the skull.

- *Contre-coup* injuries. Haemorrhages can develop at the side opposite to the point where the brain impacts with the inner surface of the skull. This is due to vacuolation within the brain as it is thrown forward.
- Haemorrhaging leading to ischaemia. The haemorrhaging resulting from damage to the brain by the bolt and by the coup and *contre-coup* effects will cause an increase in intracerebral pressure. This will not be immediate, but if the haemorrhaging is severe the rise in pressure will be sufficient to reduce the flow of blood in the capillaries within the brain. In this situation, the brain would be starved of oxygen and unconsciousness would be sustained.

When an animal is stunned by concussion and then slaughtered, it is possible to assess brain dysfunction in some detail from its cranial nerve reflexes. There are 12 pairs of cranial nerves which converge on the ventral surface of the brain. They do not pass to the brain through the spinal cord, and so a positive cranial nerve reflex is not complicated by the possibility that it was a spinal reflex which did not involve the brain. In addition, cranial nerve reflexes do not rely on a patent spinal cord for expression of the reflex response, and so they are not complicated by severance or damage to the spinal cord during the slaughtering procedure. In summary, a positive cranial nerve reflex demonstrates that the pathway it takes through the brain is functioning. It does not directly discriminate between consciousness and unconsciousness, but it assists in getting an overall picture of the degree of brain dysfunction. Negative cranial nerve reflexes are good indicators of impaired midbrain or brainstem activity and unconsciousness. Several tests involving cranial nerves are used in meatworks:

- The *corneal reflex* involves touching the cornea and watching for an eyelid blink. Point stimulation of the cornea is less likely to provoke a positive response than wiping the finger over the surface of the cornea. A positive corneal reflex can occur in both conscious and unconscious animals and so it does not distinguish these two states. A persistent negative response indicates a profound state of brain dysfunction and unconsciousness.
- The *palpebral reflex* involves touching an eyelid and watching for an eyelid blink. The interpretation is similar to the corneal reflex.
- *Normal rhythmic breathing* after stunning or sticking indicates that the medulla in the brain and also the spinal cord plus nerves which control breathing movements in the body are still functioning. Its presence is helpful in indicating a functioning brainstem, and calls for immediate appraisal of whether a stunned animal is in fact unconscious. Its absence indicates either that the brainstem is not functioning or that the activity of the medulla is being overridden by seizure activity. False negatives can occur if the spinal cord has been severed or concussed, and this possibility must not be overlooked.
- A number of tests can be conducted on any animal where there is a

suspicion that it may be conscious. *Jaw tension* can be assessed by prising the jaws apart manually. There is little point in trying to assess this in a convulsing animal, but it is helpful in assessing responsiveness in the relaxed state. A completely relaxed jaw, especially one which does not try to bite the hand, is a good indicator of a profound state of brain dysfunction and unequivocal unconsciousness. A *nose prick* with a needle or an *ear pinch* with finger and thumbnail can be used to provoke recoil. In poultry, *pulling the head* down firmly would provoke head withdrawal in a conscious bird.

Other tests have been used for evaluating brain dysfunction, but not all of them are practical as routine measures. They include responsiveness to a threatening gesture (such as rushing the back of the hand towards the eyes) or to pinching of the tongue, pupillary reflex (pupil closure in response to shining a pencil-beam light into an eye), or startle or facial response to a sudden noise. In profound forms of brain dysfunction these reflexes are all negative and unconsciousness can be inferred provided the muscles and the afferent and efferent nerves which execute the response are still capable of working and are not preoccupied with other stimuli.

This last point is quite important because it can complicate judgement about whether or not an animal is conscious. Take, for example, the situation with decapitation. We do not know whether the head is conscious or unconscious for a brief period after it has been detached from the body. Reports on the spontaneous behaviour of decapitated heads in humans and animals have indicated that the skin and muscles undergo spontaneous quivering, twitching and grimacing behaviour; the exact behaviour varies between different parts of the head (Loye, 1887). There were no responses to pinching the tongue or to loud noises directed into an ear, but we cannot tell whether this was because the animal was indeed insensible or whether the nervous barrage created during decapitation was overriding the ability of the head to respond to these stimuli.

Testing reflex responses in an electrically stunned animal is complicated by convulsive behaviour. It is also difficult if the animal is electrically immobilized before sticking. When an electroimmobilizing current is passed through the body, the muscles contract whilst the current is flowing and this masks tests of reflex responses.

The first account of electrical stunning comes from Abildgaard (1775), who stunned two chickens. In fact he went further than that. He stunned them, induced heart failure and then resuscitated the birds with a subsequent current. The first chicken was a hen:

> which at the first shock, directed from a single vessel (Leyden jar) on the head, I prostrated it, so that the hen lay entirely dead without any feeling nor could it be aroused by any stimulant; indeed another shock, now having been given on the head in vain, I believed myself to have been mistaken in the hope of resuscitation; for the hen remained dead even though shocks on the

> head had been repeated. Little contented with this success, I tried the electric shock directed through the breast to the dorsal spine, nor in vain; for having been left on the ground it raised up suddenly and quietly walked on its feet.

A cockerel was put through the same procedure, and when it received the defibrillating current it flew off and in the process knocked over Abilgaard's jar, breaking it and bringing further trials to an end.

Since Abilgaard's experiments, electric currents have been used in a variety of ways to stun animals and to relieve pain. Electric currents are not inevitably painful. When used correctly they can in fact eliminate pain. From work in laboratory animals it is known that stimulation of particular parts of the brain with small currents (about 3 mA) will induce insensibility to pain (analgesia). Two regions in the brain which are particularly responsive are the mesencephalic central grey matter and the paraventricular grey matter (Mayer and Liebeskind, 1974). One nucleus within the mesencephalon, the periaqueductal grey (PAG) nucleus, is particularly responsive to alleviating pain when it is electrically stimulated. Patients suffering from intractable pain due to cancer or back problems have had electrodes implanted in the PAG and been able to stimulate the electrodes using about 3 volts whenever the pain became intolerable. Following the stimulation, pain relief has lasted for about 5 hours (Hosobuchi, 1986; Young and Brechner, 1986). This form of pain control is known as *electroanalgesia*. When sheep are electrically stunned, electroanalgesia lasts for 10 minutes or more (Gregory and Wotton, 1988a).

Electroanalgesia has been applied in other ways. For example, applying a current across a nerve in the body can be used to block the signals conveyed in that nerve. This is known as transcutaneous electrical nerve stimulation (TENS), and it creates tingling sensations in the place of pain. It has even been effective in providing relief from phantom limb pain when applied to the intact limb on the other side of the body to the amputation (Carabelli and Kellerman, 1985). Intractable pain has also been controlled using electrodes implanted surgically in the spinal column. The patient has been equipped with a portable stimulator which he or she operates by titrating the appropriate current level from a radiotransmitter control panel to achieve analgesia (Sheally *et al.*, 1970). However, from our perspective, it is very important to note that if the current was too high it caused additional pain. Clearly, controlled electric currents have been used, with tremendous benefits, for relieving pain in humans, but when electroimmobilizing currents are applied to animals we are not in the same position of easily knowing whether we are applying too little current or whether it is in fact too much and causing additional discomfort from an electric shock. When a high current is used it immobilizes the animal by making it rigid and its behavioural responses are suppressed.

When electric currents are applied at low levels to the skin in a conscious human, there is no stunning effect. At very low currents there are tingling sensations and sometimes a sensation of warmth. As the current is increased it stimulates muscle contraction and a sense of shock. A human who is holding on to an electrode may be prevented from releasing the electrode because of the muscle contraction in the hand. When the current is applied to other parts, the body may be repelled by the motion involved in the sudden muscle contraction. The feeling of shock is due to two effects. Firstly, there is the direct activation of nerves near the point of contact, which conduct a barrage of pulses to the brain. Secondly, there is the violent jerk of the muscle contraction.

In the past, electroanaesthesia has been used in surgery for humans and animals. It usually involved titrating a high frequency current into the patient through electrodes attached to the head, and maintaining the current throughout the operation. The patient would be unconscious, insensible to pain and breathing spontaneously.

Another application for electricity is in electroconvulsive therapy (ECT), which is used in psychotherapy for humans. Like electrical stunning, it induces unconsciousness. When it was introduced in 1938 it was used without any anaesthetic. Now, the patient is anaesthetized in order to reduce the severity of the muscle contractions when the current is applied and so reduce the risk of broken bones. Provided the current is passed through the head, and does not flow through the heart, there is only a low risk of ventricular fibrillation. For example, in cats the minimum dose (in coulombs) that will cause a cardiac arrest is more than 57 times the minimum dose that will produce convulsions.

When electric currents are applied to the head and sufficient current flows through the brain, there is prompt unconsciousness and the shock effect is not perceived. When electrical stunning was first introduced in the 1930s it was thought that it produced unconsciousness by restricting the flow of blood in the brain. Since then it has been learned that blood flow in the brain actually increases; instead, unconsciousness occurs in a similar manner to that produced during a *grand mal* epileptic seizure. The epileptiform activity in the brain is brought about by the release of excitatory amino acids into the extracellular space (Cook *et al.*, 1992). These amino acids, which include glutamate, act on cell receptors which elicit depolarization of the nerve cells in the brain by allowing calcium entry. When there is sustained depolarization ('depolarization shift'), the nerve cells undergo repetitive epileptiform discharges. Termination of these discharges is brought about by the release of inhibitory neurotransmitters, including gamma aminobutyric acid (GABA). When the epileptiform discharges occur we can be confident that the animal is insensible. It takes about 0.2 seconds from the time the stunning current starts to the onset of the epileptiform discharges (Cook *et al.*, 1995). This is virtually instantaneous.

Electrical stunning causes brain dysfunction in a different way to concussion. In concussion, responsiveness in the brain is brought to an abrupt halt, whereas responsiveness in certain regions of the brain is increased following electrical stunning. This increase applies to nerve impulses coming into the brain, but subsequent processing of these signals is disrupted. The increased responsiveness can be seen in the epileptiform activity of the EEG (see Fig. 13.5), and this indicates a disordered metabolism and electrical activity which we are confident could not support conscious activity.

The physiological basis in electrical stunning is that it induces epilepsy. One of the theories on how the epilepsy is induced is as follows. The electric current that is applied to the head affects the reticular formation (RF) which is situated in the mesencephalon and the brainstem. Normally, features of RF activity would modulate responsiveness within higher structures of the brain, but electrical stunning blocks that inhibitory input. Removal of the inhibitory signals from the RF makes the cortex more responsive, and nerve impulses which are detected at the primary cortex are highly exaggerated (epileptiform). If the hyper-responsiveness and epileptiform activity extends to other regions of the cerebral cortex, and especially to regions where interpretation occurs (association cortex), then consciousness is lost. It is thought that this involvement is equivalent to an epileptiform EEG in up to 50% of the cerebral cortex. Epilepsy is terminated by reinstatement of the inhibitory signals and involves the neurotransmitters gamma amino butyric acid (GABA) and glycine. Chapter 13 describes the conditions that are necessary for achieving epilepsy in the brain during electrical stunning.

Intense physical activity in the carcass following electrical stunning can be a problem for staff safety, and sometimes it causes a carcass to slip out of its shackle. There are two types of physical activity: rigid (tonic) and kicking (clonic). While the electric current is flowing, the body of the animal is rigid. The brain is being stimulated and electrical impulses pass down the spinal cord causing a tonic muscle contraction. During this phase the hindlimbs are flexed, and the animal would fall to the ground if it was free-standing when the current was switched on. If high currents are applied, the forelimbs may go into extension, and this indicates that the strength of the extensor muscles overrides that of the flexor muscles. When the current flow stops, the generalized tonic contraction usually continues for a short period (e.g. 10 seconds) and then the convulsive (clonic) phase sets in. Carcass kicking can be particularly severe during this phase when high-voltage electric stunning is used.

The convulsions are driven by activity in the RF of the brain. The RF also entrains the whole brain in epilepsy. However, the convulsions are not proof of epilepsy in the brain as there are some instances where convulsions have been independent of epileptiform activity in the cortical EEG (Bergmann *et al.*, 1963). It is more accurate to say that the convulsions and the epilepsy usually involve dysfunction of the same brain structure and so they are very closely linked. A useful behavioural event to watch for when inspecting electrical stunning is the return of rhythmic breathing movements. This coincides with the end of epileptiform activity in the brain. Often it coincides with the end of the carcass kicking. It indicates that hypersynchrony emanating from the RF has ended, and some of the normal medullary function has been reinstated. This means that other features of brain function will probably be recovering and so in this situation the return of normal rhythmic breathing should be regarded as a prelude to the resumption of consciousness.

Running movements can occur during the clonic convulsive phase of electrically-induced epilepsy. These are due to activation of subthalamic locomotor regions. They take over once the tonic (rigid) phase of electrical stunning has ended. The behaviour arising from this activity should be distinguished from escape behaviour in otherwise unstunned animals when evaluating the effectiveness of electrical stunning. This can be done by watching for simultaneous breathing and righting activity.

If the stunning current only passes through the spinal cord, as might happen when the electrodes are placed across the neck instead of the head, and an epileptiform seizure is not produced in the brain, the subsequent behaviour of the animal would be quite different. Instead of showing a phase of tonic activity followed by clonic activity, it would only show a short period of tonic activity (Esplin and Freston, 1960). At low currents it might vocalize and show escape behaviour.

Electric currents can also be used to induce a ventricular fibrillation in the heart. In practice, they are used to stun and stop the heart simultaneously with a single current application. The currents necessary to induce ventricular fibrillation have been worked out for poultry, but they are not so clearly defined for the redmeat species. The way that current causes a ventricular fibrillation depends on the following.

- The pathway that the applied current takes through the body, and hence the proportion of the current that passes through the heart.
- The region of the heart that receives the current. In pigs, current reaching the apex of the heart is most likely to induce a ventricular fibrillation (Roy *et al.*, 1987).
- The phase of the heartbeat cycle which coincides with the start of the current flow through the heart. The heart is most susceptible to electrically induced ventricular fibrillation during ventricular repolarization (T wave of the electrocardiogram).
- The frequency and waveform of the electrical current. High frequencies are less likely to induce a ventricular fibrillation (Gregory *et al.*, 1991) and, from experience with judicial electrocutions, high-voltage DCs have been less effective than high voltage ACs.
- The species. As a generalization, the hearts in species which have fast intrinsic heart rates are less readily fibrillated with electric currents.

If heart failure occurs before an animal loses consciousness, the animal may experience some discomfort and this could include muscle pains if the muscle is metabolically active. This type of pain is due to ischaemia and a build-up of extracellular H^+ and K^+. Angina is one example of such pain in humans. The pain can develop in both cardiac and skeletal muscle, and in cardiac muscle it can also be induced by the release of bradykinin. To minimize the chance of ischaemic pain developing following stunning, it is essential to stun the animal before or at the same time as inducing a cardiac arrest. Failure to stun the animal before passing current through the body would also inflict an unpleasant electric shock.

Currents of very short duration (less than 1 second) are less likely to induce a ventricular fibrillation than currents applied for longer periods. Increasing the current from 3 to 12 seconds has no effect on the prevalence of ventricular fibrillation (Gregory and Wotton, 1988b). The likelihood of ventricular fibrillation in sheep rises as the current passing through the chest increases, up to a maximum of 6 A. Beyond about 8 A, the chance of experiencing a ventricular fibrillation declines, and with about 24 A fewer than 5% of the sheep will be fibrillated (Ferris *et al.*, 1936). It is unnecessary to use more than 1.5 A to stun sheep.

When an animal is stunned through the head there is a prompt fall in heart rate whilst the current is flowing (Fig. 4.3). This is probably due to two effects. Firstly, when current flows there is a violent spasm throughout the body and this drives blood from the muscles. This causes a brief rise in systemic blood pressure, which in turn causes a reflex slowing of the heart through activation of the vagus nerve. Secondly, the stunning current itself may directly activate nuclei in the brainstem which initiate a decrease in heart rate through the vagus nerve. When the stunning current is switched off, heart rate rapidly rises to above-normal rates. At high stunning currents there can also be strong activation of the sympathetic nervous system. In pigs, this can cause secretion of a thick saliva, lacrimation and, in boars, ejaculation without erection.

If the electric current is passed simultaneously through the head and body (e.g. with head-to-back stunning), the current can simultaneously stun the animal and induce a ventricular fibrillation (Gregory and Wotton,

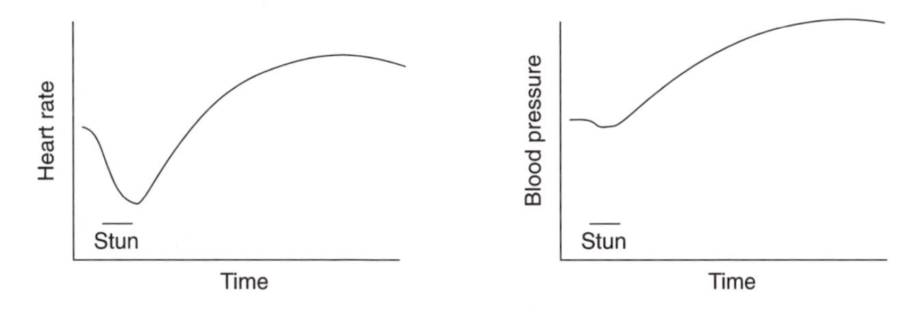

Fig. 4.3. Heart rate and blood pressure responses during and after head only electrical stunning.

1984b). When the heart is fibrillating, the heart muscle continues to contract but it quivers instead of beating rhythmically. There is no pumping action and cardiac output is zero. Arterial blood pressure promptly falls and this can be useful in reducing leakage of blood through any blood vessels that rupture during the spasm that occurs with the onset of current flow (Petersen *et al.*, 1986). In this way, head-to-back stunning can be an effective way of reducing the prevalence of blood splash. It is unusual for the fibrillating heart to return spontaneously to rhythmic beating, except in smaller species such as the rabbit.

The frequency of the electric current that is usually used for stunning sheep and pigs is 50 or 60 Hz. High frequency currents are sometimes used, especially in the poultry industry. *High frequency electrical stunning* currents produce a less intense physical spasm in the body during current flow, but the clonic phase can be more pronounced at very high frequencies. High frequency currents (greater than 500 Hz) are less potent than 50 Hz currents at activating brain metabolism, and the time to recovery of brainstem reflexes following high frequency electrical stunning is quicker. Depending on the species, high frequency stimulation of the spinal cord produces more pronounced limb extension than limb flexion. If high frequency currents are applied to the body without inducing unconsciousness, they produce less sensation of shock in comparison with low frequency currents of equal strength.

A second electric current is sometimes applied to an animal after it has been electrically stunned and before or whilst it is bleeding out. This may be done as part of an *electroimmobilization* procedure. The purpose of electroimmobilization is to control convulsions and avoid injury to staff. It is only needed where carcass kicking poses a safety risk – for example, when large cattle are electrically stunned without inducing a cardiac arrest (as in halal stunning in Australia and New Zealand). There have been concerns from the welfare perspective that the immobilizing current could be used to mask the return of consciousness and so, at worst, an animal might be immobilized but conscious during bleeding out. This concern could be evaluated by not applying the electroimmobilizing current or by switching it off as soon as sticking has been performed, and closely examining the animal for any spontaneous or response signs of consciousness. Additional safety precautions may be required when conducting this trial, such as applying the current if severe convulsions developed.

Spinal discharge is used in some lamb meatworks as a way of controlling carcass kicking. A current is applied to the carcass for a brief period (about 5 seconds) during the early stages of bleeding. The purpose is to activate and exhaust the spinal cord. Spinal discharge is usually applied as a separate system from the stunning current, but it is likely that head-to-back stunning, which involves applying current through the brain and chest of the animal during stunning, also produces a spinal discharge effect. Animals which are stunned with a head-to-back current show less carcass kicking than animals stunned with the same current applied through the head only.

One disadvantage of head-to-back stunning in pigs is vertebral *compression fractures.* These cause haemorrhages and can make carcass splitting difficult if there is a dislocation within the vertebral column. Experience with ECT in humans showed that vertebral compression fractures have been more common in well built muscular patients than in less well-developed subjects, and that it was greatly influenced by restraint and the posture of the patient before the current was applied (Hemphill and Grey Walter, 1941). The same applies to pigs, and the fractures are due to dorsal hyperflexion of the neck and back during the sudden jerk at the onset of current flow.

Another system involving the application of electric currents is *electrical stimulation* of the carcass after sticking. It is used as a way of accelerating post-mortem muscle metabolism, and so allowing rapid chilling without producing tough meat. When low voltage electrical stimulation is used, the current is applied during bleeding; when high voltages are used, they are often applied either after the bleeding tunnel or on the dressing line. When conducted after the carcass has been bled, the procedure is not a concern from the welfare perspective.

Carbon dioxide is used for stunning pigs, salmon and, to a limited extent, chickens. To humans it is a mildly pungent gas when inhaled at high concentrations, and at concentrations above 30% it causes breathlessness through activation of the medulla in the brain (Gregory, 1995a). At low concentrations it acts as a stimulant in the sympathoadrenomedullary nervous system, but with prolonged exposures or high concentrations it is a toxicant and suppresses heart rate and blood pressure.

Slaughter

After the animal has been stunned, it must be bled out. In the redmeat industry this is called *sticking* and in the poultry industry it is called *neck cutting* or killing. The term that is sometimes used by lawyers and scientists is exsanguination. The purpose of bleeding out the carcass is to remove its blood and to kill the animal whilst it is in a stunned state. The aim should be to deflect blood away from the brain to stop the delivery of oxygen. This must be achieved by either cutting both carotid arteries in the neck or puncturing the main vessels in the chest which supply the carotid arteries. Experience in humans has shown that when blood flow to the brain is arrested by occluding both carotid arteries, the time to loss of consciousness is on average 7 seconds (Rossen *et al.*, 1943). This may be preceded by a glowing sensation in the head, tingling sensations in the hands and feet, blurring of vision and mild respiratory stimulation. In a small percentage of subjects, blocking off the carotid arteries causes shooting pains in a limb, before the loss of consciousness. It is essential that the time to loss of brain function following sticking is rapid, and that the animal does not regain consciousness.

When an animal bleeds out there is a fall in blood pressure, and this activates the sympathoadrenomedullary nervous system. Noradrenaline is released from the sympathetic nerve endings, and from the adrenal medulla along with adrenaline. During the initial stages of bleeding this results in splenic contraction, cardiac acceleration and peripheral vasoconstriction. The exposure to adrenaline is very brief but it may add to the other physiological stressors that occur before sticking which help to stimulate muscle glycogenolysis. The adrenergic responses are followed by dilation of the pupil and eventually relaxation of the jaw and other muscles in the carcass as nervous activity subsides. Gagging (inspiratory spasms) may or may not occur, depending on which stunning method preceded the sticking. Bacteria can pass from the sticking knife to the red offal via the bloodstream, and so it is important to use a clean knife (Mackey and Derrick, 1979).

Normally only half the total blood volume is lost during bleeding at slaughter. The remaining blood is present throughout the carcass, and especially in the viscera. Electrical stimulation of the carcass does not affect the elimination of blood from the meat.

Blood splash is a defect where blood capillaries in the carcass have ruptured, resulting in bleps of blood appearing in the meat. It is a common post-mortem finding in humans and animals that have died from accidental electrocution. The way in which blood splash is produced has not been clearly demonstrated, but it depends on a high blood pressure in association with strong muscle contractions. The following theoretical explanation is plausible. During electrical stunning most of the muscles in the body are activated simultaneously. This is an abnormal situation. Normally, during a movement, one set of muscles contract whilst counteracting muscles relax. When all the muscles contract together during passage of the stunning current, the muscles act against each other. In extreme cases it leads to either tearing of the muscle at the ligaments or tearing deeper in the muscle, which results in haemorrhages that appear as blood splash when the meat is sliced. In many cases it is those muscles which are being stretched whilst they are contracting that are most prone to blood splash. During electrical stunning it is the strongest contracting muscles which determine overall posture. In the hindleg, the muscles causing flexion of the limb contract more strongly during electrical stunning. Muscles which would normally control extension of the leg and propulsion whilst the animal is running, such as the semitendinosus and semimembranosus, are stretched by the leg flexion during stunning, whilst at the same time they are being stimulated to contract. The semitendinosus and the semimembranosus are particularly prone to blood splash in pigs.

Glissando electrical stunning was at one time used for controlling blood splash, but it is now regarded as being inhumane. It minimized the initial spasm at the start of current flow by gradually raising the current over a period of about 3 seconds. This technique is likely to be inhumane because the animal would not be stunned immediately. Instead, it would experience an electric shock before it had enough current to render it unconscious.

Capillary haemorrhages can also occur in tissues such as the brain which do not have any skeletal muscle, and in some situations capillary rupture may be due to direct effects of the stunning current on smooth muscle tension within the blood vessels.

In some countries the spinal cord is severed after the animal has been stunned. This is very common in poultry slaughter and it used to be common in sheep abattoirs. At the time the spinal cord is cut, there is a brief body spasm, and in birds this can be seen from the sudden lifting of the wings as they pass through the automatic neck cutter. Thereafter the body is usually still. Cutting the spinal cord disconnects the brain from the body and so it removes all pain innervation to the brain except through the cranial nerves. This is only of value if there is a risk that the animal could regain consciousness, and since this should not be allowed to happen, severing the spinal cord is not justified. If the spinal cord is cut in an unstunned animal there can be a period of violent physical activity. This is not reflex activity, but instead it is initiated by spontaneous activity from within the spinal cord, which would otherwise be suppressed by inhibitory signals descending from the brain. The part of the spinal cord which synchronizes this convulsive activity lies within the cervical and thoracic region and is known as the central pattern generator.

Cutting the spinal cord without any preceding stunning used to be a common slaughtering method for cattle. It is called *puntilla*, spear pithing or neck stabbing, and it is still used in some countries. The head of the animal has to be positioned with the chin flexed towards the underside of the neck. This causes the oval hole (foramen ovale) between the back of the skull (occipital bone) and the first vertebra (atlas) to enlarge. A knife is plunged into the foramen ovale to cut the spinal cord. The animal drops to the floor with the knife in position, and the slaughterman re-works the knife across the spinal cord to make sure that it is completely severed. In this situation the animal is paralysed except for the muscles in the head. Blood continues to flow to the head through the carotid arteries, and if these are not immediately cut the animal will eventually die from being unable to breath. The nerves supplying the muscles in the chest, diaphragm and abdomen which control breathing movements are no longer activated by the spinal cord. According to one observer (Dembo, 1894) who tested the responses of an animal which had its spinal cord cut without being immediately bled:

> when I moved my fingers at a certain distance from its eyes the animal closed them energetically; the same was the case when I lifted my fist. The respiratory movements of the nostrils continued, although they were very feeble. A few oxen stunned [*sic*] in this way licked salt from a piece of bread, and one of them, in the presence of witnesses, even did me the honour of accepting

> bread and salt from my hands. In short, my observations led me to the conclusion that after having received the stab in the neck the animals remain in full possession of their consciousness.

This method is not condoned except when it is used as a pithing method after the animal has been stunned electrically or by concussion.

Chapter 5

Muscle Structure, Exercise and Metabolism

MUSCLE ANATOMY AND FIBRE GROWTH

When considering muscle metabolism it is often helpful to consider the individual muscles in detail, especially in terms of their main fibre type, their location and the way they act with respect to their points of insertion or attachment to the skeleton. This gives a better understanding of the function of an individual muscle and the situations when it is used most. This in turn allows us to anticipate which muscle could develop inferior quality when the animal performs particular behaviours. It is not possible to go into much detail on the anatomical aspects in this book, but information on the position and points of insertion of individual muscles can be found in standard textbooks (e.g. Brown *et al.*, 1978). For our purposes the approximate location of the main muscles mentioned in this book are shown in Fig. 5.1.

When a muscle is particularly well developed in one animal compared with another, it could either have more muscle fibres (hyperplasia) or larger muscle fibres (hypertrophy). Muscle enlargement during normal growth occurs through hyperplasia and hypertrophy. After birth, hyperplasia occurs through recruitment of pre-existing undeveloped muscle cells (satellite myocytes). Hypertrophy occurs as the individual myofibres expand. Muscle enlargement from regular exercise during rearing is thought to occur through both hyperplasia and hypertrophy of recruited myofibres, but often the average fibre diameter remains unaltered (James and Cabric, 1981). Hyperplasia involving division of recruited myofibres can occur postnatally – for example, during regeneration following an injury to muscle.

The growth rate for an individual muscle is determined by the difference between its rate of anabolism and catabolism. Muscle catabolism occurs during normal growth but, clearly, it is slower than the rate of anabolism if the animal is putting on muscle weight. The enzymes in muscle

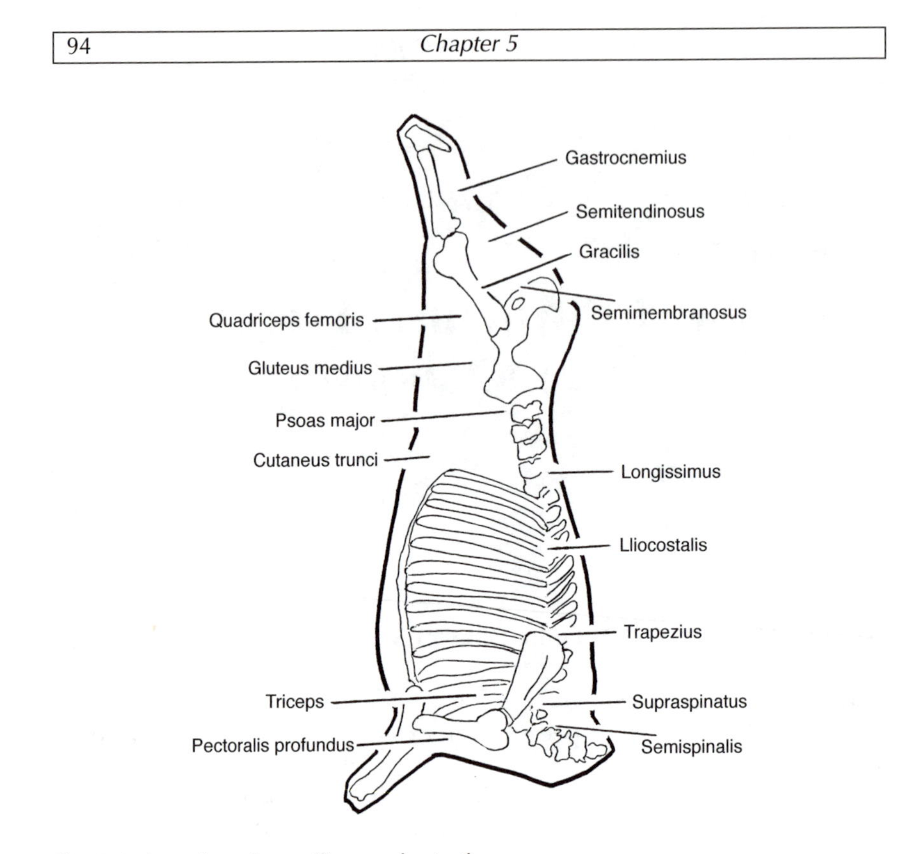

Fig. 5.1. Location of specific muscles in the carcass.

that allow catabolism are important in tenderizing meat once the animal has been slaughtered, and their role in meat toughness is discussed later in this chapter.

MUSCLE METABOLISM

When an animal is taken to slaughter there are several factors which could promote muscle metabolism. Firstly, there is the tension and excitement of the journey, followed by the activity that can occur in the holding pens. Then there is the activity involved in moving to the stunning point, and finally there is the stunning procedure itself, which causes muscle tension during the contraction at stunning and during the convulsions that follow. All this activity uses energy as ATP and CP in the muscle (see Chapter 6) and this in turn affects subsequent meat quality. Of all the stressors that livestock and fish experience before slaughter, excessive exercise is the one that has the most predictable effect on meat quality.

Unnecessary *exercise* is a common outcome of poor preslaughter management. It is provoked by fear or alarm in the animals; by poor technique or facilities during mustering, yarding or catching; during fighting between animals in holding pens; by swimwashing animals before slaughter; and when animals attempt to escape whilst being driven or handled. Exercise is a common sequel to distress and stress in livestock, but taking exercise is not necessarily distressing. It is only when there is excessive exercise leading to breathlessness, extreme fatigue, muscle cramps and muscle soreness that exercise itself becomes a direct cause of suffering. It is more appropriate to consider exercise as a common outcome of stress which has important effects on product quality.

To understand how preslaughter exercise stress affects the animal and subsequent meat quality, it is helpful to first look at the underlying features of muscle structure, muscle contraction, myofibre type and muscle metabolism. Muscle is made up of fibres which are held together by interconnecting connective tissue sheaths. The muscles are separated from each other and from other tissues by a *fascia* of connective tissue. This fascia contains pain receptors which are activated when they are stretched excessively. For example, this occurs when muscle is bruised. The bruise causes swelling under the fascia, the pain receptors are activated and a nociceptive signal is transmitted to the brain, where it may be interpreted as pain.

The fibres within a muscle are made up of myofibrils (Fig. 5.2). The myofibrils are enveloped by tubules, which have the appearance of a stocking net. Within the myofibrils there are two types of protein myofilament: actin and myosin; these are the basic structural components which perform *muscle contraction* (Fig. 5.3). The myosin filaments have side branches which extend laterally to the actin filaments and they have an ATP molecule in the terminal position. When a nerve impulse reaches the sarcolemma of

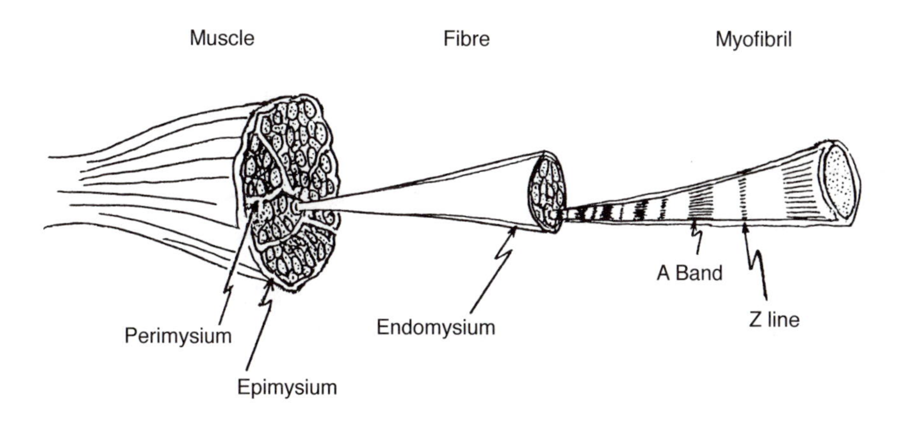

Fig. 5.2. Structure of a muscle.

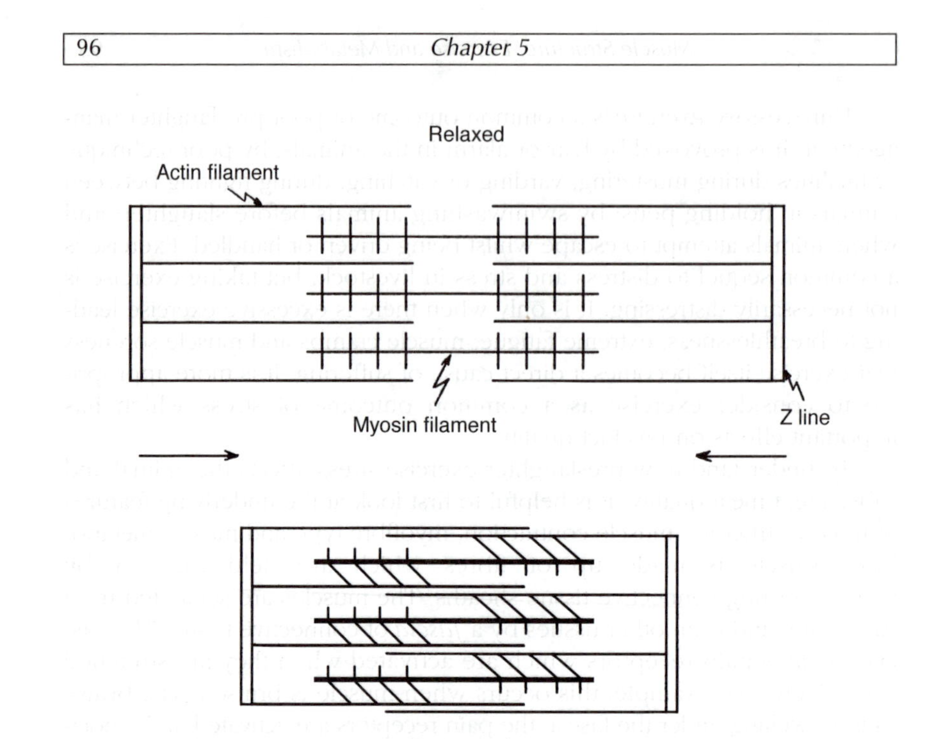

Fig. 5.3. Muscle contraction according to the sliding filament theory – sarcomere shortening. During contraction, the actin and myosin filaments slide over each other, and the Z lines are drawn towards each other. This occurs through the myosin side-branches repetitively making and breaking contact with the adjacent actin filament; each time an actomyosin bond is formed, myosin ATPase is activated and ATP is broken down. During relaxation, the myosin has to be reloaded with an ATP molecule; if no ATP is available (as occurs after slaughter) the side-branches remain attached to the actin filaments and the muscle stays in rigor.

the muscle, it spreads through the tubule system and depolarizes the sarcoplasmic reticulum of the cells. The sarcoplasmic reticulum releases Ca^{2+} into the sarcoplasm, and from there it binds to troponin molecules in the actin myofilaments. The binding of Ca^{2+} to the troponin allows the side branches of myosin to bind to actin to form actomyosin (Fig. 5.4). During this binding process a region of the myosin myofilament is exposed which bears an ATPase enzyme. This enzyme causes the terminal ATP to be broken down to ADP + P_i, with the release of large amounts of energy. Part of this energy is used in re-orienting the myosin side branches. They twist, swivel and collapse and in so doing cause the actin to slide over the myosin in one direction or the other. If the actin slides towards the Z line, the myofibre shortens; if it slides away from the Z line, the myofibre lengthens. Both the shortening and the lengthening involve a contraction process that

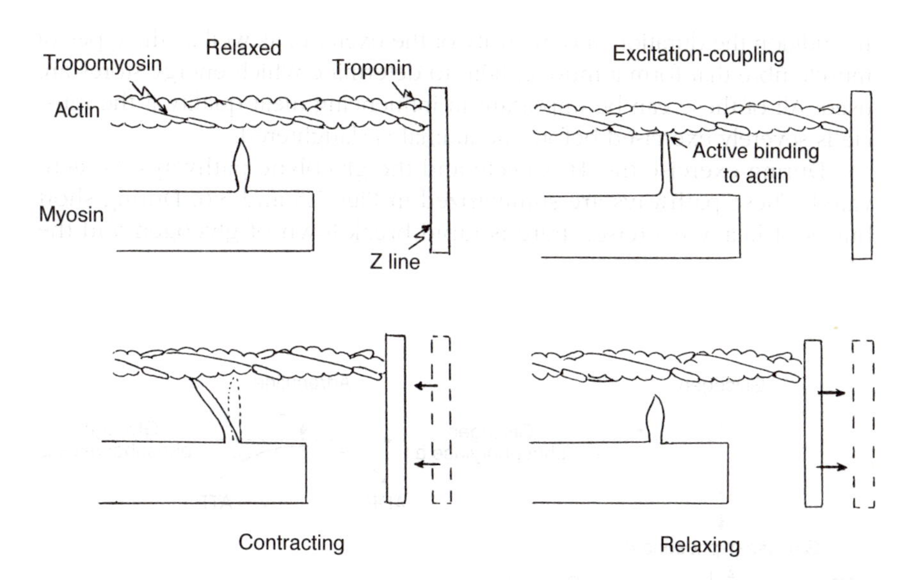

Fig. 5.4. Muscle contraction according to the sliding filament theory – actomyosin formation. During excitation-coupling, Ca^{2+} is released from the sarcoplasmic reticulum and binds to troponin, which then activates an actin site to accept the terminal ATP molecule of the myosin side-branch. During contraction the ATP molecule is broken down, releasing energy which swivels the side-branch, causing the actin to slide over the myosin. This creates tension and causes the muscle to contract. During relaxation, Ca^{2+} is released from the troponin and is taken up by the sarcoplasmic reticulum. The actomyosin bond is released and the muscle is restored to its original dimension.

uses energy and ATP. When the nerve impulses stop, Ca^{2+} is unbound from the troponin and passes back to the sarcoplasmic reticulum. The ATPase in myosin is no longer active, no more ATP is broken down and the muscle relaxes. The ability of a muscle to contract depends on the presence of ATP and on the presence of the nerve impulse or other stimulus that sets off the above process.

The ATP that fuels the contraction process can be regenerated from ADP in a number of ways:

- transfer of high energy phosphate groups from stores of creatine phosphate within muscle
- breakdown of stores of glycogen within muscle
- utilization of glucose supplied by the blood stream
- utilization of fatty acids (VFAs and FFAs) supplied by the bloodstream
- utilization of free fatty acids derived from fat which is stored in the muscle.

The physiological state of the animal (e.g. fed or fasted, physical fitness) can help to determine which of these fuels contribute most to ATP regeneration.

In addition the duration and intensity of the exercise, as well as the types of muscle fibre that form a muscle, help to determine which energy stores are used. All of these can be important in influencing meat quality if the muscle is severely exercised before the animal is slaughtered.

During exercise the TCA cycle and the glycolytic pathways are activated. These pathways are summarized in Figs 5.5 and 5.6. During short bursts of heavy exercise, there is rapid breakdown of glycogen and the

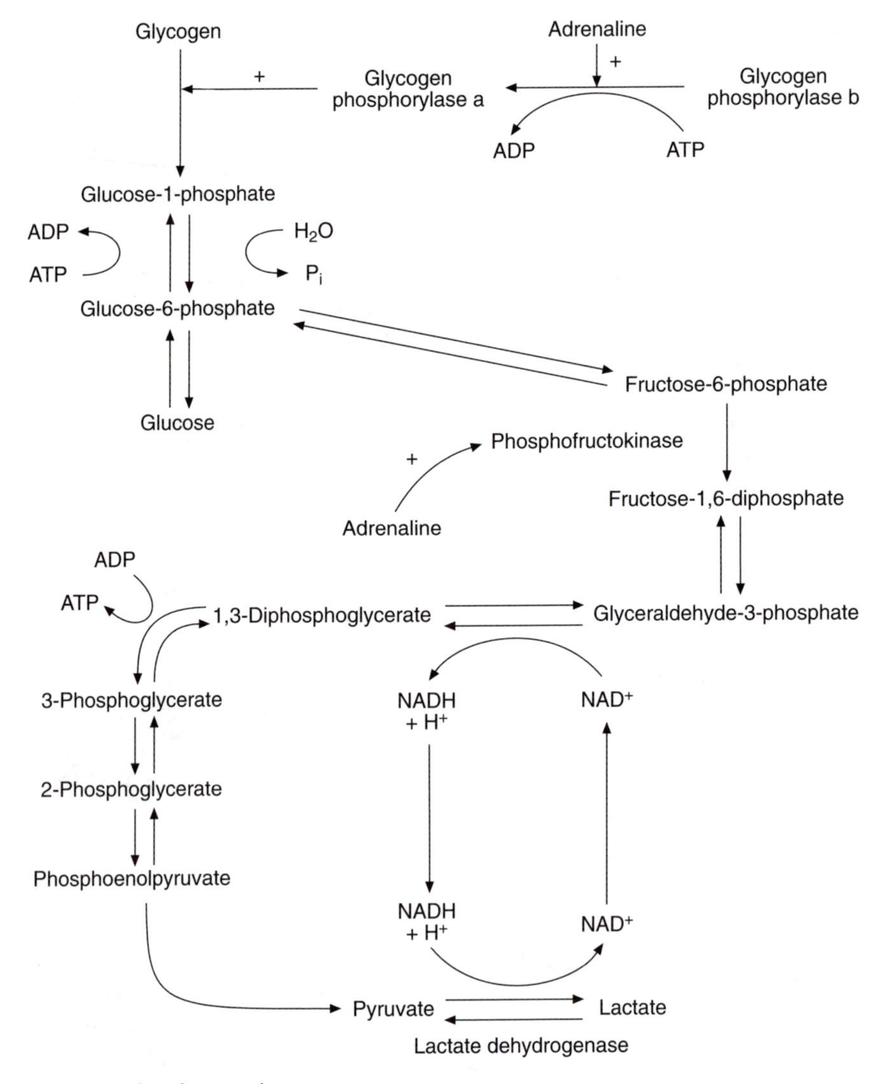

Fig. 5.5. Glycolytic pathway.

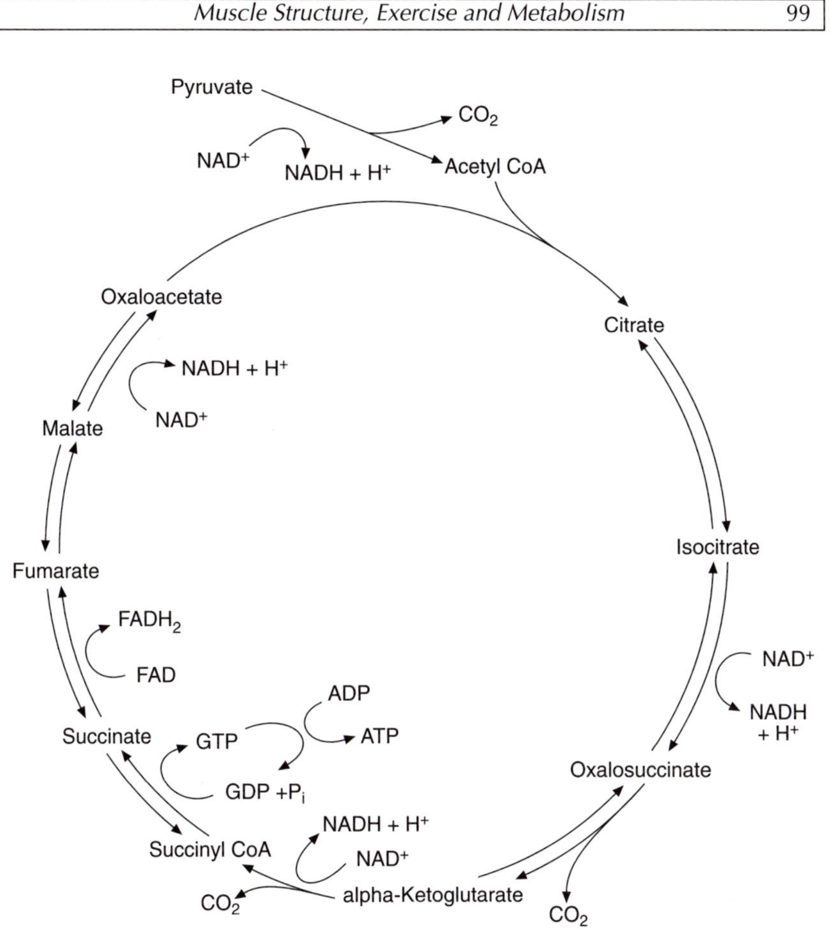

Fig. 5.6. TCA cycle.

production of large amounts of lactic acid through the glycolytic pathway (Fig. 5.5). Lactate and H^+ enter the bloodstream and in mammalian species their blood levels are useful indicators of the severity of the exercise. During heavy exercise, the pH in the muscle of the live animal may fall to 6.3, and in extreme circumstances to as low as 5.9

Glycogenolysis in muscle is initiated by exercise and by adrenaline released from the adrenal medulla. Glycogenolysis does not depend on adrenaline, as glycogen stores in muscle can be depleted by exercise alone. For example, when young bulls were given propranolol (a beta-adrenergic receptor blocking agent which inhibits the glycogenolytic action of adrenaline) before being mixed, the exercise stress still resulted in muscle glycogen depletion and in the dark-cutting beef condition (McVeigh and Tarrant, 1981).

Glycogen is broken down in the glycolytic pathway to pyruvate (Fig. 5.5). Pyruvate can either be used for generating ATP in the TCA cycle (Fig. 5.6), or it is converted to lactate. This difference is important in terms of the efficiency of energy use, as the two systems capture different amounts of energy. When 1 mol glucose is oxidized to 2 mol lactate, there is a fall in free energy of 47 kcal. However, 3 mol ATP (21 kcal) is produced in this process by transferring energy to ADP. If, instead, glucose oxidation proceeds to CO_2 and H_2O through the TCA cycle, the fall in free energy is 686 kcal, with 252 kcal conserved as ATP (36 mol at 7 kcal per mol ATP). In terms of the metabolism of the contracting myofibre, it is less efficient to convert glucose to lactate than to oxidize it to CO_2. Only 21 kcal energy is conserved within the myofibre as ATP when 1 mol glucose is converted to lactate, whereas 252 kcal is conserved when the same amount of glucose is converted to CO_2.

The release of CO_2 from exercising muscle into the bloodstream stimulates panting when it reaches the brain; the increased heat generated by the contracting muscle initiates vasodilation, and sweating or panting (depending on the species). The sense of *fatigue* that accompanies exercise is not due to low levels of glycogen in the muscle. Instead, it is due to a build-up of end-products of muscle metabolism which activate afferent nerves which, in turn, convey signals to the brain where they are interpreted as fatigue (Saito *et al.*, 1989). It is not certain which metabolite is mainly involved in this type of chemoreception, but it could be either phosphate, lactate, H^+ or K^+.

The conversion of glucose to lactate occurs when the muscle is hypoxic, or when there is an excess of pyruvate. *Lactate formation* from pyruvate does not require oxygen, whereas the conversion of 1 mol glucose to CO_2 requires 6 mol oxygen. Oxygen delivery, from myoglobin in the muscle and haemoglobin in the blood, is essential if the muscle is to continue to refuel its ATP reserves rapidly and in an energy-efficient manner using the TCA cycle. The oxygen consumption rate at which lactate starts being produced by exercising muscle is a useful indicator of physical fitness in humans. Physically fit individuals can maintain an aerobic metabolism during exercise for longer before their muscle changes to lactate production. In addition it has been found that pigs which were familiar with physical exercise and had been subjected to a training schedule before slaughter showed considerably lower blood lactate responses during exercise stress than untrained pigs (Fogd Jørgensen and Hyldgaard-Jensen, 1975). They were also less prone to developing PSE (pale soft exudative) meat when they had been slaughtered. Sleep deprivation before a bout of exercise is likely to lead to a higher lactate response during the exercise.

There are two reasons why training and fitness are associated with lower plasma lactate responses to exercise. Firstly, when lactate concentrations are elevated, fit individuals clear the lactate from the bloodstream more rapidly. The liver is the main site for lactate uptake, but it can also be metabolized in cardiac and skeletal muscle in some species. In addition, fit individuals can sustain aerobic metabolism for longer when they exercise and so they produce less lactate.

There are three ways in which the muscle glycogen reserves in an animal can be managed:

- reducing preslaughter exercise and stress;
- supercompensation;
- allowing repletion of glycogen.

During training, human athletes often boost their muscle glycogen reserves by a process known as *supercompensation*. This involves switching during strenuous training, and shortly before a competition, from a low carbohydrate to a high carbohydrate diet. The total muscle glycogen content can be doubled. A form of supercompensation is used at some abattoirs where pigs are fed a sugar solution whilst in the lairage waiting to be slaughtered. This provides them with additional reserves of glycogen in their muscle and helps to prevent dark, firm, dry (DFD) meat.

In cattle, *repletion of muscle glycogen* following exhaustive exercise takes at least 24 hours and can take up to 48 hours. The rate of repletion in a muscle depends on the predominant fibre types in the muscle. In the laboratory rat, red-fibred muscles have greater blood flow rates and so these muscles receive larger amounts of glucose after feeding. This allows the red-fibred muscles to replete glycogen at a faster rate than the white-fibred muscles.

Muscle can use other substrates besides glycogen and glucose during a stress response. When animals which have been fed take exercise, glycogen is utilized initially; if the exercise is sustained, the muscle switches to *FFA utilization*. The way in which an animal is fed just before a period of exercise can affect the type of substrate that the muscle uses. As a general rule, circumstances that favour elevated plasma FFA help to spare the utilization of muscle glycogen (Costill *et al.*, 1977). In monogastric species, carbohydrate intake results in greater reliance on plasma glucose and muscle glycogen and less reliance on intramuscular fat and plasma FFA. Fasting before the exercise results in greater reliance on muscle fat and on plasma FFA. Feeding high fat diets before exercise can help to improve exercise tolerance, by sparing glycogen.

The contribution that glycogen makes to metabolism during fasting declines as the oxidation of fatty acids increases. When a 60 kg pig goes without feed, it derives its energy initially from what is absorbed from its gut. As this declines, energy is mobilized from the liver; when this is depleted, it is derived from adipose tissue. The total energy that is stored as glycogen and fat in the pig's liver is about 310 kcal (Table 5.1). A 60 kg resting pig loses energy as heat at a rate of about 80 kcal per hour, and so the reserves in the liver do not last for long even when it is resting. Free fatty

Table 5.1. Energy stores in the pig.

	Energy (kcal)	
	Glycogen	Fat
Muscle	1200	9400
Adipose tissue	0	140,000
Liver	80	230

acids (FFA) start to be mobilized from adipose tissue after 16 hours fasting in resting pigs (Fig. 5.7) (Gregory *et al.*, 1980).

A potentially important issue for meat quality is whether animals that are using FFAs in their muscle instead of glycogen are more prone to developing anaerobic metabolism and a preslaughter acidosis. During aerobic metabolism the rate of consumption of oxygen during glycogen and FFA utilization are similar – even though, on a molar basis, FFA utilization consumes more oxygen. When 1 mol glucose is completely oxidized, 6 mol oxygen is used. The corresponding rates of oxygen use for other substrates are: acetate 2 mol, acetoacetate 4 mol, beta-hydroxybutyrate 4.5 mol, FFA (e.g. palmitate) 23 mol. However, when 1 mol palmitate is completely oxidized, 980 kcal are conserved and the ratio of energy conserved : oxygen used is the same as that for glucose. So, when animals utilize FFAs when they are stressed, they are neither more nor less likely to develop an oxygen deficit than animals which are utilizing glucose. When bulls in the fed state take to fighting during the preslaughter period, they utilize FFA as well as glycogen from liver and muscle. They are capable of maintaining an aerobic metabolism without becoming lactacidotic even when the exercise is severe enough to induce high pH_{ult} meat (Warriss, 1984).

During short bursts of strenuous exercise, ATP is broken down to ADP and to AMP, which can be deaminated to ammonia and inosinic acid (IMP) by the action of AMP deaminase. IMP concentrations can increase from less than 10 to about 3500 nmol g^{-1} wet weight of muscle during intense exercise, and a rest period is needed to allow IMP to be reaminated to AMP. IMP can contribute a flavour-enhancing effect when meat is cooked, and so on a theoretical basis if the animal is slaughtered immediately following severe exercise its meat may develop enhanced flavour. There are reports which show that preslaughter stress has improved meat flavour in pigs (Lewis *et al.*, 1967), but the exercise was severe and the effects on flavour were small. IMP does not accumulate in muscle during moderate exercise, but its production may be enhanced if the muscles become hypoxic or ischaemic. Muscles that have a high proportion of alpha white fibres are generally more prone to IMP accumulation and this may be linked to their reduced capacity to regenerate ATP from AMP during exercise.

In mammalian species, the *ammonia* that is produced during IMP formation enters the bloodstream. The ammonia concentration in the blood

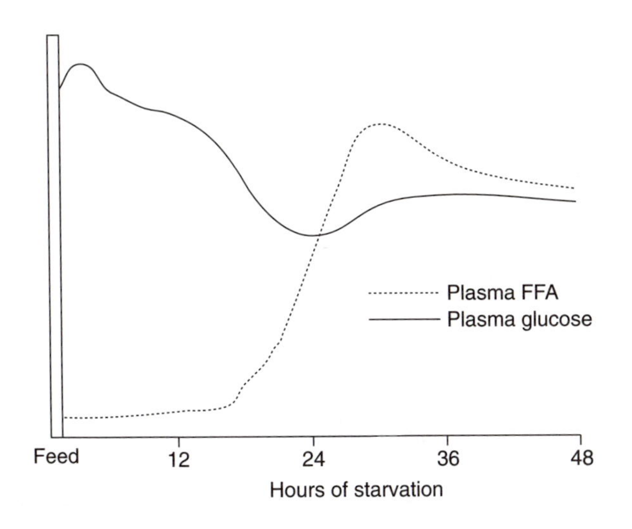

Fig. 5.7. Changes in plasma FFA (free fatty acid) and glucose concentrations during fasting in pigs.

can be used as an indicator of severe exercise. During prolonged exercise, blood ammonia will continue to rise long after blood lactate concentrations have plateaued through failing glycogen reserves. However, in physically fit animals ammonia production is likely to be less, because they are less prone to depleting ATP and accumulating AMP in muscle. In some fish species, ammonia is metabolized within muscle and it is not used as an exercise stress indicator.

Different muscles also have different *muscle fibre types*. The muscle fibres can be classified into three main types according to their contractile and metabolic characteristics:

- β-red – slow twitch oxidative
- α-red – fast twitch oxidative
- α-white – fast twitch glycolytic.

The properties of the three types are summarized in Table 5.2. Alpha fibres contract rapidly and are involved in phasic contractions that occur during bursts of activity. Beta fibres contract tonically and are involved in the continuous contractions that are used in posture. The red fibres are equipped for oxidative metabolism, whereas white fibres rely more on the glycolytic pathway. The red fibres have high myoglobin concentrations and a relatively high capillary blood flow, which helps to maintain oxygen supply. Their capacity for oxidative metabolism is reflected in the large number of mitochondria in each fibre, and by the high levels of the TCA cycle enzyme succinic dehydrogenase, which is used histochemically to distinguish these

Table 5.2. Main properties of the three types of muscle fibre.

	β-Red	α-Red	α-White
Colour	Red	Red	White
Contraction speed	Slow	Fast	Fast
Contractile action	Tonic	Phasic	Phasic
Myoglobin concentration	High	High	Low
Capillary density	High	Intermediate	Low
Fibre diameter	Small	Small/intermediate	Large
Number of mitochondria	High	Intermediate	Low
Glycogen storage	Low	Intermediate	High

fibres. Red fibres can utilize fatty acids more effectively than can white fibres, and they store more lipid.

Different muscles have different proportions of the three types of fibre (Table 5.3). Postural muscles (such as the trapezius in the shoulder) have a high proportion of beta red fibres, whereas muscles involved with breathing movements (such as the cutaneus trunci) and running (such as the semitendinosus) have a higher proportion of alpha white fibres. Some of the physiological and meat quality consequences of fibre type are as follows.

- Animals which are fasted mobilize body fat as FFAs. Free fatty acids are used as an energy source by red-fibred oxidative muscles.
- White-fibred muscles are better equipped to obtain energy by anaerobic metabolism than are red-fibred muscles. They tend to hold more energy in a readily utilizable form (e.g. CP and ATP), and during exercise and post-mortem metabolism they produce more lactate and a lower pH_{ult} than red fibres.
- Postural muscles which are rich in red fibres tend to be continuously active. Their sustained activity in the live animal makes them more susceptible to depletion of energy reserves when energy supply from the bloodstream declines. So, these muscles are more prone to becoming glycogen depleted during fasting (Wittmann *et al.*, 1994).
- Muscles that are used during exercise and are rich in white fibres do not necessarily show glycogen depletion during fasting if they are inactive. If, on the other hand, they are active and the animal is fasted at the same time, they are more prone to glycogen depletion (Fernandez *et al.*, 1995).
- Double-muscled cattle have a higher proportion of alpha white fibres in their muscles and are more prone to developing high blood lactate levels during severe exercise.
- During prolonged activity the intracellular pH of the muscle gradually declines. As the muscle becomes more acid, the force and velocity of contraction declines and fatigue sets in. Fast-contracting muscle fibres are more sensitive to this effect than slow-contracting fibres.

Table 5.3. Proportion of fibre types in some different muscles.

	β-Red	α-Red	α-White
Pig			
Longissimus	10	14	76
Semipinalis capitis	39	20	41
Trapezius	43	34	23
Cattle			
Semitendinosus	8	26	66
Cutaneus trunci	7	28	65
Semimembranosus	13	31	56
Gluteus medius	26	22	52
Longissimus	25	25	50
Triceps longus	22	32	46
Psoas major	52	15	33

- White-fibred muscles are more likely to exhibit rapid post-mortem glycolysis than muscles that have a predominantly oxidative type of metabolism.
- White-fibred muscles can exert strong tensions and are able to contract and relax rapidly. Red fibres can maintain a sustained but weaker contraction for a long time. White-fibred muscles usually have shorter sarcomere lengths when in rigor than red-fibred muscles.

In most fish species, between 75 and 80% of the muscle is white muscle. These are predominantly fast-twitch glycolytic muscles, and they allow the fish to perform short bursts of vigorous activity. Red muscle is present as a thin triangular strip running the length of the fish under the lateral line. It is an aerobic slow-twitch oxidative muscle which is recruited during long-term steady-state swimming.

Figure 5.8 helps to summarize the key energy reserves that are used during the preslaughter period. There are three important energy substrates for muscle: glycogen, glucose and fatty acids (Fig. 5.8). If a fasted animal is unable to mobilize body fat to supply muscle with FFAs, the muscle instead relies on glycogen and blood glucose for its energy. These carbohydrates only last for a limited period and so the risk of high pH_{ult} meat increases as the period without feed lengthens. The importance of sustained fat mobilization has been demonstrated by Lister and Spencer (1983). They treated sheep either with an intravenous infusion of isoprenaline, which is an adrenergic β-agonist that stimulates lipolysis and muscle glycogenolysis, or with isoprenaline plus MPCA (methyl pyrazole carboxylic acid). MPCA inhibits lipolysis without having any direct effect on glycogenolysis. There was also a saline control. The main findings are shown in Table 5.4. In addition, they monitored plasma glucose, FFA and lactate concentrations, all of which were higher in the sheep treated with isoprenaline than in those

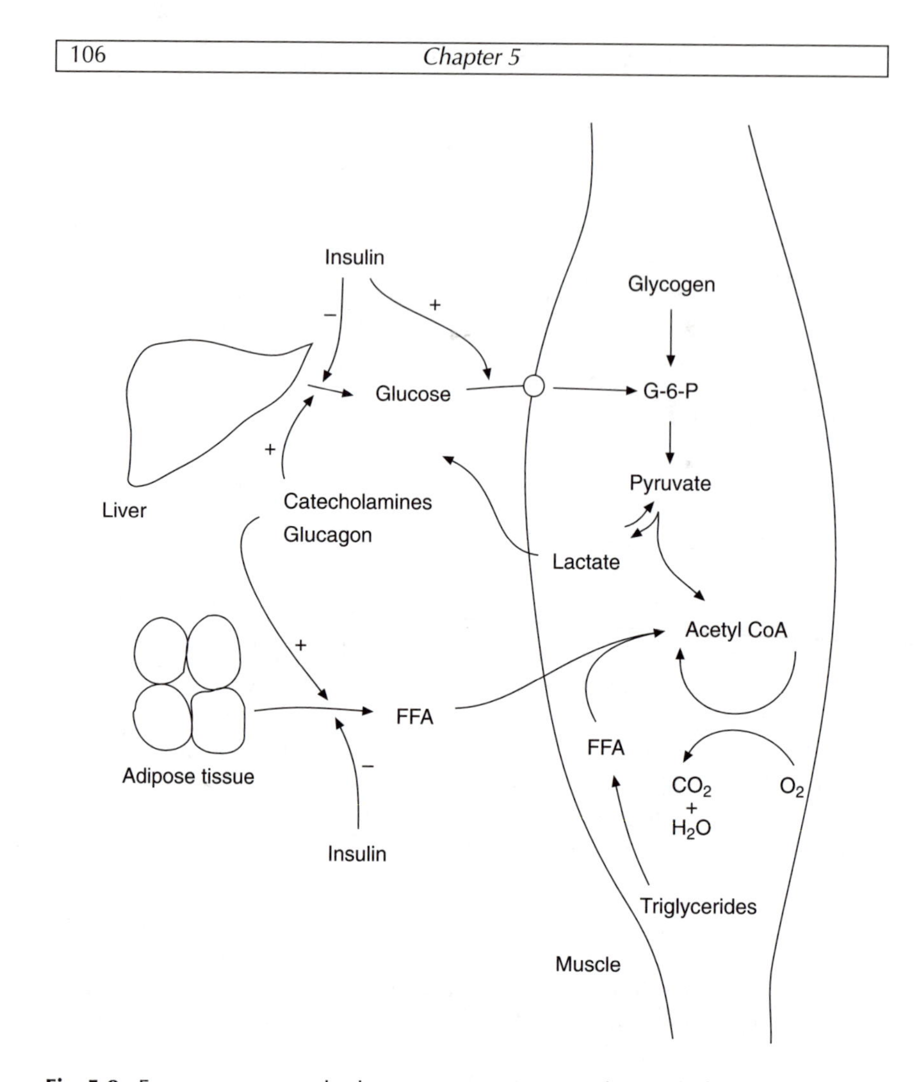

Fig. 5.8. Energy sources and substrates supporting muscle metabolism.

treated with isoprenaline plus MPCA. Isoprenaline alone resulted in a halving of muscle glycogen concentration, whereas isoprenaline plus MPCA virtually depleted the muscle glycogen. As a result, pH_{ult} was high and the dark-cutting condition was more pronounced in the sheep which were unable to mobilize body fat. It is not known whether failure to mobilize or utilize body fat adequately is a common problem in sheep, but, it has been observed in fat sheep in Australia which had been grazing good pasture and were subsequently fasted. By comparison, sheep off poor arid pasture were adapted to mobilizing their body fat, and coped with the fast more effectively by sustaining fat mobilization and using their body fat reserves (Richards *et al.*, 1991). In humans and laboratory animals, ability to mobilize

Table 5.4. Effect of isoprenaline or isoprenaline plus MPCA infusion on meat quality in sheep.

	Saline control	Isoprenaline	Isoprenaline plus MPCA
Muscle glycogen at slaughter (mg g^{-1})	10.4 ± 3.1	5.5 ± 0.8	1.2 ± 0.3
Muscle pH_{ult}	6.03 ± 0.07	6.07 ± 0.04	6.55 ± 0.05
% Sheep showing dark-cutting	0	0	100

and utilize FFA is reduced in physically unfit individuals. Exercise training overcomes this and it increases the mobilization of intramuscular lipid during bouts of exercise.

FFA utilization within muscle is limited by the rate of entry of the FFA into the mitochondria. The transfer of FFA from the sarcoplasm into mitochondria is controlled by carnitine acyl transferase, an enzyme that is located in the walls of the mitochondria. The activity of this enzyme is low in muscle of unfit or untrained animals; physical training helps to increase its activity, and also reduces the likelihood of developing high blood lactate levels during severe exercise. Lipolysis is impaired when there is a lactacidosis, and so this is another cause for exercise intolerance and reduced ability to mobilize fat.

Chapter 6

Post-mortem Muscle Metabolism and Meat Quality

Post-mortem muscle metabolism is important in contributing to the following meat quality defects:

- pale, soft, exudative (PSE) meat;
- dark-cutting beef (DCB);
- dark, firm, dry (DFD) pork;
- tough meat;
- abnormal meat colour;
- excessive drip.

PSE, DCB and DFD meat are stress-related conditions. PSE meat occurs in pigs and turkeys. In pigs it is common in particular breeds which are known as stress-sensitive (SS) or halothane-positive (*nn*) genotypes. This chapter focuses on some of the key features in post-mortem muscle metabolism which lead to these meat quality problems, and so helps to explain how preslaughter stress influences meat quality.

When an animal is slaughtered, its muscle continues to metabolize energy, contract and produce heat. Some of the energy is used to power the convulsions, muscle twitching (fasciculations) and rigor contractions which occur in the carcass, and some is used in non-contractile biochemical changes. During muscle contraction, adenosine triphosphate (ATP) is utilized and it forms adenosine diphosphate (ADP) and free phosphate (P_i). ATP breakdown provides the energy needed for the contractions. ATP is also utilized in pumping mechanisms that regulate the concentration of ions in the cell.

ATP is resynthesized in two main ways. The first is from an energy store which is in the form of creatine phosphate (CP). Creatine phosphate passes on a high energy phosphate group to ADP, forming ATP, in a reaction that is catalysed by the enzyme, creatine phosphokinase (CPK):

$$CP + ADP \leftrightharpoons ATP + C$$

CPK is present in large amounts in muscle. In the live animal its leakage into the bloodstream can be a useful indicator of damage to muscle membranes or excessive activity of the muscle.

The other way in which ATP is resynthesized is through the mitochondrial respiratory chain. This involves an electron transport system which is catalysed by NAD-linked dehydrogenases, flavoprotein dehydrogenases and cytochromes (Fig. 6.1). Every time the electron transport chain is activated, three molecules of ATP are produced from three molecules of ADP and P_i, and one atom of oxygen is incorporated into water. It is important to note that this way of regenerating ATP requires oxygen.

The electron transport chain is linked to other metabolic processes as follows. In the sarcoplasm of the cell, the end product of the glycolytic pathway is pyruvate. After pyruvate enters a mitochondrion it joins the tricarboxylic acid (TCA) cycle as it is converted to acetyl CoA (see Fig. 5.6). This reaction is linked to the respiratory chain through NAD. For each molecule of pyruvate that is converted to acetyl CoA, one atom of oxygen is incorporated into water and three molecules of ATP are resynthesized from ADP. The conversion of isocitrate to oxalosuccinate fuels the respiratory chain in the same way, but in the case of the oxidation of succinate to fumarate the reaction is linked to a flavoprotein instead, and only two molecules of ATP are formed from ADP.

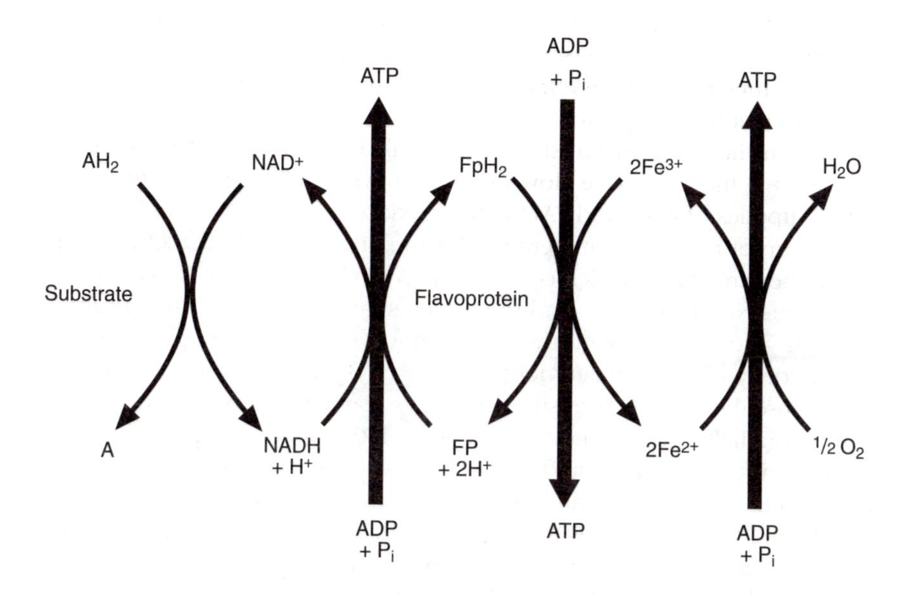

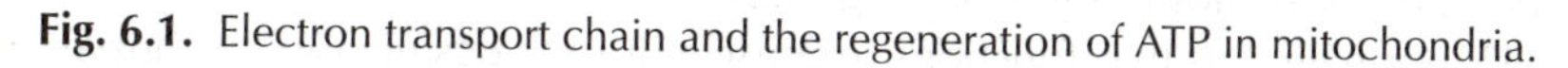
Fig. 6.1. Electron transport chain and the regeneration of ATP in mitochondria.

The relevant features of the above are that the reactions which are catalysed by the NAD-linked dehydrogenases and the flavoprotein dehydrogenases form a necessary link between the electron transport chain, which regenerates ATP, and the oxidation of metabolic fuels derived from carbohydrates, fats and proteins. It is the electron transport chain and the need to regenerate ATP which drives the whole system during post-mortem muscle metabolism.

The glycolytic pathway helps to fuel the TCA cycle and hence the electron transport chain. Exchange between glycolysis and the TCA cycle only occurs when pyruvate leaves the sarcoplasm, enters the mitochondria and is converted to acetyl CoA. This is a one-way process, which acts as a valve, maintaining the direction of flow of energy towards the TCA cycle. After slaughter, glycolysis is no longer fuelled by glucose derived from the bloodstream and instead it relies predominantly on the glycogen that is stored in muscle. FFA utilization post-mortem is greatly reduced in comparison with that occurring in the live animal, as there is limited ability to translocate FFA from the intramuscular lipid stores to the mitochondria post-mortem.

During death there are three processes which cause the normal metabolic processes in living muscle to slow down and eventually stop:

- depletion of oxygen;
- depletion of substrate;
- inhibition of enzymes.

When an animal is stuck, the blood supply to its muscles stops. The muscles no longer receive oxygen and the respiratory chain instead depends on the reserves of oxygen that were in the tissues at the time the animal was slaughtered. When these reserves are used up, the electron transport chain ceases to function. ATP resynthesis will continue for a short period from the store of creatine phosphate.

When the electron transport chain fails through lack of oxygen, the reactions in the TCA cycle slow down and eventually stop through inadequate supplies of NAD and FAD in their oxidized forms. This would lead to a build-up of pyruvate if it were not for the presence of lactic dehydrogenase in the sarcoplasm which converts the pyruvate to lactate. In so doing, it reoxidizes NADH to NAD, and the replenishment of NAD allows a further burst of glycolysis through the continuation of the reaction catalysed by glyceraldehyde 3-phosphate dehydrogenase. Thus, whilst anaerobic conditions cause the TCA cycle to stop, glycolysis continues. Glycolysis eventually comes to a halt through one of two effects. Either there is depletion of substrates (glycogen, glucose and hexosephosphates) or the build-up of acidity in the form of lactic acid inhibits the enzymes in the glycolytic pathway.

Putting these processes together, we can see a pattern in the depletion of ATP, CP and glycogen, and the accumulation of lactic acid in muscle during the early post-mortem period (Fig. 6.2).

ATP normally has two functions in muscle. It provides energy for muscle

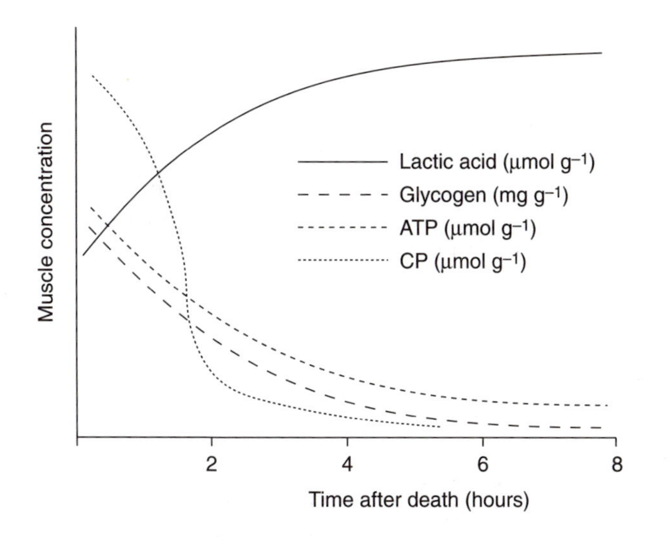

Fig. 6.2. ATP, CP, glycogen and lactic acid changes during post-mortem muscle metabolism (after Tarrant *et al.*, 1972).

contraction, which occurs when actin and myosin filaments interlock by sliding over each other. The contraction process is normally initiated by Ca^{2+}, which is released into the sarcoplasm when the muscle is stimulated by a nerve.

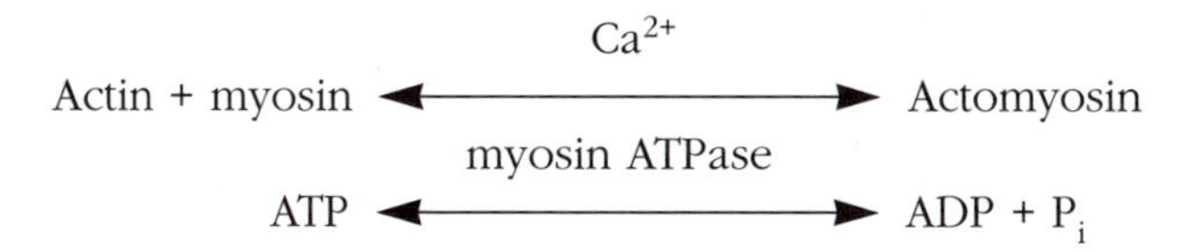

ATP also provides energy that operates two ionic pumps within the muscle cell. These pumps reduce the concentration of Ca^{2+} in the sarcoplasm; one of the pumps is present on the sarcoplasmic reticulum and the other in the mitochondria. As the ATP level falls post-mortem, the ionic pumps start to fail. There is insufficient energy to operate the pumps and the Ca^{2+} level in the sarcoplasm gradually rises. When the Ca^{2+} level exceeds 10^{-6} M, the Ca^{2+} activates the muscle to contract. At this stage there is insufficient ATP to reverse the contraction by pumping the Ca^{2+} out of the sarcoplasm, and so the muscle remains in a contracted state. This permanent contracted state is known as *rigor*. The severity of rigor is important in influencing the toughness of meat. Once rigor has set in, the toughness it creates can only be released by breaking up the myofibres. Disruption of the myofibres can occur enzymatically during normal ageing of meat, or mechanically when a steak is beaten before cooking.

When an animal is stressed before slaughter, the reserves of glycogen and ATP at the time of slaughter are likely to be low. This means that ATP depletion is likely to occur shortly after the animal is killed, the sarcoplasmic Ca^{2+} levels will quickly rise and so rigor will set in earlier. A characteristic feature of carcasses from animals that have been severely stressed immediately before slaughter is that they enter rigor sooner. A simple way of distinguishing this in different carcasses is to select an appropriate point in the slaughterline, and to lift a forelimb of each carcass as it passes that point.

If muscle glycogen levels became depleted during a preslaughter stress, the muscle may have to switch to using free fatty acids as an energy source instead. The free fatty acids are utilized by breaking them down to acetyl CoA, which feeds into the TCA cycle, providing the muscle with much needed energy. The presence of acetyl CoA inhibits the conversion of pyruvate to acetyl CoA and glycolysis is greatly reduced. A common feature of aerobic but glycogen-depleted muscle is that all the glycolytic intermediates are suppressed except for pyruvate, which is either normal or has built up to higher than normal levels.

In some situations the metabolites in muscle provide a better indication of stress than measuring metabolites and hormones in blood. This is because the change in concentration in some metabolites in muscle provides an integration of stress over a longer period. Table 6.1 summarizes some commonly used measures of muscle exhaustion.

An important feature of glycogen-depleted muscle from stressed animals is that it has insufficient glycolytic substrates to allow the muscle to acidify properly when the animal is slaughtered. Failure in acidification can be measured from the pH of the meat 24 hours after slaughter. This is known as the ultimate pH, or pH_{ult}. A high pH_{ult} (e.g. greater than 6.0) indicates that the muscle was glycogen-depleted at slaughter, that the animal was metabolically stressed before slaughter and that the meat is likely to be *dark-cutting* (i.e. DCB or DFD pork). Dark-cutting meat is objectionably dark in colour and it is prone to microbial spoilage.

The pH of the muscle at the time the animal is bleeding out is called the *initial pH* of the muscle. A low initial pH indicates either that there has been intense stimulation of the animal or muscle just before stunning, or that

Table 6.1. Measures of exercise stress or exhaustion in muscle and meat.

Muscle (immediately after slaughter)	Meat (24 hours after slaughter)
↓ Glycogen	↑ pH_{ult}
↓ ATP	Dark colour
↑ Lactate	

stunning itself caused excessive activation of the muscle as convulsions. The initial pH is also sometimes called the $pH_{5\ min}$. The importance of stress during the minutes before slaughter on initial pH was demonstrated experimentally by Bendall (1966), when pigs had nervous transmission to their muscles blocked with curare just before they were slaughtered. This resulted in a high initial pH (Fig. 6.3).

A third measure of pH which is important in meat science is the $pH_{45\ min}$. If the rate of post-mortem metabolism is accelerated, the $pH_{45\ min}$ will be lower than normal. At the same time the lactate concentrations in the muscle will be higher. In pork, if the pH at 45 minutes is less than 6.0 the meat is likely to be PSE, and $pH_{45\ min}$ measurements are often used as a way of classifying pig carcasses for PSE during commercial slaughtering operations. PSE meat can also be detected from the rapid onset of rigor, from the amount of drip released from the cut surface and from the reflectance (brightness) of light from the cut surface. In poultry, post-mortem glycolysis is relatively rapid and so the $pH_{15\ min}$ is measured instead of the $pH_{45\ min}$.

PSE meat is particularly common in SS breeds of pig. These animals have an unusually reactive muscle metabolism. They develop PSE meat

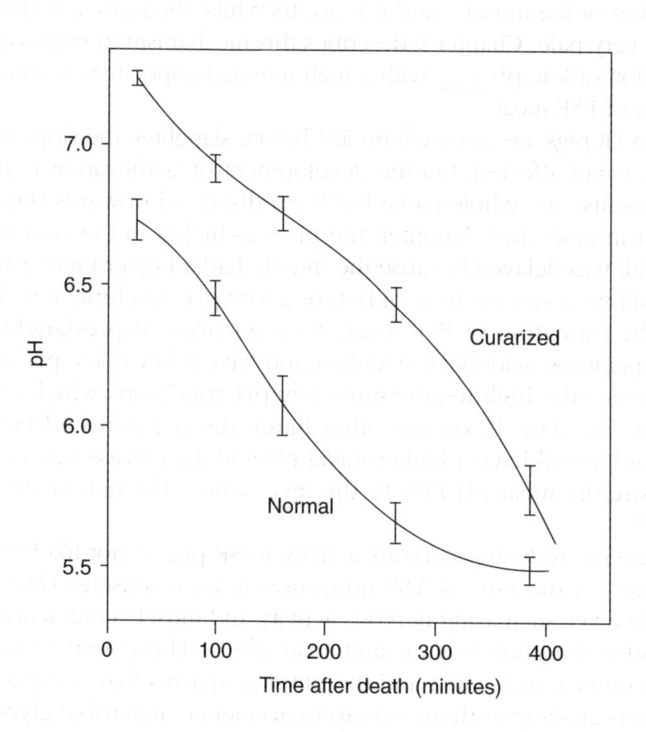

Fig. 6.3. Effect of pre-treatment with curare on post-mortem muscle pH decline in pigs.

even when handled and transported in a gentle manner. An example of their super-sensitivity is the response that they show to anoxia. Anoxia causes rapid ATP depletion in their muscle, whereas it has less effect in stress-resistant (SR) pigs (Lister *et al.*, 1970). Even when SS pigs are totally relaxed before slaughter and have no muscle contractions (for example, following treatment with curare), they still have accelerated muscle ATP utilization when bled out, in comparison with SR pigs (Sair *et al.*, 1970). Their muscle has a higher resting rate of metabolism and it is unusually sensitive to even the mildest stimuli. The effect of preslaughter handling stresses on their muscle metabolism can, however, be blocked with carazolol, the β-adrenergic receptor blocking drug, which suggests that a large part of their excessive responsiveness during normal preslaughter procedures is mediated through the sympathetic nervous system (Warriss and Lister, 1982).

When an animal is slaughtered, muscle metabolism is stimulated through the release of Ca^{2+} into the sarcoplasm. In SS genotypes, the sarcoplasmic reticulum and mitochondria fail to extract (sequester) Ca^{2+} at a fast enough rate to control the accelerated metabolism. In extreme cases, SS pig carcasses can develop rigor before the slaughterfloor staff have had a chance to do the evisceration. The accelerated glycolysis results in rapid acidification of the muscle, and if it occurs whilst the muscle is still warm it becomes very pale. Chapter 9 describes this mechanism in more detail. The combination of low $pH_{45\ min}$ with a high muscle temperature is critical in the formation of PSE meat.

When SR pigs are given curare just before slaughter, the slope of the pH fall curve is not affected, but the development of acidification in muscle is altered because the whole curve has been displaced upwards (Fig. 6.3). At any point in time after slaughter, the pH was higher in the curarized pigs. The pH fall was delayed because the muscle had a higher initial pH. If such a delay allows a carcass to cool before a low pH develops, it will help to reduce the formation of PSE meat. To summarize, if preslaughter stress causes a pig to be acidotic at slaughter and have a low initial pH, it is likely to experience the high temperature–low pH conditions which cause PSE meat (see Fig. 9.6). If, on the other hand, the pig is rested before it is slaughtered, it will have a higher initial pH and the carcass has a chance to cool before the meat pH falls to the level where the risk of PSE meat is increased.

In general, reducing nervous activity in SR pigs is not likely to have a large effect on the rate of ATP utilization in their muscles (McLoughlin, 1974). However, increasing nervous activity and muscle contractions immediately after slaughter has an immense effect. The extent to which the muscles contract and twitch and the physical spasms that occur during the convulsions at slaughterhouses help to accelerate anaerobic glycolysis. In extreme situations they can cause a low pH at a high muscle temperature, and this leads to PSE meat. For this reason, excessive contractions following stunning or during electrical stimulation of the carcass can cause PSE meat in pigs and turkeys.

Ischaemia (failure of blood supply) during bleeding out can help to accelerate ATP depletion in muscles. This is due to reduced resynthesis of ATP because of an inadequate supply of oxygen to the tissue, rather than an increased utilization of ATP by muscle. Before slaughter, muscle contractions are more important than hypoxia in causing low initial pH values in meat (McLoughlin *et al.*, 1973).

Fish that are severely exercised during the catching procedure go into rigor more quickly than fish that have less exercise. Exercised fish also have a shorter rigor duration before they start softening during the resolution of rigor. Unlike beef, lamb and pork, exercise-stressed fish do not usually produce high pH_{ult} meat. Instead, they tend to have a low pH_{ult}. This is because, in live fish, lactic acid accumulates within the muscle, and often persists through to the post-mortem period.

Meat tenderness is influenced by three factors:

- The chemical nature and amount of connective tissue in the meat. For example, forequarter cuts have more intermuscular connective tissue, which makes them tougher
- The extent of rigor. A strong rigor can cause tougher meat
- Meat ageing. When left to age, meat softens enzymatically.

Immediately after slaughter, meat is tender and has a low shear force when it is compressed. The toughness that is present in this pre-rigor meat is influenced by its connective tissue and marbling content. However, once the meat goes into rigor, these two components together only account for 20% of the variation in meat tenderness (within an aged muscle). Variation between muscles is more likely to be explained by differences in their connective tissue content, especially if there is inadequate trimming.

Theoretically, chronic stress during rearing could affect meat texture by altering the ratio of myofibres to connective tissue. There are two ways in which this could occur. In long-term exercise-induced muscle hypertrophy there is an increase in the ratio of myofibrillar to connective tissue proteins and the meat is more tender (Aalhus *et al.*, 1991). Alternatively, if there is no hypertrophy and instead the chronic stress is associated with catabolism of muscle protein, the meat may end up tougher (Bramblett *et al.*, 1963). This may also explain why animals that are severely fasted before slaughter, as a way of reducing excessive carcass fatness, are reputed to produce tougher meat.

As rigor develops, the muscles shorten and they become tougher. The conditions under which the carcass is held are important in influencing the extent of rigor and subsequent toughness. There are five ways in which the extent of rigor can be affected:

- **Rigor shortening** – removal of muscle from the carcass before rigor has set in, allowing excessive shortening of the myofibres during rigor contraction. This can occur during hot deboning and in early portioning of poultry breast fillets.

- **Heat shortening** – combination of high temperature and acid accumulation in muscle leading to an excessive contraction as rigor sets in.
- **Cold shortening** – excessive cold-induced muscle contraction during rigor, which occurs when a carcass is rapidly chilled.
- **Mechanical stimulation** – mechanically induced rapid post-mortem glycolysis leading to heat shortening (e.g. plucker-induced toughness in poultrymeat).
- **Thaw shortening** – delayed, excessive contraction during thawing which occurs in meat that was frozen pre-rigor.

In pigs and poultry, acute stress can lead to tougher meat through heat shortening. If the animal is exercised and gets hot before it is slaughtered, the combination of a high temperature and a low pH leads to an early, stronger rigor. In practice this can occur in pigs which develop PSE meat, and in poultry it develops in birds that flap their wings excessively before slaughter.

The relationship between pH_{ult} and meat toughness is curvilinear (see Fig. 8.5). At low or high pH_{ult} values the meat is more tender; it tends to be toughest at an intermediate pH_{ult} (Purchas, 1990). The effect of preslaughter stress, and muscle glycogen depletion, depends on the extent to which it affects the pH_{ult}. If, as often happens in stressed cattle, the pH_{ult} is only slightly raised, the meat may end up marginally tougher. Part of this effect is due to greater sarcomere shortening during rigor in meat which develops an intermediate pH_{ult} (Purchas and Aungsupakorn, 1993; Olsson *et al.*, 1995). If, on the other hand, the animals are stressed to exhaustion and the pH_{ult} is very high, the meat will be more tender (Chrystall *et al.*, 1982).

As meat ages it loses some of the strength that developed during rigor. This relaxation is known as *resolution of rigor*. It is not a true relaxation, as the myofilaments do not slide apart. Instead, the meat is partly digested by calpain enzymes and the myofibres break up, particularly through solubilizing of the Z lines in the sarcomeres.

The calpain enzyme system has three components: a low calcium-requiring enzyme (μ-calpain), a high calcium-requiring enzyme (m-calpain) and a calpain inhibitor (calpastatin). Meat tenderness can be explained by this system in a number of situations. Ruminants have higher calpastatin activities than non-ruminant species, and this probably explains why the rate of tenderization is slow in beef and lamb. Addition of calcium to meat can help to activate the calpains and make the meat more tender. The activity of both calpains is greater at high pH_{ult} values (Cena *et al.*, 1992) and this partly explains why meat from severely stressed animals is often more tender. Genetic differences in meat texture are partly due to differences in calpastatin activity in the meat (Koohmaraie *et al.*, 1995). Giving β-agonist growth promoters to the live animal results in tougher meat through increased calpastatin activity. Similarly, intravenous infusion of adrenaline for 7 days before slaughter resulted in increased calpastatin activity (Sensky *et al.*, 1996).

In both redmeat and whitemeat species, if the animals are stressed and muscle is glycogen-depleted before slaughter, and if ATP is rapidly depleted post-mortem, the pH of the meat will be elevated and Ca^{2+} levels will rapidly increase because of failure in ATP-powered calcium re-uptake mechanisms. The combination of high pH and high Ca^{2+} concentration usually enhances the calpain activity. Meat from severely exhausted animals is likely to be more tender because of this.

Ways that are used for tenderizing meat post-slaughter include:

- **Tenderstretch** – holding muscles in a stretched position before they go into rigor (as in hip suspension of the carcass).
- **Ageing** – endogenous enzymatic breakdown of myofibrillar proteins post-rigor (also known as conditioning).
- **Hot conditioning** – holding the carcass for up to 24 hours at a high temperature to encourage calpain-induced tenderization.
- **Electrical stimulation** – electrically induced accelerated post-mortem ATP utilization, which prevents cold shortening.
- **Mechanical tenderization** – mechanical tearing and disruption of myofibres post rigor (e.g. beating a steak before cooking).
- **Chemical tenderization** – injection of papain before slaughter to break down the myofibres enzymatically after slaughter.
- **High-temperature cooking** – solubilizing the collagen.

Meat colour is measured from its L-, a- and b-values. L is its lightness, which is directly proportional to its luminous reflectance. The a-value is its redness value; meat with a high a-value would be red. The b-value is a measure of its yellowness. PSE pork and meat from heat-stressed poultry have high L-values and low a-values. Dark-cutting beef has low L-, a- and b-values (Purchas and Grant, 1995). If a piece of normal beef and DCB are sliced very thinly across the fibres of the meat and the two slices are then placed on a white background, the slice of DCB appears to be more translucent than the normal beef. This is measured objectively in its lower reflectance (L-value). The reasons for the dark colour in high pH_{ult} meat are described in the section below on myoglobin. On cooking, dark-cutting semitendinosus can remain slightly darker but because of its high pH the myoglobin does not denature readily and the meat remains redder in colour than beef with a normal pH (Hawrysh *et al.*, 1985).

Dark-cutting beef should not be confused with three other conditions which cause dark discoloration in beef. These are darkening of the meat surface due to desiccation, exercise-induced changes in haem pigments in the muscle and brown discoloration which develops on exposure to the atmosphere. Desiccation causes darkening because the muscle pigments become more concentrated as water is lost. It can be controlled by using appropriate packaging. Allowing young bulls to exercise whilst they are growing, instead of being confined to cubicles with tethers, causes their meat to have a higher pigment concentration and to be darker (Ramsgaard Jensen and Oksama, 1996). Browning in uncooked meat is due to the formation of metmyoglobin. The rate of oxidation of myoglobin to metmyoglobin is pH dependent. For example, the rate of autoxidation in air doubles with a decrease in pH from 6.6 to 5.4 (George and Stratmann, 1954). This means that high pH_{ult} meat is less prone to metmyoglobin formation.

In some veal markets there is a preference for pale meat, and the methods used for producing the pale colour are contrary to good welfare. Calves that are grown for producing white veal are fed milk substitute that has a low iron content. The haematocrit in their blood is closely related to the haem iron content in the muscle ($r = 0.8$ to 0.9), which suggests that the intensity of colour of muscle is related to the degree of anaemia in the calf (Charpentier, 1966). In extreme situations, anaemia is a weakening and debilitating disorder.

The post-mortem chemical reactions involving *myoglobin* have a profound effect on meat colour. Normally, myoglobin is oxygenated to oxymyoglobin shortly after meat is cut, and the fresh meat changes from purplish-red to a bright red. This process is known as blooming, and the bright red colour is synonymous with freshness. High pH_{ult} meat does not bloom when it is cut; instead, it remains a dark colour. The reasons for this are as follows. The proteins in high pH_{ult} meat are above their isoelectric point and this favours stronger water retention by the meat. The greater water retention makes the meat more turgid and firm, and it has a less open structure. This reduces the penetration of oxygen when the meat is cut. Poorer oxygen penetration reduces the oxygenation of myoglobin (dark purplish-red in colour) to oxymyoglobin (bright red colour), and so high pH_{ult} meat remains darker in colour. This effect may not be evident after cooking. During cooking, myoglobin and oxymyoglobin are denatured to brown pigments. However, at high pH, myoglobin is more heat stable and less prone to being denatured. So, the dark purplish-red pigment in high pH_{ult} meat is also more likely to persist during cooking. In summary, high pH_{ult} meat is dark in colour when it is uncooked and it retains more redness when it is cooked, in comparison with normal pH_{ult} meat.

Preslaughter stress can also enhance the rate at which myoglobin turns green in vacuum-packaged meat. Meat from severely stressed animals is more prone to putrefying, and the mechanisms behind this are explained in Chapter 7. When it goes off, H_2S is liberated from the sulphur-containing amino acids and combines with myoglobin to form sulphmyoglobin, which is green in colour. Sulphmyoglobin formation only occurs when the meat pH is above 6.0 (Nicol *et al.*, 1970).

The *water-holding capacity* of meat is a measure of the strength with which it retains water. It can be assessed by pressing a slice of meat on to a filter paper and measuring the spread of moisture out of the meat in terms of the area that is covered. The mechanisms that influence water retention are described in Chapter 12, and the relationship between pH_{ult} and water-holding capacity is shown in Fig. 12.1. This relationship is fundamental in the link between preslaughter stress and weight loss from meat as water. Meat which develops a high pH_{ult} retains charges on its proteins which hold water electrostatically, whereas at a normal pH_{ult} the proteins are near their isoelectric point where they lose their charge and do not bind water so strongly. Water-holding capacity is reduced in PSE meat, which can release considerable amounts of fluid as drip. The drip acts as a good medium for bacterial growth; it is unsightly; and in wholesale cuts it contributes to weight loss and reduced yield.

Meat juiciness can be affected by fat content and the amount of moisture left in the meat after it has been cooked. If a carcass is excessively lean (e.g. a pig carcass with a P2 backfat thickness of 8 mm), the meat is less juicy. The reason for this is best explained by analogy with hamburger manufacture. If fat is added in varying amounts to a batch of ground hamburger meat, juiciness improves as the fat level increases from 9% to 20% (Table 6.2). The fat imparts a self-basting effect during cooking and molten fat gives *succulence*, provided it is not burnt off during cooking. Tenderness can improve with the increase in fat content simply through a dilution effect. The fat is more tender than ground lean and so the more fat there is, the more tender the product. Over this range of fat content (9–20%), flavour is not likely to be affected. The juiciness of meat is spoilt if the meat is cooked to dryness, and when meat is being overcooked its water-holding capacity can influence the stage at which juiciness is lost. High pH_{ult} meat is less prone to loss of moisture during cooking than normal pH_{ult} meat, and so with prolonged roasting or grilling it will retain its moisture for longer and this could, theoretically, delay the point at which it loses juiciness. Whilst high pH_{ult} meat can retain moisture and juiciness, PSE pork is less likely to be juicy than normal pork (Sayre *et al.*, 1964).

Raw meat has a salty, metallic *flavour*. The meat-like flavour develops as the meat is being cooked and it is largely due to the formation of Maillard

Table 6.2. Effect of fat level in hamburgers on their eating quality.

	Fat in hamburgers		
	9%	20%	28%
Juiciness	7.2^{a}	10.5^{b}	11.3^{b}
Tenderness	9.6^{a}	11.8^{b}	13.1^{c}
Flavour	9.9^{a}	9.3^{a}	9.0^{a}

Subjective score ratings were used.
$^{a–c}$ Columns without a common superscript letter were significantly different at $P = 0.05$.

reaction products and caramellized products. Inosinic acid (IMP) helps to enhance flavours within meat. Different cooking methods result in different meat-like flavours. Meat cooked in a microwave oven or meat that is stewed has less meat-like flavour compared with roasted, fried or grilled meats. This is because the cooking temperature is lower during microwave cooking and stewing, and there is less surface browning. High cooking temperatures are usually associated with stronger flavours. Part of this effect could be due to the formation of more Maillard reaction products and part could be due to the greater release of IMP (Cambero *et al.*, 1992).

Maillard reaction products are formed on heating amino acids, peptides, sugars, sugar phosphates, nucleotides and nucleosides. Functional groups on meat proteins, lipids and carbohydrates also take part in Maillard reactions. Amino acids and reducing sugars combine to form N-sugar amines which are modified by elimination of water and the amine group to deoxyreductones, deoxyosones and aldehydes. These contribute meat-like flavours, along with products belonging to the furan, furanthiol, furanone and ethanethiol groups of compounds, and they all help to provide character impact (Bailey, 1992). Sulphur-containing Maillard reaction products are thought to be particularly important in providing meat-like aromas. Cooking conditions that favour Maillard reaction product formation also appear to favour the formation of mutagenic compounds on the surface of the cooked meat (Holtz *et al.*, 1985).

Warmed-over flavours (WOFs) can displace meat-like flavours when meat has been cooked and then stored for 48 hours or more in a refrigerator. Paint-like, cardboard and oxidized flavours take its place. These flavours are formed in a similar manner to the oxidative rancidity that develops in frozen meat, except that they occur much more rapidly. Some Maillard reaction products can inhibit WOF development by acting as antioxidants. Pro-oxidants that favour WOF formation include ultraviolet light, iron and activated oxygen species such as superoxide and hydroxyl radicals.

There are three counteracting ways in which animal welfare and meat flavour could theoretically be linked. Firstly, if preslaughter stress exhausted the animal and reduced the level of glycolytic intermediates in the muscle, there would be fewer hexose and triose aldehyde groups available for the formation of Maillard reaction products. This would result in the meat being more bland. Secondly, if the stress caused extensive conversion of ATP to AMP, there could be enhanced meat flavour. This would be due to the gradual conversion of AMP to IMP post-mortem through the action of AMP aminohydrolase which is present in fresh meat. IMP has a flavour-enhancing effect, but during prolonged storage this is lost as the IMP is degraded to inosine. The third way is by enhancing oxidative rancidity and the formation of WOFs. When animals are forced to take strenuous exercise, the subsequent susceptibility of the muscle to develop lipid peroxidation is increased (Alessio *et al.*, 1988). The mechanism is as follows. During exercise, oxygen uptake by muscle increases by up to 200 times its resting rate.

The oxygen helps to regenerate energy by oxidative phosphorylation in the mitochondria. However, about 2–4% of the oxygen escapes from the respiratory chain as superoxide (O_2^-). Superoxide is converted to toxic hydroxyl radicals ($OH^\bullet$) by the Haber-Weiss reaction, as follows:

$$H_2O_2 + O_2^- \longrightarrow O_2 + OH^- + OH^\bullet$$

Hydrogen peroxide is needed for this reaction and it is produced from superoxide by dismutation reactions in the mitochondria and microsomes. Hydroxyl radicals are important because they cause peroxidation of unsaturated phospholipids in cell membranes with the formation of lipid peroxides, which in turn give rise to hydroperoxides, carbonyl compounds and hydrocarbons, all of which contribute to rancid flavours. This process can be inhibited by either chemical reduction of the oxidized membrane lipids (e.g. with vitamin E), $OH^\bullet$ scavengers (e.g. thiourea), complete removal of superoxide by dismutation to H_2O_2 and O_2 (e.g. with superoxide dismutase), or removal of H_2O_2 (e.g. by catalase, or glutathione peroxidase). Thus, pre-feeding rats with vitamin E or injecting them with superoxide dismutase helps to reduce muscle lipid peroxidation during severe exercise stress (Goldfarb *et al.*, 1994; Radak *et al.*, 1995). Protecting muscle from hydroxyl radical injury also helps to reduce the muscle soreness that can develop after strenuous exercise (Ørtenblad *et al.*, 1997).

Research into the effect of preslaughter exercise on meat flavour has not produced any consistent findings. However, in general, high pH_{ult} beef has less beef-like flavour and high pH_{ult} lamb has less distinct aroma. If bruised tissue which is rich in haem iron is included in mince, there is a risk that the added iron will act as a pro-oxidant and favour oxidative rancidity and WOF formation.

Broilers reared at low stocking densities have been found to produce thigh meat with a stronger odour (Farmer *et al.*, 1997), and broilers raised with a reduced intestinal flora have been found to have a weaker breast meat flavour. It is possible that these effects are due to differences in the litter, which may impart flavours to the meat through the skin.

There is a growing consumer trend away from fresh meat and towards processed meat products. An important technical feature which influences the appearance and eating quality of processed meats is the way in which the meat pieces bind and hold together. Clearly, nobody wants a hamburger that falls apart when it is cooked. It should also have an appropriately meaty mouth-feel. A large component in the mouth-feel of meat is due to the alignment of fibrous proteins. This makes the mechanical and chewing properties highly directional, or *anisotropic*. In particular, the strength of fibres when pulled along their length is much greater than pulling at right angles to their length. When unprocessed meat is chewed, the initial stages are the breaking down of the epimysium and perimysium (see Fig. 5.2). In later stages of chewing, an appreciation of the anisotropic nature of the fibres develops. In manufactured meats the aim is to retain these anisotropic properties but to lose the connective tissue structures. In practice this is achieved by trimming the larger pieces of connective tissue and cutting the meat into sufficiently small pieces to disrupt the intramuscular connective tissue. The cut pieces are then stuck together again.

The main adhesive used in sticking the pieces together to make a re-formed meat is myosin. During the manufacturing procedures soluble myosin is extracted and coats the surface of the pieces of meat. When the re-formed meat is cooked, the myosin forms a gel that binds to adjacent meat particles, holding them together. The binding can be ruptured in one of three ways:

- Gel can be pulled apart – tensile fracture.
- Gel can break by sliding apart – shear fracture.
- Gel or meat can break by tension or shear – cohesive fracture.

The strength of the gel can be important in influencing the shape or deformability of the product as well as its holding-together properties during cooking. High pH_{ult} meat is likely to produce strong myosin gels, whereas PSE meat produces weak myosin gels.

Chapter 7

Cattle

Knowing the ancestral behaviour of a species is helpful in understanding the behaviour and needs of animals kept in modern farming conditions. It can help us to understand, but not necessarily solve, some of the welfare problems in today's farming. Cattle have been domesticated for over 6000 years. In their wild state they were grazing and browsing animals, without a fixed territory but with strongly developed herd behaviour. The calves were protected by the herd for a large part of their early life. If threatened by a predator, the herd would have behaved in much the same way as Cape buffalo do today when stalked by a lioness. The horned adults, and in particular the bulls, defend the herd by facing outwards towards the danger whilst the herd makes an escape. The strong herd and maternal bonds helps to explain why there can be so much emotional upheaval when a dairy calf is separated from its mother.

The systems used in cattle production fall into six main categories: dairy farming, beef breeding herds, semi-intensive grazing systems, bobby calf production, veal farming and intensive fattening units. The beef breeding herds approach the social and to some extent environmental conditions in which ancestral stock would have evolved. The calves are reared by their mothers and the only contacts they have with humans are either aversive (e.g. parasite control, dehorning, branding) or neutral events. They often become fearful of humans and this can lead to difficulty in handling them at meatworks, and even to aggressive outbursts when they are mustered or handled in confined spaces. Fractious behaviour and unpredictable escape behaviour inevitably lead to bruising. This can be prevented by familiarizing the calves at an early age with the presence of a human. One study showed that calves receiving as little as 10 days non-aversive *handling* during the first 3 months of life was sufficient to make them easier to handle later on (Le Neindre *et al.*, 1996). In the absence of this familiarization training, certain breeds are less suited to extensive farming systems because of their erratic temperament when handled. In one county in England, where there has been a gradual change from traditional British breeds to Continental breeds, the police marksman for the county is now called out to shoot an animal that has escaped and 'gone wild' about once every month (personal observation). This is thought to be an increasing problem which is a throwback to ancestral behaviour.

Other welfare problems that can occur in cattle are summarized in Table 7.1. The focus in this chapter is on those issues which have a bearing on beef or veal quality. *Dystocia* (difficult calving) causes stress and pain for the cow and is a common cause of death in calves. It can be caused by inappropriate matching of the size of the calf's parents. If the calf is oversized through selection of a large muscular bull, or if the pelvic opening of the cow is too small, the cow has difficulty in expelling the calf. Large muscular breeds of bull are chosen because of the rapid growth potential and hindquarter conformation of their offspring. The risks of dystocia with this shape of animal are greatest in cows that are calving for the first time and in purebred sireline herds where the genes of both the bull and the cow combine to produce a large calf. This risk is managed either by ensuring the cow is not overfat at calving (as this would increase the risk of dystocia further) or by removing the calf surgically by Caesarian section.

Dystocia is common in breeds such as the Belgian Blue, Blonde d'Aquitaine, Charolais and Piedmont which show *muscular hypertrophy*. These breeds have additional muscle in their hindquarters. This is recognized in the live animal from the bulging hindquarters and in the surface

Table 7.1. Stress and welfare issues in cattle.

	Dairy cow	Beef breeding herd	Semi-intensive beef grazing systems	Feedlots	Veal units	Bobby calf production
Dystocia	√	√				
Cow–calf separation	√				√	√
Mastitis	√					
Lameness	√					
Metabolic and digestive disorders	√			√ *	√ *	
Poor body condition/ underfeeding	√ *	√ *				√
Social stressors	√		√ *			
Dehorning/disbudding/ docking	√	√				
Castration		√ *	√ *	√		
Hot-iron branding		√ *		√ *		
Handling		√	√	√	√	√
Transport	√		√	√	√	√

* Only applies to particular systems, countries or regions.

crease between the gluteobiceps and the semitendinosus. The animals are valued for producing carcasses with large cuts of meat in the rump and round joints. The expanded muscle mass is associated with a reduced proportion of red-fibre muscle and an increased proportion of α-white glycolytic fibres, which are larger. This difference in muscle fibre type is important because it influences the animals' metabolic responses to stress. During intense muscle activity and when exposed to heat stress, they have an increased capacity to produce lactic acid. When they are severely stressed, lactic acid production can be excessive; the muscles become rigid; there is hyperthermia and panting and in extreme situations the animal may die. During a stress crisis these animals have a very clumsy, stiff hindleg gait because the muscle above the stifle joint (quadriceps femoris) becomes rigid. The excessive muscle contractions cause high plasma CPK and K^+ levels as well as lactate, and the urine may be pale brown from the presence of myoglobin, which is excreted if there is muscle damage. Fortunately, this reaction is rare, but when it occurs it is very unpleasant for the animal (Holmes *et al.*, 1973):

> One animal which collapsed was in great distress, unable to rise, and exhibiting signs of heat stress (extreme panting), despite being hosed down repeatedly. This panting may have been due to respiratory compensation for lactic acidosis ... When she attempted to rise her front legs appeared to function normally but her hindlegs appeared stiff and incapable of movement. About 10 hours after the exercise the heifer appeared to be in great pain. At intervals, muscular spasms gripped her entire body for about 15 seconds, during which breathing ceased. Relaxation was followed by a moan, and renewed panting.

This heifer developed a rectal temperature of 40.3°C and she had the same type of stress crisis as that seen in SS pigs that have muscular hypertrophy. These animals are usually handled very carefully because of their high commercial value and their sensitivity to stress.

Other problems that develop in cattle breeds with muscular hypertrophy include dystocia, stillbirths, poorer calf survival and enlargement of the tongue, which in calves causes difficulty with suckling. Some of the breeds or strains have smaller pelvic openings and they require more assistance during calving and more Caesarian deliveries. In one study involving nine breeds of bull used on Friesian cows, the prevalence of difficult calving was highest in the Charolais-cross calvings and lowest in the Hereford-cross calvings (Everitt *et al.*, 1978) (Fig. 7.1).

In central Europe the carcasses from cattle with muscular hypertrophy have much higher butcher value than normal cattle because of the greater size and lean content of the retail cuts and because the meat is reputed to be tender. These breeds do not have a reputation for producing well marbled meat, nor do they produce high pH_{ult} meat. Conversely, they sometimes have a rapid post-mortem muscle glycolytic rate and produce a

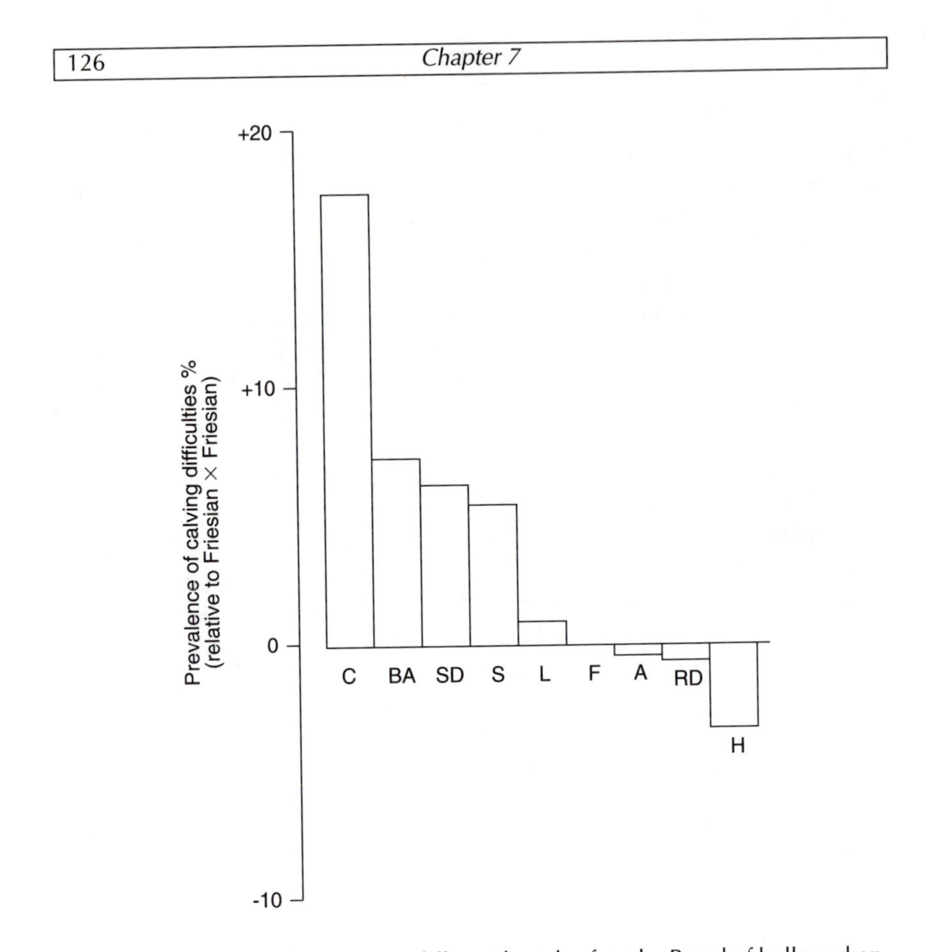

Fig. 7.1. Prevalence of dystocia in different breeds of cattle. Breed of bull used on Friesian cows: C, Charolais; BA, Blonde d'Aquitaine; SD, South Devon; S, Simental; F, Friesian; L, Limousin; A, Angus; RD, Red Devon; H, Hereford.

slightly paler meat, but this does not raise any problems with marketing their meat.

Mastitis is an important welfare problem in the dairy farming industry. It can be painful for cows when associated with inflammation and swelling of the udder. Meatworks are generally very reluctant to accept cows with advanced black udder (gangrenous mastitis) because of the risk of contaminating the surface of the carcass with pus during udder removal. Other forms of mastitis may be tolerated, but the decision as to whether the carcass is fit for human consumption depends on whether bacteria have invaded the body from the udder when the animal was alive. This is determined at meat inspection by examining the lymph nodes. The lymph nodes are inspected for their colour, size and consistency. By looking at the nodes which receive lymph from particular parts of the body, it is possible to determine how far the disease has spread and which parts of the carcass may harbour the microorganism. In some types of mastitis the bacteria can be present in the meat. Where microbiological examinations have been done, 14% of carcasses from cows with mastitis had bacteria in their foreleg meat, whereas it was only 3% for cows without mastitis. Of the bacterial isolates, 60% were *Clostridia* (Schuppel *et al.*, 1996). In conclusion, mastitis is a disease which is of welfare importance and it can be associated with contamination of cull cow carcasses by undesirable bacteria.

In parts of Africa and Asia it is common to see emaciated animals presented for slaughter, especially when there has been a drought. In temperate climates, emaciation in stock that are presented for slaughter is more common in the winter and early spring (Evans and Pratt, 1978), especially in years when there has been a feed shortage. *Emaciation*, or poor body condition, has nine distinct features in the live animal (see Fig. 2.2). In the carcass, the muscles are depressed instead of being well filled. What little fat that is present is wet, gelatinous in appearance and sloppy to the touch and does not set when the carcass cools. This is because the fat contains more water and less lipid than usual. It is self-evident from the absence of muscle that the carcass may be virtually worthless in high value markets, and that the animal must have gone through periods of hunger to reach an ultimately weak and lethargic state. In spite of this, such animals are slaughtered on a regular basis in poorer countries for the export canning industry and for home consumption. Emaciation is one of the more common causes of condemnation in bobby calves. Characteristic features include the absence of perirenal, pericardial and omental fat, and the fat tends to be pink instead of white. In addition, the bone marrow in the femur is gelatinous instead of fatty (Schoonderwoerd *et al.*, 1986).

There are a number of on-farm husbandry procedures that are used routinely but which are painful for the animal and affect the value of the carcass. *Hot-iron branding* is used on some North American farms as protection against theft. On some feedlots it is a requirement imposed by the insurance company. It is also used widely in Africa, whereas in parts of Europe it is considered inhumane and is illegal. Studies that have used the heart rate response as a measure of the stress and pain associated with the procedure have shown that the initial rise in heart rate was slightly higher during the application of the hot-iron brand in comparison with a freeze-brand, but the heart rate rise following freezebranding remained high for longer (Lay *et al.*, 1991). One interpretation that has been made from this is as follows. Third-degree burns, such as the ones produced with hot-iron branding, often cause pronounced physical recoil and alarm at the time they are inflicted, but if the tissue is burnt quickly and severely the nerve endings in the skin are damaged and the tissue loses its sensitivity. Severe chilling or freezing of tissue causes less reaction initially but it produces a delayed throbbing pain as the tissue warms up and circulation of blood is restored. The conclusion from the heart rate responses is that hot-iron branding probably causes a brief intense pain at the time of application, whereas freezebranding causes a delayed, more protracted pain.

The part of the skin that has been hot-iron branded is unusable for leather making. Location of the brand on the hide is important. The traditional area – the rump – puts the brand right in the middle of the most valuable part of the hide. The shoulder is almost as bad. The neck and lower leg cause less wastage, as these areas are easily trimmed. In one survey in Africa, 32% of the hot-iron brands were at a site which caused devaluation of the hide.

Another painful procedure performed routinely on young cattle is *horn disbudding*. This is done either with a hot-iron cautery or with a scoop dehorner. The cautery burns out the horn bud and surrounding skin, whereas the scoop dehorner quickly cuts the bud, with some overlying skin and underlying bone. Depending on the country, these procedures may or may not be done with a local anaesthetic. The likely pain and distress with these two methods have been compared from the plasma cortisol responses in the calves. In one study it was found that local anaesthetic blocks the immediate cortisol response to both methods, but after the anaesthetic effect has worn off the calves which were scoop disbudded had a large late plasma cortisol rise; the cautery disbudded calves did not have a late rise in their cortisol levels (Fig. 7.2) (Petrie *et al.*, 1995). The conclusion is that when a short-acting local anaesthetic is used, the burning action of the cautery gives pain relief after the anaesthetic has worn off, whereas the scoop method does not.

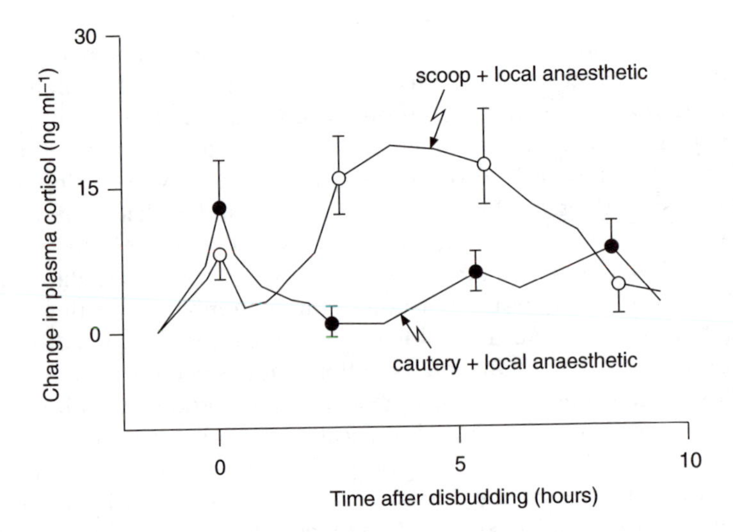

Fig. 7.2. Comparison of two methods of disbudding on plasma cortisol concentrations in calves.

Disbudding is a necessary procedure – without it, cattle can do considerable damage to each other and to animal handlers. The horns cause carcass bruising and damage to the hide. It is important to use methods (such as cautery with local anaesthetic) that minimize pain and distress, and to develop better alternatives in the future. Sawing off the tips of the horns once they have grown has not been effective in preventing bruising. The only effective alternative at the moment is to breed cattle which are naturally polled.

Castration is performed either by applying a tight rubber ring around the scrotum above the testes, or by cutting out the testes with a sharp blade, or by crushing the spermatic cord and associated blood vessels through the scrotum using an emasculator. Castration with a Burdizzo emasculator or with a sharp blade causes a rapid increase in plasma cortisol which remains elevated for up to 8 hours. This response is larger in old calves than in young animals, and it is recommended that these methods should only be done during the first 3 weeks after birth. The rubber ring method gives a smaller immediate rise in plasma cortisol, but it produced behavioural changes over the following 7 weeks which indicated irritation or pain. These changes in behaviour including licking the scrotum, turning the head towards the hindquarters, alternate lifting of the hindlegs, abnormal posture and slow movements of the tail. From a welfare perspective, the emasculator is the preferred method.

Castration is mainly performed to allow safe handling and to control unwanted breeding in mixed sex groups of cattle. There are growth-rate advantages from not castrating, as bulls grow faster and are leaner than steers. The additional muscle in bull carcasses is largely in the low-priced cuts in the neck, thorax and forelimb.

A large number of cattle are fattened every year in *feedlots* in Africa, America, Asia and Australasia. Feedlots have a poor public image in some parts of America and Europe, but this is more to do with pollution and the aesthetics of mass production than with animal welfare. Keeping cattle in feedlots is not inevitably inhumane. As with all farming systems, it has particular welfare problems but, with care, these can be managed. The problems that can arise are:

- stress associated with transporting weaner calves to the feedlot;
- harsh treatment when the calves join the feedlot (vaccination, branding, castration, dehorning, hormone implantation);
- poor adaptation to new feed on entry to the feedlot, leading to lacticacidosis, rumenitis, liver abscesses and enterotoxaemia;
- shipping fever;
- difficulties in detecting sick cattle within large groups, leading to failure to treat animals with a disease or disorder;
- inadequate drainage, leading to boggy conditions when wet;
- irritation from heat, flies and dust – inadequate shelter.

There are two types of feedlot: those that buy in weaner calves and take them through to slaughter, and those that buy in forward store cattle or cull cows and fatten them for up to 4 months or so. Weaner calves are prone to developing stress-associated disorders when they join the feedlot. In North America a large number come off range conditions and are trucked long distances (sometimes up to 1500 km) to the feedlots in the grain-growing regions. They may be put through a number of stressful procedures such as castration and branding on the day they arrive, and then they are mixed with unfamiliar animals and given an unfamiliar feed. These stressors combine to suppress the immune system, and as a result they can develop a respiratory infection known as shipping fever. The length of the journey is not necessarily the most important stress (Cole *et al.*, 1988). The combined effects of weaning, mustering, marshalling, loading, unloading and handling on arrival at the feedlot are more significant.

Heat stress is a problem at feedlots where there is inadequate shade. It can be made worse if there is a problem with stable flies, as these make the cattle bunch together and the crowding reduces convective heat loss. Both heat and flies can reduce the animals' appetite and depress growth rate, and when they occur together they have a synergistic effect (Campbell, 1988). If cattle are sent for slaughter under hot conditions, their meat quality is not usually affected. For example, in one study it was found that trucking bulls at 36°C and 65% relative humidity for 4 hours had no effect on the prevalence of dark-cutting beef.

One of the main problems with large feedlots is maintaining good animal health. Shipping fever is one of the more important diseases and it causes substantial economic loss in the North American feedlots. It is usually caused by a *Pasteurella* infection in the lungs following a stressful introduction to the feedlot. The problem is probably made worse by dust. From studies in laboratory mice, it is known that high dust levels in the air increase the risk of *Pasteurella* infection. The particle size of the dust is important, as small particles (3 μm and less) tend to pass through to the alveoli of the lungs whereas larger particles (5 μm or more) are trapped in the upper respiratory tract. Dust levels in the air at feedlots can be very high, especially in the early evening at the end of all the day's activity, and the average particle size is usually in the range of 2.5–3.5 μm. The calves depend on their immune and physical defence mechanisms to rid themselves of this type of dust, and there is greater likelihood of infection if their immune system is suppressed by a stressor. Some feedlots use water sprinklers to reduce dust inhalation.

At some feedlots a meatworks is situated alongside the feedlot unit. This makes it quicker and easier to transfer the cattle to the point of slaughter, and if there is no mixing and only a short holding period at the meatworks, preslaughter stress can be reduced to a level that is as low as could ever be hoped for. Where preslaughter stress is low it is unusual to find any dark-cutting beef in either bulls or steers. In that situation, steer meat is slightly more tender than meat from bulls, and it has a lower cooking loss and less pronounced sour and browned flavours (Jeremiah *et al.*, 1988b; Purchas and Grant, 1995). This is opposite to the situation where the animals are stressed – bulls have a high pH_{ult} meat which is more tender and has less flavour than meat from steers. To summarize: meat from young bulls would normally have a slightly lower eating quality (in terms of tenderness and flavour) than meat from steers, but because bulls are more prone to getting excited and stressed before slaughter the tenderness of their meat is often improved. In terms of the appearance (colour) and keeping quality of the meat, there is no difference between bulls and steers when they are unstressed, but bull beef is inferior when they have been stressed.

Grain-fed beef can be slightly paler in colour and have a stronger beef fat odour and flavour than grass-fed beef (Melton *et al.*, 1982; Crouse *et al.*, 1984). This flavour from grain-fed cattle is preferred in the North American market in comparison with the slightly sourer flavour of beef raised on fescue pastures. When cattle are raised on grass and finished on grain, the flavour change that occurs with grain feeding takes about 2 months to develop.

Feedlots are not common in Europe. Cattle are either fattened on summer pasture, or on conserved feeds indoors whilst on concrete, slatted concrete or straw-covered floors. On *hard floor surfaces* cattle can show behavioural difficulties in getting up and lying down. Some animals experience discomfort and in some cases pain during these simple activities, but this does not usually show itself as an abnormal gait. Laminitis and arthrosis of the joints are the main causes of this problem, and these are more common in fast-growing cattle. It is aggravated by mounting behaviour and by falls on slippery floor surfaces.

Many feedlot steers are implanted with or fed a *growth-promoting hormone* or agent. The objective with growth-promoting agents is to increase growth rate without producing too much fat or any undesirable effects on meat quality. The growth promoters are positioned under the skin of the animal's ear so that it will not leave any residues in the meat. Zeranol is one of the most widely used growth promoters. It does not have any pronounced effects on meat quality, but some people with sensitive palates can detect a slight increase in the intensity of sour flavours and a decrease in some of the beefy aftertastes (Jeremiah *et al.*, 1988a,b). The increase in growth rate by growth promoters is achieved either by increasing the rate of anabolism in muscle, or by decreasing the rate of catabolism. The exact mechanism depends on the growth promoter that is used. In the case of the β-agonist growth promoters, the improvement in growth rate is achieved by reducing the rate of catabolism in muscle. This is due to inhibition of the catabolic enzymes (calpains) responsible for myofibrillar breakdown. In this situation there is a risk that the meat from these animals will not tenderize during ageing and so it will be tougher. Normally the calpains in muscle would remain active after an animal has been slaughtered; they continue to break down myofibrillar proteins after the muscle has gone into rigor, and this helps to tenderize the meat. Overdosing cattle with β-agonists could lead to dark-cutting meat, as many of the compounds which inhibit calpain activity have actions similar to those of adrenaline.

In some meatworks, *papain* is injected intravenously shortly before slaughter. This helps to tenderize the meat. This procedure has been criticized on welfare grounds because the injections are sometimes given in an unprofessional manner, involving unacceptable mishandling of the animals.

The most important welfare problems for cattle in the tropics and in some subtropical regions are *heat stress* and starvation during droughts. Providing shade and ample water and selecting the appropriate breed are the best ways of managing heat stress. Shade can be provided with a row of trees planted in a north–south alignment. Some farmers feel that these shade-belts encourage cattle to spend more time loafing in the shade instead of grazing and putting on weight, but research experience does not support this view. The hotter an animal becomes, the more its appetite is suppressed. In one study in Louisiana, beef herds were provided either with no shade or with the opportunity to shelter in wooded pasture. The calves and cows that had shelter grew faster (McDaniel and Roark, 1956). The stock with no shade spent more time standing instead of lying, presumably trying to lose more heat by convection. In feedlots, shade encourages cattle to eat more and drink less.

Cattle breeders in hot climates usually incorporate genes from *Bos indicus* in their breeding programme to help offset the risk of heat stress. There are two mechanisms they can select for: firstly, appropriate coat and skin colour, and secondly, the ability to sweat.

Black surfaces absorb more heat than light-coloured surfaces, and they absorb much of the heat at the outermost layer. So, cows with dark coats absorb more of the sun's heat in their hair. In doing so they gain more heat than a pale-coated animal and so they are more prone to heat stress. Pale coats reflect a higher proportion of the sun's heat, but some radiation also passes through to the skin. If a pale-coated animal also has a pale skin, the sun's ultraviolet rays can penetrate deep into the skin and cause skin cancer. If the skin is dark, the outermost layer of the skin absorbs these rays; as this layer is due to be shed as dead cells, the risk of skin cancer becoming established is reduced. The ideal combination is a pale-coated, dark-skinned animal.

By choosing a *Bos indicus* type, the cattle breeder is selecting an animal that sweats a lot. A well adapted tropical breed can lose twice as much heat by sweating in comparison with a European breed, without having to pant. The disadvantage in choosing a tropical breed such as the Brahman is that the animals have a poorer carcass conformation, and in particular a poorly developed eye muscle in the loin; also their meat is often tougher, because it has a lower calpain activity.

Dehydration during transport before slaughter is a common occurence in hot climates. In Australia many cattle are trucked over 1000 km to meatworks in Western Australia and south Queensland. In one study (Wythes *et al.*, 1980), steers were trucked by road and then by rail over a total distance of 1420 km. The animals lost 10% of their liveweight, but 40% of that was recovered when they had a chance to drink. Rehydration increased the hot carcass weight from 369 kg to 383 kg, and part of this gain was due to a rise in the water content of the muscle. In other situations, dehydration occurs in cattle which are sold through an auction market (saleyard) instead of being sent direct to a meatworks. Dehydration is easily recognized by the amount of competition at the water trough once the animals arrive at the holding pens. The cattle will rehydrate quickly if they are allowed to drink before they are slaughtered, but if they are not given this opportunity the meat is likely to be drier, darker and tougher (Jones *et al.*, 1990). In Australia, periods of drought have been linked with periods of darker meat.

In hot climates it is common for stock to carry a lot of dust in their coats. Dust is easily transferred to the carcass during hide removal, and this is controlled by *spraywashing* the cattle before slaughter. Spraywashing can stir the animals up, depending on how it is done and whether the floor gets slippery, but it has not been shown to cause dark-cutting beef.

In pastoral farming systems cattle develop diarrhoea in the spring when the grass is particularly lush. This leads to faecal soiling of the hindquarters and faecal soiling of other animals in the truck when they are transported to the meatworks. The emotional stress that occurs during transport induces defaecation and this adds to the problem. The contamination of the skin, which is a hygiene problem in some countries, is sometimes managed by spraywashing the stock. Springtime diarrhoea is more severe in cattle than in sheep because cattle have a relatively short colon. The colon is responsible for absorbing water from the digesta before it is excreted. The short colon in cattle, combined with the rapid transit through their colons of a low-dry-matter, poorly bound digesta, causes the diarrhoea.

Genigeorgis (1975) reported that cattle in Brazil carry greater concentrations of *Clostridium perfringens* type A in their caeca when transported by rail in comparison with truck, and that the levels were higher on dry days compared with rainy days. The reasons for these differences were not clear, but they could be important in view of the fact that enterotoxigenic *Clostridium perfringens* can enter the bloodstream and pass to muscle, mesenteric lymph nodes, kidneys, liver and spleen. The risk of such systemic infections is said to be increased if the animals are not fasted preslaughter and if they are exhausted. Grau *et al.* (1968) found a high incidence of *Salmonella* in cattle railway wagons, saleyards and abattoir holding pens in Australia. In this situation cattle are continually exposed to this group of bacteria during the preslaughter period. Preslaughter fasting causes *Salmonella* to proliferate in the rumen, and the longer the time from farm to slaughter, the greater is the chance that an animal will carry *Salmonella* in its rumen.

Preslaughter fasting, water deprivation and transport lead to liveweight and carcass *weight loss*. Typically, cattle lose about 7% of their liveweight during the first 12 hours, 9% after 24 hours and 11% by 72 hours. For a 48-hour fast, up to 8% of carcass weight can be lost but it is usually much less than this. From the meatworks' perspective there are two aims in fasting cattle before slaughter. The first is to reduce the weight of the rumen contents, so that there is less risk of breaking the rumen when it is removed. The second is reducing the passage of intestinal contents during transport and lairage, otherwise other animals will become contaminated. Dry, firm faeces are preferred to wet, loose faeces as they do not spread so far.

As a general rule a 470 kg liveweight steer will lose about 1 kg of stomach contents and 0.25 kg of intestinal contents per hour during the first 24 hours of fasting (Bass and Duganzich, 1980). During fasting the moisture content of the gut contents rises, and for the 1 kg per hour decline in stomach contents only 400 g of that loss is water, whereas in a fed animal, there is normally about 850 g of water in every 1 kg of stomach contents. Fasting in bobby calves for 24 hours results in a carcass weight loss of about 5%.

DARK-CUTTING BEEF

Beef becomes dark-cutting as a direct result of stress before slaughter. It is caused by any situation which leads to exhaustion of glycogen in the muscle before the animal is killed (Tarrant, 1989b). Glycogen depletion leads to reduced post-mortem glycolysis and a high pH_{ult}. Some of the conditions which cause *dark-cutting beef* will be described, but before embarking on this it is useful to consider the quality aspects of this type of meat. In its extreme form, dark-cutting beef is purplish-black, firm in texture and dry and sticky to the touch. In terms of appearance, its most objectionable feature is the abnormally dark colour which is similar to that seen when beef has been cut and the surface has been allowed to dry out over a long period. The retailer rejects this type of meat irrespective of the cause, and so valuable parts of the carcass which have this condition no longer realize a good price. Instead, they have to be discounted as manufacturing beef or sold at a reduced price to the catering trade. Producers of manufactured meats (e.g. pies and burgers) will accept dark-cutting beef provided it has been stored properly. Some meat manufacturers specialize in using dark-cutting beef, because they benefit from its higher water-holding capacity.

The greater water-holding capacity of dark-cutting beef has the following benefits:

- smaller losses of weight as drip from fresh meat;
- less weight loss when frozen meat is thawed;
- lower weight loss during cooking.

When meat is cut into primals, joints or portions, the meat surface acquires bacteria. From this time onwards the meat is going to start spoiling through the effects of the bacteria (Gill and Newton, 1981). Before the meat is cut up, the deep tissues contain few microorganisms, if any, and *spoilage* is usually limited to the outer surface of the carcass. As long as it remains whole, the storage life of a dark-cutting carcass is similar to that of a normal beef carcass.

After the carcass has been deboned, the meat is usually stored at 0–5°C. At these temperatures the types of microorganism that grow on the surface and the storage life of the meat are determined by the pH, the availability of readily utilizable substrates and the availability of water at the meat's surface. A high pH is associated with faster bacterial growth and decomposition of the meat. Dry surfaces are associated with retarded bacterial growth. The bacteria that cause meat spoilage prefer moist conditions with a near neutral pH.

When dark-cutting beef has been cut open, it is prone to rapid spoilage by bacteria. Part of the reason for this is that the high pH allows bacteria to grow faster. Of greater importance is the low level of glucose and glycolytic intermediates (Newton and Gill, 1978). These are present in normal meat, but are greatly reduced in dark-cutting beef (Fischer and Hamm, 1981). Most of the bacteria which develop on meat preferentially use glucose for their growth. When glucose is exhausted, they convert to using amino acids instead. Ammonia and putrefactive amines are produced, giving spoiled meat its characteristic odour. In dark-cutting beef, glucose and glycolytic intermediates are exhausted before the animal is slaughtered and so any aerobic spoilage bacteria that are present start degrading the amino acids straight away. Shelf life is correspondingly short.

Theoretically, spoilage could be delayed by applying glucose to the carcass or meat surface. This provides the bacteria with their preferred substrate and it delays the production of spoilage odours. In legal terms, however, meat treated with glucose would be classed as a processed meat instead of a fresh meat, and this would decrease its value. Whether a 'processed' meat could be converted back to a 'fresh' meat by rinsing off the glucose with a water spray is not clear.

Dark-cutting beef can develop a different type of microflora from normal meat. The major aerobic spoilage microorganisms on fresh meat are the pseudomonads. This group of bacteria is unaffected by pH within the range occurring in normal and dark-cutting meats, but it is affected by glucose availability. On the other hand, *Alteromonas putrefaciens* cannot grow at the pH (5.5) of normal meat; it is only likely to grow on dark-cutting meat.

Spoilage can occur to a limited extent on the surface of fat. It is not so pronounced as spoilage on lean meat as less protein is available to the bacteria. The fat itself is not degraded, but water-soluble solutes on the surface are used by the bacteria. The surface of fat tissue is less moist than the cut surface of meat and so bacteria do not grow so fast. However, growth will be faster if water condenses on the carcass because warm air is allowed into the chiller or fridge. Similarly, spoilage on the surface of the fat can occur if the fat surface in packaged products is bathed in drip that originates from muscle.

In practice, the storage life of fresh meat can be extended by vacuum packaging. This deprives the bacteria of oxygen and so only a limited number of bacterial species will be able to grow. It is used particularly for beef primals sent from the southern to the northern hemisphere. Normal meat can be stored at chill temperatures for more than 10 weeks under the anaerobic conditions provided inside these packs, whereas in aerobic non-packaged beef the shelf life is only 3–4 weeks. With vacuum-packaged high pH_{ult} beef, the time to spoilage is often less than 4 weeks. The contents of the pack turn green and when the pack is opened it gives off a putrid odour. It does not need many packs to arrive in this condition to cause a whole consignment to be rejected.

With normal pH_{ult} meat, most of the anaerobic bacteria that are found on vacuum-packaged meat are glucose users; they do not produce ammonia from amino acids, as the main deamination pathways require aerobic conditions. The total counts of bacteria in this product are high, but with hygienic processing the types of organism are harmless. The microflora is usually dominated by anaerobic lactobacilli. These bacteria are beneficial as they compete with and inhibit spoilage anaerobes. If there is insufficient glucose present on the meat surface to allow a large culture of lactobacilli to develop, a different microflora could get established. The facultative anaerobes that often develop on dark-cutting beef are *Yersinia enterolitica, Enterobacter liquefaciens* and *Alteromonas putrefaciens. E. liquefaciens* produces spoilage odours and *A. putrefaciens* is responsible for *greening of meat* (Newton and Gill, 1980). Greening occurs when H_2S is produced as a breakdown product from sulphur-containing amino acids. The H_2S converts myoglobin (red) to sulphmyoglobin (green). Commonly, the greening is seen as a green drip (green weep) and as green discoloration of the surface of the fat.

A high pH_{ult} in meat can favour the growth of bacteria in the clostridial genus which cause *bone taint.* For this to occur in practice, there has to be a combination of circumstances including incorrect chilling or freezing (case hardening) plus the presence of these particular anaerobic bacteria. These combinations do not often occur and so the bone taint condition is rare. It can be detected by inserting a knife into the carcass or joint down to the bone and then smelling the tip of the blade after it has been withdrawn. If there is bone taint, there is an unmistakable sewage-like odour.

When meat is bought for manufacturing purposes the buyer must keep in mind the potentially short storage life of dark-cutting beef. If the meat or manufactured meat product is frozen, this may not be a major risk, but otherwise adequate chilling and a rapid turnover are essential.

High pH_{ult} beef has less *flavour* than normal pH_{ult} beef when the meat is grilled or fried, but this difference is less noticeable if the meat is roasted or casseroled. Beef of normal pH is generally more acceptable than dark-cutting beef because beef eaters prefer a stronger beef flavour. A possible explanation for the bland flavour of high pH_{ult} beef is that it contains less glucose and glycolytic intermediates and hence potential for producing Maillard reaction products. At high cooking temperatures these normally join with amino acids or peptides in Maillard reactions to create the basic meaty flavour of well-cooked meat. The flavour components produced in these reactions are responsible for meat-like flavours as distinct from species-specific flavours and odours, which are present in the fat.

A piece of uncooked dark-cutting beef is firm in *texture* but it is not usually tough when sliced with a knife. On cooking, it is usually more tender than beef with an intermediate pH_{ult} (e.g. 5.8). The relationship between pH_{ult} and meat toughness in beef is the same as that shown for lamb in Fig. 8.5. As pH_{ult} increases above 6.2 the meat becomes progressively more tender, and this effect is due to greater calpain activity in the meat at the higher pHs. The increased toughness with increasing pH_{ult} between 5.4 and 6.2 is associated with a decrease in sarcomere length in the individual fibres. This suggests that at low pH the extent of muscle contraction during rigor development is important in determining meat toughness. The relationship between pH_{ult} and sarcomere length in the pH_{ult} range of 5.4–6.2 depends on the temperature of the muscle before it goes into rigor. The higher the temperature, the greater is the contraction of the sarcomeres, but the higher temperature appears to favour hot-conditioning and better resolution of any toughness (Olsson *et al.*, 1995). Dark-cutting beef cannot be made more tender by pre-rigor tenderstretching, or electrical stimulation, or by ageing. Since there is limited ageing-associated tenderization in dark-cutting beef, there is little point in hanging dark-cutting carcasses for long periods.

Electrical stimulation of carcasses from unstressed steers helps to prevent toughness that is due to cold shortening. In carcasses from stressed cattle it has no effect on meat tenderness. In general, carcasses from stressed cattle would not be prone to cold shortening if the ability to regenerate ATP has been reduced by the stress.

Juiciness in beef has two components: an initial impression of succulence during the first few chews and a sustained wetness during mastication. No consistent differences in overall juiciness exist between high pH_{ult} and normal pH_{ult} beef.

The most important cause of dark-cutting beef is the sex of the animal. Bulls are more prone to producing dark-cutting beef than steers, heifers or cows (Graafhuis and Devine, 1994). In different countries the prevalence of dark-cutting beef in steers and heifers varies between 1 and 13%; in cull cows it is 6–14%, and in bulls it is 10–59%. The *causes of dark-cutting beef* within bulls are listed in Table 7.2. Over-excitement leading to excessive exercise is the main factor. In practice, the novelty and stresses of handling, transport, mixing with unfamiliar animals and lairaging will set this off

Table 7.2. Causes of dark-cutting beef in bulls.

Main causes	Contributory causes
Mixing unfamiliar bulls leading to aggressive behaviour:	Young, lean lightweight animals
mounting	Long transport journeys
butting	Fasting
chasing	
Overnight holding at meatworks	

(Tarrant and Grandin, 1993). A predisposing factor that influences how the animal will react to these situations is what the animal is used to. When bulls from socially stable groups are kept separate from other cattle, there is a lower risk of dark-cutting beef (Bartos *et al.*, 1993). If unfamiliar bulls are mixed, many of them can be expected to produce dark-cutting beef and in particular the aggressive, dominant animals (Warriss, 1984). Familiarity with humans and with handling are also important. In New Zealand the prevalence of dark-cutting beef is particularly high. The bulls are kept on pasture all the year round. They are handled regularly when moved to fresh paddocks but they do not have such close contact with humans in comparison with Scandinavian countries, where they are grazed in the summer and tethered in barns and hand-fed during the winter. The close attention and management that those animals receive when kept indoors makes them considerably less excitable and easier to handle when it comes to sending them for slaughter. Some animals are head-haltered the entire time from leaving the farm up to slaughter; if they were mixed, they would probably experience considerable social stress because of their previous isolation. In New Zealand the bulls are often younger, with less finish; they are kept in groups during the preslaughter period and so they are able to fight and exhaust themselves.

Besides tethering, a more common way of avoiding preslaughter mixing and exercise in some European countries is to keep the bulls in individual pens at the meatworks. The penning is arranged as series of parallel races with gates fitted about every 3 m. The animals are penned overnight inside the races and this has been particularly effective in solving high pH_{ult} meat problems at some works. At one slaughterhouse for example, it was found that the prevalence of dark-cutting beef fell from 47% to 8% when the lairage was changed from group penning to individual penning.

When young bulls are penned together for the first time they spend the first 12 hours fighting. This includes butting, mounting, pushing and chasing each other about the pen. As the horns are usually absent they tend to butt with the crown of the head. This is the most effective means of hurting an opponent and it causes carcass bruising. The butts are not usually aimed at the head. They are directed at the neck, shoulders, flank, or round, but when the opponent defends itself there is head-to-head pushing. The pushing develops into a trial of strength and in these contests animals lose their footing if the floor is slippery. The bulls also chase each other in an attempt to mount, which is often assumed to be a form of domination but could in fact be play behaviour.

The exercise associated with mounting behaviour would be expected to deplete glycogen in the muscles in the body that are most active: iliocostalis, longissimus lumborum (caudal end), semitendinosus, gastrocnemius and gluteus medius. Adrenaline would also be secreted during mounting behaviour, but because it is distributed throughout the bloodstream, it would be expected to affect all the muscles in the body. An adrenaline-type stress would therefore be expected to lead to more generalized dark-cutting in the carcass, whereas exercise stress is more muscle specific. Within a muscle, the fast-acting muscle fibres are more likely to be affected by the preslaughter exercise than slow types.

The prevalence of dark-cutting beef is lower in heavyweight bulls, presumably because they are more placid (Fig. 7.3) (Puolanne and Aalto, 1981). This effect has been noted for bulls that are penned individually and in bulls that are penned in groups. In addition, dark-cutting beef is less common in fatter animals. The lighter, lean type of animal is more frisky. Dark-cutting could be an occasional problem in plants that specialize in heifer or cull cow beef if there are animals that are in oestrus (Kenny and Tarrant, 1988). Isolating these animals or slaughtering them as soon as they arrive can preempt the problem.

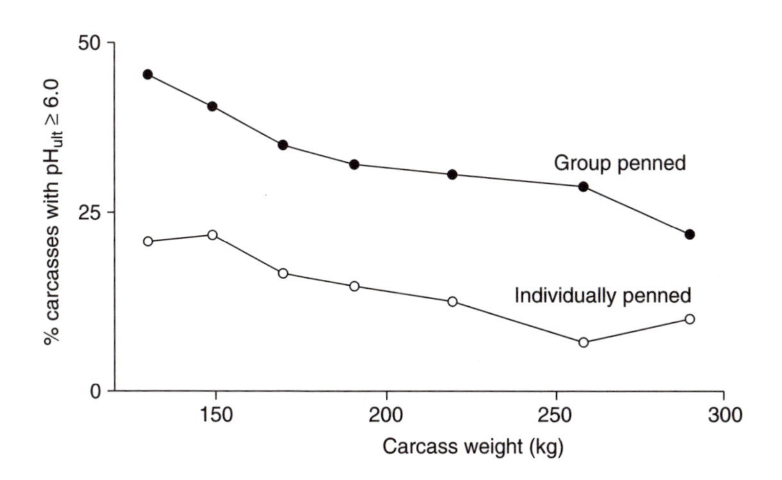

Fig. 7.3. Prevalence of dark-cutting beef in bulls according to liveweight and whether they were penned in groups or individually.

In countries where herd size is small, the cattle are collected from several farms in order to make up a truckload which is taken to the slaughterhouse. This has two consequences: it tends to increase the distance and duration of the journey and it increases the likelihood of mixing unfamiliar stock. Transport distance sometimes influences the prevalence of dark-cutting beef, and an example of this is shown in Fig. 7.4 (Puolanne and Aalto, 1981). If unfamiliar bulls are mixed together in the truck, they may not fight during the journey but there is a strong likelihood that they will not settle down when held in the lairage. One of the first steps that should be taken when trying to reduce the prevalence of dark-cutting beef is to ensure or check that the cattle are not being mixed at any stage before slaughter.

Fasting alone does not cause appreciable loss of muscle glycogen and so it is not a potent stimulus for producing dark-cutting meat. If it is accompanied by exercise, glycogen can be depleted and the meat will have a high pH_{ult}. When animals are allowed to feed after preslaughter mixing stress, complete recovery of muscle glycogen can take a long time – between 2 and 4 days in the study by Warriss *et al.* (1984). Resynthesis of muscle glycogen can be faster in red muscles than in white muscles, but this does not have any practical significance in preventing dark-cutting beef.

Various attempts have been made to modify bull behaviour in the lairage besides penning them individually. Switching the lights out is not particularly effective in preventing night-time activity. The animals become accustomed to the dark and still manage to mount each other, though it may

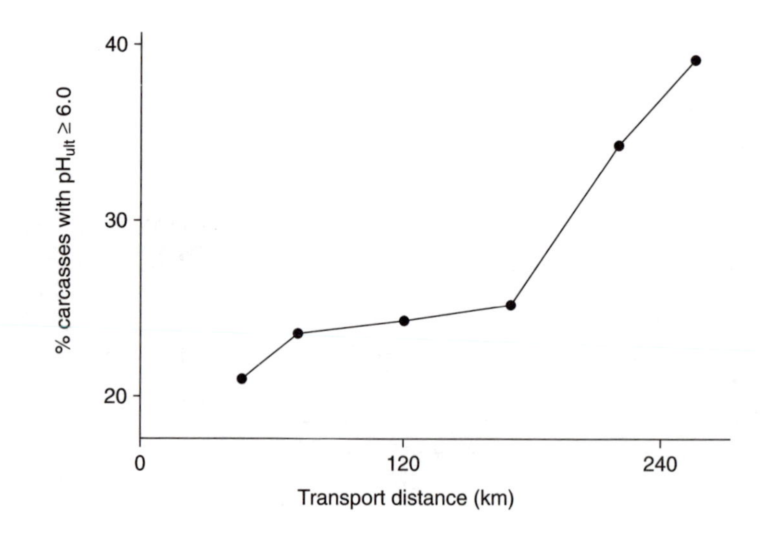

Fig. 7.4. Effect of preslaughter transport distance on the prevalence of dark-cutting beef in bulls.

be more haphazard. If an overhead electric grid is installed which delivers a brief high-voltage discharge when touched by an animal's head, then mounting will be reduced. When this has been combined with darkness, dark-cutting beef has been completely prevented.

Another way of preventing dark-cutting beef is to slaughter the bulls on the day they arrive at the plant. In the example shown in Fig. 7.5, those bulls that were kept overnight and slaughtered the next morning had the highest prevalence of dark-cutting beef (Puolanne and Aalto, 1981). Bulls that are penned separately and slaughtered 8–12 hours after arrival at the plant can also develop dark-cutting beef, so presumably exercise stress is not the only reason for this condition.

The way the cattle are herded to the slaughter point has an important influence on how stressed they will be when they are killed. This procedure is too brief to cause much depletion of muscle glycogen, and so it does not have much bearing on meat quality. However, it will influence how stressed the animals are when they are loaded into the stunning pen, and this in turn can affect the ease with which they are stunned. *Electric goads* are used for driving cattle at this point. In general their use should be limited to the final race that leads to the stunning pen (they help to prevent cattle from refusing to move) but it should be kept in mind that a good substitute is a yard broom. Electric goads should not be needed elsewhere, and if they are, this

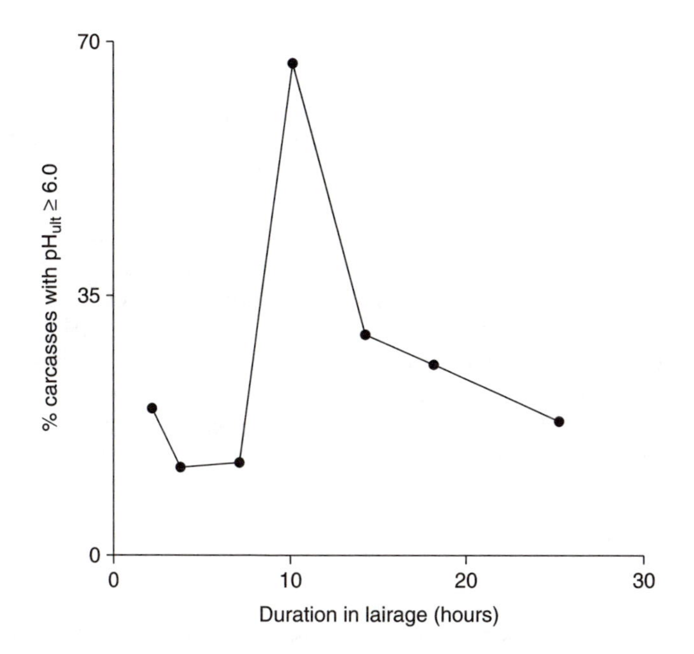

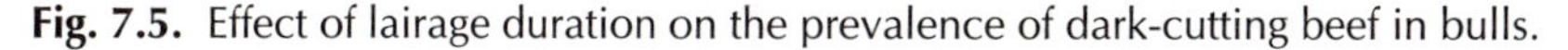
Fig. 7.5. Effect of lairage duration on the prevalence of dark-cutting beef in bulls.

is a poor reflection on the design of the facilities or the standard of stockmanship.

When cattle are confined in the race, and in particular when they are confronted with the stunning pen, they can show the following behavioural responses.

- **Fear** – backing along the race. Refusing to move, with the head lowered, and head shaking.
- **Alarm** – struggling, bellowing, head shaking, defaecating.
- **Submission** – standing with head lowered and extended forwards. Kneeling. Striking an animal which is in this state is pointless as it makes it more submissive.

The fear, alarm and submission responses usually develop from a period of refusing to move (freezing) when the animal recognizes that there is no way out of the stunning pen except from the way it came. Few stunning pens avoid this by having 'through vision' at the front of the pen; instead, a goad is used to get the animal to move into the pen. Without the goad there is a risk that the animal will recognize its predicament and refuse to move. Even this does not always work. Occasionally there will be an animal which will go down into submission and its refusal to move holds up the dressing line. In this event it is pointless to goad the animal repetitively. It is best to stand back for a minute, let the animal decide that it wants to get up, and then continue.

VEAL

Veal production has been a controversial welfare topic within Europe and North America. There are two types of production: white veal and pink veal. Most of the white veal is produced in France, where it fetches a high price in the luxury restaurant trade. For veal to be white, the calves must have low myoglobin levels in their muscles. In times gone by this was achieved by periodically bleeding the calves to reduce their iron levels. In modern white veal units it is done by feeding them a low-iron milk substitute and confining them in crates or narrow pens so that they do not exercise. The calves are grown to about 160 kg liveweight in North America and up to 360 kg in Europe. The welfare problems with white veal production are as follows.

- Calves are deprived of solid feed. This can lead to: (i) stereotypic licking, sucking and tongue rolling behaviours; (ii) hairballs in the gut from obsessive licking.
- Confinement in a crate. The calf may be unable to sit down and stand up easily, adopt a normal sleeping position, turn around, take exercise, play, and experience normal contact with other calves.

- Low iron intake can cause low blood haemoglobin levels and clinical anaemia.
- Incidence of diarrhoea and pneumonia can be abnormally high.

When the calves are sent to the meatworks some have difficulty in walking. This is because they may have never walked before and because they may be weakened by anaemia. To allow for this, one veal works in Europe has a tractor and chain permanently at the unloading bay which is used for drawing any animal off the truck that is unable to walk off by itself. Trunkfield *et al.* (1991) demonstrated that veal calves reared in crates had higher plasma cortisol responses to preslaughter handling and transport than calves reared in group pens, which may also be a reflection of the greater difficulty they experience in moving. There have been several attempts to ban white veal production in the EC by imposing standards on veal producers which would only allow pink veal production, but because of commercial interests they have not been successful.

In pink veal production the myoglobin levels in the muscle are higher. The milk substitute usually contains adequate iron and the calves may be raised in groups in pens that allows exercise and social contact. At the meatworks, pink veal can be made paler by electrically stimulating the carcass. This accelerates the rate of post-mortem acidification. If this occurs whilst the carcass is still hot, the meat develops a paler colour at its cut surface in the same way as PSE pork becomes pale. This does not produce veal with the same whiteness as farmed white veal, and it is not accepted as an alternative in the white veal market. Part of the reason for this is because the meat processor has to be cautious about how the carcass is stimulated. If the carcass is overstimulated it will lose more weight as drip. In practice, the processors aim to achieve a 3-hour pH of 6.1 in the loin. This combination allows some paleness without producing excessive drip. Toughness is not usually a problem in veal, but Fernandez *et al.* (1996) reported that a long transport duration in 120 kg white veal calves caused tougher meat, without being associated with any effect on pH_{ult}.

Bobby calves are a by-product of the dairy industry. They are usually 4–5 days old when slaughtered. The vells (abomasum) are sold for extraction of rennet, which is used in cheese making, and the skins are always in demand for making quality leather goods. The dressed carcass is of low value, the meat having a small portion size which fails to meet the needs of the high value veal market. Much of the bobby calf meat is sold as ground veal for making hamburger patties.

Besides the ethical concern that some people have about slaughtering an animal that is so young, there are three common welfare problems in the bobby calf industry:

- separation from mother;
- inconsiderate handling and inadequate feeding;
- preslaughter dehydration and starvation.

Inadequate feeding and inconsiderate handling stem from the fact that the animal has little commercial value. If it was worth more, there would be greater incentive to care for the animal. In some countries there is a legal requirement that bobby calves must be at least 4 days old or have a dry navel before they can be sent for slaughter. The reason is that calves less than 4 days of age do not withstand the journey so well. This was shown when calves were trucked at either 1, 2, 3 or 4 days of age and then, instead of being slaughtered, they were grown on (Fig. 7.6). The younger the animal when it was trucked, the higher was the subsequent mortality, until they reached 4 days of age.

Even though bobby calves have a short life it is important that they receive colostrum within the first 12 hours of birth. This helps them to fight off diseases such as diarrhoea, which can develop before they are slaughtered. On the day they are despatched from the farm they should be fed shortly before the journey. This prevents them from becoming weak through lack of feed, which in turn makes it easier to move them on to and off the truck and through the holding pens. Calves have not developed following behaviour by the time they are 'bobbied' (sent for slaughter) and so they are difficult to handle and herd, even when well fed. This is made worse if the calf came from a cow which was induced to calve with the injection of corticosteroids. Induced calving is common in countries that concentrate on summer milk production for the export of processed dairy products. Induced calves are physiologically and behaviourally immature,

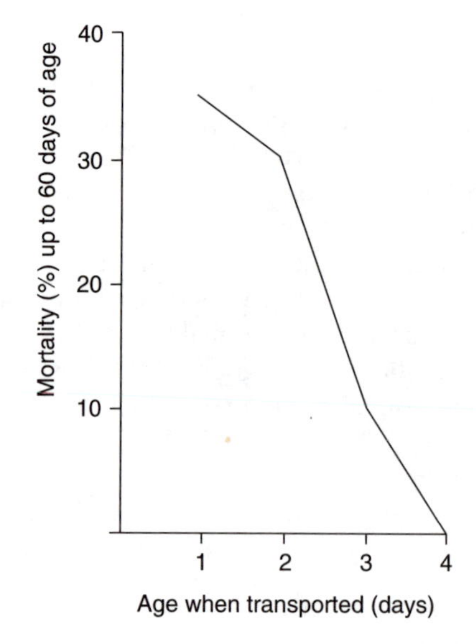

Fig. 7.6. Effect of age at transport on subsequent mortality in calves (Barnes *et al.*, 1975).

and are particularly difficult to handle in a meatworks. In many instances forced movement of calves is used, which causes particular problems during unloading. The calves are liable to fall over, especially if the ramp is steep, and this contributes to carcass bruising.

Since calves receive their feed as a liquid, fasting and dehydration usually go together. Few bobby calves have learnt how to drink from a trough by the time they are bobbied and so they do not usually rehydrate when they get to the meatworks. Dehydration is made worse if the calf is scouring. Dehydration can be recognized in the live animal from a tight skin which is not pliable, a dry mouth and sunken eyes. Skin pliability is tested by lifting a skinfold with the fingers. If the calf is dehydrated the skin feels thick and tight and is difficult to lift. On letting go, it falls back slowly. The tightness of the skin makes flaying more difficult. Skin removal tends to be difficult in calves anyway, and dehydration makes it worse.

Calves and large cattle which are sold through an auction market before slaughter are more prone to developing dehydration. They are also more likely to be lethargic from physical exhaustion. Lethargy can be recognized in cattle if they soon lie down once they have been put into a pen. They also spend more time resting instead of standing.

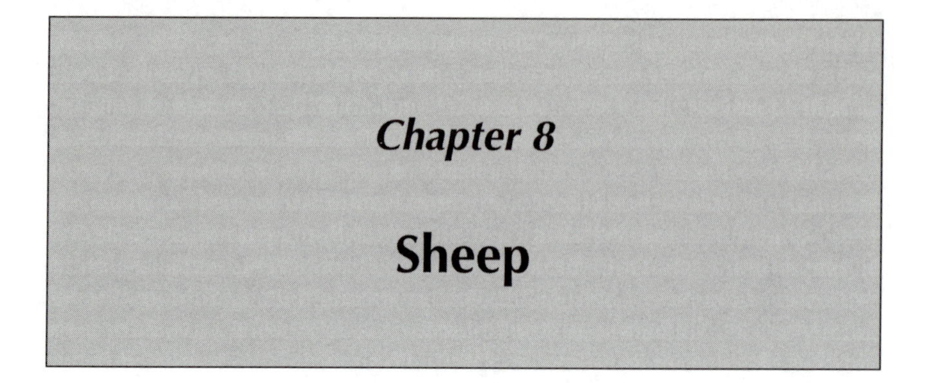

Chapter 8

Sheep

The stresses and welfare problems that occur in sheep are as follows:

- Chronic stress
  - ewe hypothermia;
  - underfeeding;
  - ewe hyperthermia;
  - disease;
  - lameness.
- Acute stress
  - dystocia;
  - lamb mortality due to insufficient feed and warmth;
  - dog worrying;
  - shearing;
  - pizzle dropping;
  - flystrike;
  - mulesing;
  - docking;
  - castration;
  - smothering;
  - mustering and yarding;
  - transport;
  - swimwashing and dipping.

This section considers those problems which are in various ways linked to meat quality.

The effects of on-farm *chronic stress* on a lamb's subsequent meat quality are not properly understood. From experimental work it is known that meat texture can be affected. In one study, chronic emotional stress involving fear resulted in tougher meat (Bramblett *et al.*, 1963). The mechanism explaining this was not clear, but it is unlikely that it was due to any additional exercise the lambs may have taken. Long-term physical exercise has the opposite effect; it leads to more tender meat (Aalhus *et al.*, 1991). Exercise-induced tenderness has been explained by enlargement of the muscle fibres in relation to the tougher collagen component in the meat. Little is known about the effects of *underfeeding* early in a lamb's life on subsequent meat quality, but slow growth to slaughter can be associated with high pH_{ult} meat (Pethick and Rowe, 1996). This is not invariably the case, as the way the animal responds to being handled before slaughter can have an overriding influence. Reduced feeding during the weeks leading up to slaughter can affect meat quality. The findings are probably most relevant to farming situations where there is a drought and part of the flock has to be slaughtered because of a feed shortage. Lambs that were slaughtered after a period of subsistence feeding were inevitably leaner; they had a smaller eye muscle area; their meat was darker in colour but it was slightly more tender (Jacobs *et al.*, 1973).

Some of the worst forms of chronic suffering that sheep experience are probably the feelings that accompany disease. Diseases that cause particular suffering are footrot, flystrike and facial eczema. Facial eczema is caused by a fungal toxin (sporodesmin) which is present in spores that are ingested with grass by sheep living in hot, wet climates. The toxin causes damage to the liver, which is then unable to detoxify the compound phylloerythrin (a normal constitutent of grass). Excessive intakes of phylloerythrin lead to photosensitization: the sheep develops severe skin burns from exposure to the sun, and in advanced cases patches of wool and skin slough off. The condition can be very painful, especially in recently shorn sheep which have limited protection from the sun. Another effect of damage to the liver is jaundice. In severe cases of facial eczema there is build up of bile pigments in the body and these impart a bitter flavour to the meat. The meat is also tougher (Kirton *et al.*, 1976). Some species of *Phalaris* grass contain alkaloids which cause debilitating neurological disorders when eaten by sheep. The poisoning is often fatal, but in those that survive, and are subsequently sent for slaughter, the meat can have a high pH_{ult} and an unpleasant flavour (Young *et al.*, 1994). Meat from carcasses that have been condemned for emaciation has been found to have a high pH_{ult} (Petersen, 1983).

An often underrated disorder in sheep is diarrhoea and soft faeces. It occurs in sheep affected by nematode parasites in the gut or when sheep graze lush young pasture in the spring. It can also occur when sheep are turned on to a new feed, such as changing from grass to a forage crop. Having soft faeces does not inflict any direct harm to the sheep but it has knock-on effects which create chronic and *acute stress* problems. The welfare problems created by dirtiness in sheep are:

- interference with suckling and underfeeding of lambs if the ewe is dirty;
- extra handling in crutching and dagging;
- tail docking;

- mulesing;
- swimwashing and crutching before slaughter.

Soft faeces are prone to clinging to the ewe as dags forming a black breech and these reduce wool yield. The dags on the ewes interfere with suckling by the lambs. This problem is controlled by crutching the ewes before lambing and periodically dagging them during the year if needed, all of which involves extra handling and stress for the ewes and accompanying lambs.

Soft faeces and diarrhoea in springtime are one of the underlying reasons for tail docking sheep. Docking reduces the risk of *flystrike*, which is caused by three species of fly that are particularly attracted to sheep with dirty backsides. The flies lay their eggs on sheep in the dirty breech areas. The larva that hatches out has a pair of sharp claws near its mouth which it uses to anchor itself to the sheep and to tear open the skin and muscle on the leg or rump. The larva then regurgitates digestive enzymes into the wound and later sucks up the puddle of digested tissue. Flystrike infestation is very unpleasant for the sheep, which shows a characteristic frenzied behaviour.

Crutching, docking and dipping are the three main methods for avoiding flystrike problems, all of which are stressful for the sheep, and some Australian and New Zealand wool farmers also mules their sheep. *Mulesing* reduces the risk of flystrike in the breech region and it is done in strains of Merino that have a well developed skinfold in that region, which is prone to harbouring the larvae. The skinfold is cut out, without an anaesthetic, using a pair of hand shears (blades). In more radical mulesing procedures the skin on the tail, the rump and a horizontal strip of skin below the anus or vulva may also be removed, but not all in the same animal. One of the aims with the breech cuts is to allow hair to replace the woollen skinfold that is removed, and so the cut needs to be made on the margin where wool on the outer aspect of the leg merges into hair at the groin. If the cut is too long (along the length of the leg), movement of the leg will be restricted as the skin becomes taut during healing. If the cut is too deep, muscle is removed; this would be particularly painful for the lamb, besides disfiguring its carcass and producing a hard, inedible scar tissue when it heals. There is a strong dislike of mulesing amongst the public who know about this procedure, because of its severity and the suffering it inflicts on the sheep. However, it is a well established practice amongst Merino farmers that they strongly defend on the basis that it saves a lot of suffering from flystrike. Flystrike can occur remarkably quickly and under extensive farming conditions it is not always feasible to do anything about it. Long-acting insecticides are an alternative but there is growing resistance amongst woolbuyers against their use, from an environmental perspective.

Tail docking is done in almost all breeds of sheep to reduce the risk of flystrike and to avoid the accumulation of faeces on the hindquarters. It is done without anaesthetic, with either a knife, a hot iron cautery or a rubber ring, and the male lambs may be castrated at the same time. The distress that is associated with *castration* has been assessed by measuring the lamb's plasma cortisol concentrations. It has been found that castration using a rubber ring or a knife causes significant distress for up to 4 hours. If the lambs are tail docked at the same time, and a knife is used for cutting both the tail and the scrotum, there is longer-lasting distress (about 8 hours) than when two rubber rings are used instead – one ring for the tail and the other placed around the scrotum above the testes. The conclusion is that, where castration and tailing are done together, one of the least stressful methods is to use rubber rings (Stafford and Mellor, 1993).

Besides the plasma cortisol responses, there are behavioural expressions of distress or discomfort following castration and these include frequent standing up and lying down, rolling, kicking and stamping. During the first hour after docking and castration with rings, the lamb may lie down in an abnormal posture with the neck extended, or it may stand with its hindlegs splayed behind it.

In some countries, short-scrotum castration is becoming very common. A rubber ring is placed around the scrotum below the testes, which are held up against the abdomen. The warmth of the body transmitted to the testes renders the animal infertile. The advantage of this method is that the lambs grow faster than lambs castrated by rubber ring placed above the testes (Lee, 1986).

The most common reason for castrating sheep is to prevent the check in growth that occurs when ram lambs reach puberty. At this time entire males become more active; they may eat less and growth rate declines. Castration is not necessary if the males are sold for slaughter before puberty, and many farmers have recognized this and no longer castrate sheep. Short-scrotum castration is used where the farmer wishes to maximize the early growth advantage of the entire male but needs to take the lambs on to hogget weight. Additional reasons for castration are the control of indiscriminate breeding, avoiding the oily fat problems that can occur in ram carcasses and minimizing the risk of undesirable odours or flavours in the meat. Indiscriminate breeding becomes a problem if it stunts the growth of a ewe lamb made pregnant when it is small, and if the farm loses control of its genetic selection programme.

The disadvantages of castrating are listed with the advantages in Table 8.1. Typically the growth rate advantage ranges from an additional 10–15 g liveweight per day in the ram lambs. An advantage of 10 g per day means that a ram lamb would reach a slaughterweight of 35 kg about 4 days before a wether lamb; it will be leaner and have a larger shoulder joint. Rams also have a higher collagen content in the loin meat but this is not sufficient to affect meat tenderness.

What *flavours and meat odours* can be expected in meat from ram lambs? Normally, sheep meat contains particular branched-chain fatty acids

Table 8.1. Advantages and disadvantages of castrating male lambs.

Advantages	Disadvantages
Prevents indiscriminate breeding	Wethers grow slower
Prevents stunting of young ewe lambs	Check in growth rate
Prevents weight loss in ram lambs that reach puberty	Pain of castration
	Risk of infection
Less risk of taints and oily meat	Fatter carcass

which give it a characteristic odour in comparison with beef, pork and chicken. One of these is 4-methyloctanoic acid. Differences between rams and wethers in meat odour, flavour and the levels of flavour-influencing fatty acids only become distinct when they are slaughtered at heavy weights. Entire male hoggets have a stronger mutton-like odour and flavour which is thought to be mainly due to 4-methyloctanoic acid.

Faecal soiling in the breach region is a major problem for meatworks. For some meatworks it is probably the single most important irritation. In the worst case, the sheep are wet and faecal juices run down the arm of the slaughterline staff as they hold and peel back the pelt during legging and pelt removal. In other situations, dirt from the breech is transferred to the carcass through contaminated implements and hands, or if the loosened pelt rolls back on to the carcass. These are all situations which staff endeavour to control, but standards may slip if a mob of sheep are excessively dirty and the Meat Inspection Service will call a halt to the processing by refusing to allow further dirty sheep on to the line. The only options are making sure that the sheep arrive at the slaughterhouse in a clean condition, or washing and crutching them in the holding pens. In some countries the supplier may be asked to come in and crutch the lambs if they are unduly dirty, or may be charged for a contractor to do this job, both of which are strong disincentives to supplying dirty stock in the first place. Crutching is inevitably stressful for the sheep. It may help to reduce visible soiling on the carcass but it is not necessarily effective in reducing the number of bacteria (Roberts, 1980).

Preslaughter washing is commonplace in some countries. There are three methods. Spraywashing is done for 10 to 15 minutes with lambs standing in a pen: water is directed on to their bellies from below and in some yards there is an overhead shower as well. Dunkwashing takes place in a pen fitted with an hydraulic lift that lowers the sheep into a bath for about a minute. *Swimwashing* also lasts for about a minute, during which the sheep are forced to swim the length of a 15 m waterbath. In some plants a moving conveyor tips the sheep into the swimbath and there may be another conveyor at the exit end. In New Zealand, sheep are usually spraywashed and then swimwashed, and they may be swimwashed more than once if they are particularly dirty. The procedure should be closely supervised. For example, if a sheep is facing the wrong way in the bath and tries to get out at the wrong end, it will have other sheep landing on it and it may drown. Effective intervention in this situation is essential. Swimwashing has been shown to increase the risk of bruising and it is a serious cause of high pH_{ult} meat (Petersen, 1978; Bray, *et al.*, 1989). Sheep that have been washed once may show considerable reluctance when approaching the bath a second time.

On the slaughterline the main sources of visible *carcass contamination*, when they occur, are from dirt attached to the fleece or skin, digesta from the oesophagus and mouth, rupture of the alimentary tract and leakage from the bung. Preslaughter washing leads to fewer carcasses becoming visibly contaminated with faeces (Table 8.2) (Biss and Hathaway, 1995). However, when the overall contamination of the carcass has been assessed microbiologically from standardized regions of the carcass, washing the live animal was found to produce carcasses with higher counts of bacteria (Biss and Hathaway, 1996). The dirtiest sheep microbiologically were those that had

Table 8.2. Effect of live lamb cleanliness and wool length on microbiological contamination of their carcasses (log_{10} aerobic plate counts cm^{-2} and 95% confidence limits).

	Microbiological contamination assessed at:	
Lamb condition	Pelt removal	Loading the chiller
Clean, shorn		
Washed	4.16 (3.91–4.41)	3.95 (3.69–4.22)
Unwashed	3.93 (3.66–4.18)	3.79 (3.60–3.99)
Dirty, shorn		
Washed	4.33 (4.12–4.54)	4.19 (4.00–4.39)
Unwashed	4.26 (4.08–4.44)	3.99 (3.75–4.22)
Clean, woolly		
Washed	4.47 (4.34–4.61)	4.25 (4.21–4.39)
Unwashed	3.94 (3.81–4.06)	3.91 (3.77–4.06)
Dirty, woolly		
Washed	4.63 (4.49–4.75)	4.28 (4.11–4.45)
Unwashed	4.30 (4.18–4.42)	4.12 (3.98–4.27)

been washed and had long wool. In terms of bacteria counts, washing an otherwise clean live sheep made its carcass dirtier. The conflicting conclusions between visible contamination and microbiological status is an age-old problem in the meat industry. For some reason, it is unusual in microbiological research to assess bacterial loading in visibly dirty regions of a carcass as well as doing routine sampling from standardized regions.

Preslaughter fasting helps to empty the guts before the carcass is dressed. This has two advantages. It reduces the disposal burden at the meatworks, and it makes it easier to lift or drop the viscera from the abdominal cavity without rupturing the gut wall. This in turn reduces the risk of carcass contamination. When a 28 kg lamb is fasted for 24 hours, the weight of its gut contents is reduced from 5 kg to 3 kg (Kirton *et al.*, 1971).

In the live animal, preslaughter fasting causes a reduction in rumen fermentation and less volatile fatty acids (VFA) are produced. As a result the pH of the rumen contents rises and this allows any *Escherichia coli* or *Salmonella*, spp. that are present in the rumen to multiply (Grau *et al.*, 1969). Giving fasted sheep a feed when they arrive at the works encourages further multiplication of *Salmonella* in the gut.

At abattoirs in tropical and subtropical countries, sheep and cattle are often held for several days before slaughter in pens which have an earth floor. They are fed intermittently in these pens before slaughter. Work in Australia has shown that under these conditions the fleece became contaminated with *Salmonella* within 1 day, even when there was less than 1 salmonella organism per gram of soil in the pens. The longer the sheep were held under these conditions, the more likely they were to develop a gut population of this bacteria, and the greater the risk that their carcasses would acquire the microorganism during evisceration (Fig. 8.1) (Grau and Smith, 1974). In this situation, contamination could occur through dust from the fleece, spilt digesta during viscera removal, or from faeces from the bung or fleece.

From the farmer's perspective there has to be a balance between complying with the needs of the abattoir for an empty animal and not losing too much weight during the preslaughter fast. When lambs are taken off pasture they lose up to 0.4% of their liveweight per hour during the first 24 hours of fasting. About 76% of this loss is due to the gut partly emptying itself. Carcass weight loss starts to occur between 12 and 24 hours after the start of fasting and over the first 48 hours it averages about 0.09% carcass weight per hour. In the frozen lamb trade this loss is offset by smaller losses in weight during freezing in carcasses from fasted lambs. The effects that preslaughter fasting has on eating quality of the meat are not clear, as the findings are contradictory.

Some general recommendations which apply to *mustering and yarding* sheep before slaughter are as follows.

- In hot weather, muster during the cooler times of the day.

- Muzzle any biting dogs.
- Regulate the pace according to:
  distance and terrain to be covered;
  temperature;
  mobility of any lame or sick sheep;
  mobility of the smaller lambs.
- Avoid downhill gateway smotherings.
- Avoid lamb smotherings during yarding.
- Do not yard sheep for more than 24 hours without feed and water.

Sheep are usually easy to handle if the facilities are well designed and there are sufficient staff and dogs to do the job. They show strong following behaviour, they move rapidly and generally they take good care of themselves. They will not try to escape, except as a whole mob, and their behaviour is predictable.

These qualities are apt to disappear if stockhandlers try to take on too much. As the size of a flock increases, the strength of the stimulus required to control its movement also increases. One situation where care is always needed is in driving sheep through farm gateways, particularly on fast downhill runs. With large flocks, there are ways of reducing risks.

- Ensure that gateways are not positioned in fencelines where sheep are able to have a fast run-in. Sheep move fastest when running downhill.
- Regulate the speed of the flock by positioning someone at the gateway to step in and check the flow if needed. This person can also save a sheep from being smothered if one goes down.

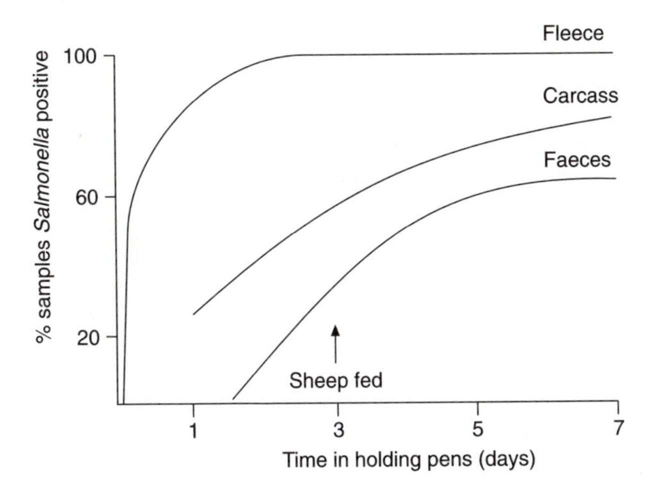

Fig. 8.1. Effect of holding time in the abattoir pens on contamination of the live animal and carcass with *Salmonella*.

Some sheep breeds have a reputation for being more active or flighty when handled in abattoirs, but this may be due to the conditions under which they are reared rather than a genetic trait. One example is the Perendale, a hill breed developed from the South Country Cheviot and the Romney. It tends to have a higher pH_{ult} meat, but whether this is because it is more active or because it usually has further to run during mustering, as it is farmed on extensive properties, is not clear (Petersen, 1984). It is best to yard the sheep for a few hours before pick-up to give them a chance to rest. Longer yarding times should be avoided on cloudless hot days.

Transport is a moderate to severe stress in comparison with other husbandry stresses experienced by sheep. Although it is not strictly valid to compare plasma cortisol responses between different experiments, the summary shown in Table 8.3 indicates that transport is not as stressful as shearing but it is more stressful than castration with a rubber ring. Not all journeys would provoke such a large cortisol response as that shown in the table, and it is important to note that cortisol levels do not usually remain elevated for the whole transport period (Fig. 8.2) (Knowles *et al.*, 1995). Levels are high at the start of the journey but after a time the sheep adapt and the levels fall to those typically seen in mildly stressed conditions (about 30 μg/l).

Metabolic stresses during transport can be relatively long lasting (Knowles *et al.*, 1995). They develop from three causes – emotional stress, fasting and exercise – and in practice fasting probably has the bigger effect. In the fed sheep, up to 80% of its energy is derived from VFAs produced in the rumen. The main VFAs are acetate, propionate and butyrate, which for a roughage feed are typically produced in the proportions 70 : 20 : 10. Nearly all the propionate is removed by the liver, where it is converted to oxaloacetate and then glucose (Jarrett *et al.*, 1976). In the fed state, approximately 20% of the metabolic energy is derived from oxidation of acetate

Table 8.3. Peak plasma cortisol concentration in sheep during different husbandry procedures.

	Peak cortisol concentration ($\mu g\ l^{-1}$)
Shearing	131
Transport	80
Part shearing	79
Castration	62
Tail docking	49
Mustering	48
Restraint	34
Laparoscopy	22

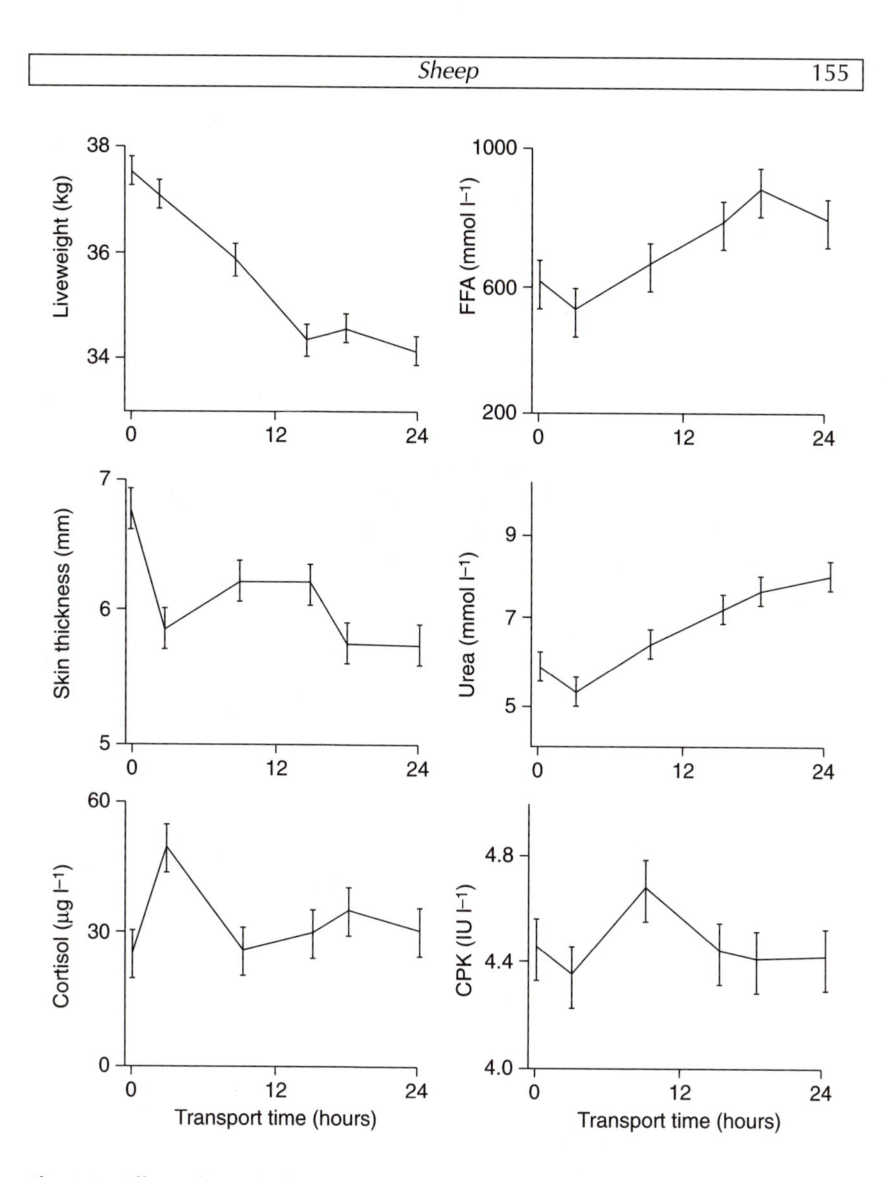

Fig. 8.2. Effect of a 24 h transport on liveweight, skinfold thickness and plasma stress indicators in sheep.

and most of the remaining energy comes from glucose. During fasting, the VFAs stop being produced in the rumen and the utilization of acetate as an energy source falls to 2%. Glucose continues to be used until the liver runs out of glycogen, which takes about 24 hours. Thereafter, plasma glucose and acetate concentrations fall, and plasma free fatty acids (FFA) take over as the main source of energy for muscle. The FFAs are derived from body fat stores where triglycerides (fat) are broken down by lipolysis to FFA and glycerol. With prolonged or severe fasting and where oxaloacetate is limiting, there is ketogenesis and a rise in levels of plasma acetoacetate and β-hydroxybutyrate. In addition, fasting leads to body protein catabolism, which is reflected in high blood urea concentrations.

During 24-hour transport, liveweight declines and plasma FFA, β-hydroxybutyrate and urea rise, which shows that reserves of glucose are limiting and instead body fat and protein reserves are mobilized to provide energy (Fig. 8.2) (Knowles *et al.*, 1995). Muscle activity, as shown by the plasma creatine phosphokinase (CPK) levels, does not necessarily increase during transport. This suggests that sheep do not usually exert themselves whilst the truck is moving, and measurements of plasma lactate levels have confirmed this. It appears that the most strenuous events for lambs over the whole preslaughter period are mustering and swimwashing (A.J. Pearson, unpublished data). Blood measurements also showed that sheep were distressed following loading but they adapted within 8 hours. They started to mobilize body reserves in the place of using glucose and acetate as energy sources after 9–16 hours. They did not perform undue exercise nor did they become dehydrated. The picture could be different in other journeys. For example, sheep have been found to develop dehydration during long journeys within Europe. In several studies it has been shown that the metabolic stresses associated with mustering and holding sheep before the journey have been as bad as the journey itself (Knowles *et al.*, 1994).

Broom *et al.* (1996) performed an interesting study in which they examined a range of plasma stress indicators in lambs that were loaded and confined for 15 hours on a stationary truck, compared with those in the same animals when loaded and driven for 15 hours on a subsequent occasion. In terms of the heart rate, plasma cortisol and plasma prolactin responses, the most stressful part of the procedure was loading the sheep on to the truck. Plasma cortisol levels were higher during the first 3 hours of the journey, in comparison with the stationary control treatment, but thereafter there was no difference.

Cold stress is unlikely to be a serious problem during transport because of the total warmth generated by all the sheep. One exception to this is for sheep on an open-top deck in high altitude or blizzard conditions. Heat stress is more common than cold stress, and it has been known for sheep to die from heat stress when left in trailers parked in the sun or in the holds of ferries. In general, mortality in sheep during transport is low (0.02%), but it tends to be highest when sheep are sold through auction markets and it is probably worst in diseased animals.

Sheep farmers vary between countries in their views as to which diseased or sick animals are *fit to travel* and which are fit for slaughter. Some take the view that the meatworks is expert at salvaging what they can from carcasses and so most diseased stock are sent in, whereas in other countries farmers appreciate that diseased sheep are low grade and their likely return does not justify sending them in. Sickness and disease are two of the most serious forms of animal suffering, and transporting sick animals imposes an additional stress which from a financial and welfare perspective is pointless. Some diseases no doubt lead to metabolic exhaustion either through chronic inappetence or stress or from a metabolic disorder. In the carcasses of these animals, the meat that is left behind after the inedible material has been trimmed is likely to have a high pH_{ult}. Emaciated sheep, and sheep that were traumatized when their truck toppled over, have been found to have high pH_{ult} meat.

The next question is: how long does it take for *recovery following transport* to occur? When hill lambs were transported for either 9 or 14 hours in northwest Europe, it was found from their blood parameters that the length of journey had no effect on their rate of recovery (Knowles *et al.*, 1993). If the sheep were allowed to drink and feed when they were unloaded, recovery occurred in three phases. During the first 24 hours the lambs rehydrated and their blood lactate levels returned to normal; during the next 24 hours the plasma FFA and blood urea levels fell in response to feeding; and between 48 and 96 hours after transport their liveweight and liver glycogen levels recovered. These findings are not relevant to the usual situation where stock are slaughtered within 24 hours of completing the journey, but they indicate how long the effects of transport stress persist.

The way sheep are handled and managed at the abattoir will determine whether they have an opportunity to recover or whether they continue to be stressed. The layout of the lairage and the proficiency of the lairage staff are particularly important in deciding how they are handled. The overall aims in the design of the holding area are to provide:

- easy unloading;
- sufficient space to house and shelter over a day's kill in the holding pens;
- a simple way of reducing the flow of sheep leaving the holding pens into a single file at the stunning point;
- the minimum of interference at the forcing pen from other activities in the holding area.

The main features of a well-designed holding area are as follows:

Unloading facilities

More than one ramp helps to maintain an even, unhurried flow of sheep into the building. The height of the ramp is adjustable hydraulically to meet the different deck heights of the trucks. The ramp is stable and has an easy-grip surface for the sheep. The height of the dock from which the ramp extends is level with the middle deck for most of the trucks, as this minimizes the steepest angle of the ramp. The count-out pen is well lit and follows directly from the ramp. In other words, there are no corners which could discourage following behaviour during unloading. The purpose of the count-out pen is to allow a check to be made on the number and condition of the sheep as they are unloaded. If a truck arrives late at night, the driver may leave the sheep in the count-out pen to be checked in the morning. This should be discouraged if the floor of the count-out pen slopes down into the building, as sheep (especially flighty animals) tend to gravitate at the bottom of the slope and they can smother.

Driving and holding area

All the sheep are housed under a roof out of the rain (wet sheep produce drip, which contaminates the carcasses during pelt removal). A steel grating floor is used because it allows easy drainage and floor cleaning. In general, sheep flow better when they pass across rather than along the direction of the surface rib of a steel grating floor, as it provides a better grip for their feet. The same floor material is used throughout the building to avoid discontinuities and interruptions in stock flow. There is a minimum of steps, visible sills and changes in the floor material between the ramp, count-out pen and holding pens, as such changes could cause the sheep to balk. Sheep also tend to balk at shadows and at lights shining through a steel grid floor from below – they have evolved to a mountain lifestyle where light from below causes them to stop and take check of the situation ('visual cliff response'). In other respects sheep are similar in behaviour to horses; they seem to trust the judgement of others in the group and follow accordingly, rather than assess each uncertainty for themselves. This means that once a mob starts to flow, following behaviour often takes precedence over wariness of objects that would otherwise cause balking.

The holding pens are arranged on a through-flow system. They are relatively long and narrow with the sheep entering at one end and leaving through the opposite end. This system makes unloading the pen easier; a stockperson or dog does not have to walk through the sheep to drive them out of the pen, and the sheep are less prone to confusion caused by sheep in adjacent pens moving in the opposite direction. The raceways are 3 m wide and the walls of the races are blanked in those regions where experience has shown that blanking helps stock flow.

In some countries dogs are used for loading and unloading the holding pens, and they are particularly useful where there are deficiencies in the design or layout of the pens. A dog may need to be muzzled or trained with an electronic training collar if it takes to biting the sheep, and this will depend to some extent on its temperament and breeding.

Forcing pens and races

The forcing pens are designed to hold about an hour's kill. The intention is to provide a continuous flow to the single-file race whilst giving the sheep time to settle after moving them out of the holding pens. Processing the sheep through the forcing pens needs to be done in a calm manner without any dogs. Too much exercise, noise and disturbance increases the overall duration of stress unnecessarily. The sheep should follow on voluntarily at every stage and ideally there should be a smooth, continuous flow of animals. The pens are only 2.5 m wide and parallel walkways are sometimes used by the operators to avoid having to move against the flow of the stock. The system used for advancing and crowding the sheep towards the single-file race involves the stockperson walking behind the sheep and closing swing gates behind the mob. Sheep in a pen in front act as a draw for sheep that are about to fill an empty pen. Lift-and-swing gates, which lift over the sheep, are fitted where appropriate and these have the advantage of causing less bruising than swing and guillotine gates. In the design shown in Fig. 8.3, a double forcing pen system is used because it ensures a continuous flow of unhurried sheep. If sheep are forced too much in the final forcing pen, some may jam together in the funnel. Ideally, they should enter the single-file race by following on, but often some prompting is needed by the operator. It is important that sheep at the funnel entrance do not turn round and this can be avoided by inclining the race upwards in a way that maintains visual contact with the sheep that are moving along the race. The race itself is six sheep long, which is a manageable length for one operator. If it is shorter, there is a risk that sheep will break back to the forcing pens. It is V-shaped, being narrower at leg height as this discourages turning or burrowing under a sheep in front. It is important that light does not shine upwards through the floor of the race, as this checks voluntary flow (visual cliff effect). At the top of the race the restraining conveyor that leads to the stunner is set slightly below the race floor. The sheep drop into the conveyor. As with all other parts in the handling procedure, critical attention to detail helps to ensure a smooth and low-stress delivery of stock to the required point.

In countries where investment in these types of handling facilities is not available, there can be difficulty in stock handling. A common procedure is for one person to select a sheep manually and pull it towards the entrance of the slaughterhouse whilst other stockhandlers drive the mob from behind. This is undoubtedly stressful for the lead sheep. In other situations movement is made easier by using *Judas sheep.* These are tame trained animals kept permanently at the meatworks to act as leaders or decoys. By driving the easily managed Judas sheep, the others can be enticed to follow. The Judas sheep has to be trained to peel off from the mob at the appropriate moment if it is to avoid being slaughtered. They have been used successfully at many meatworks, and are a good improvisation when handling facilities are poor. Some countries disallow the use of Judas sheep because they are considered to be an animal health risk: they are exposed to all the contagious sheep diseases that enter a meatworks and so they are thought to act as a reservoir for those diseases.

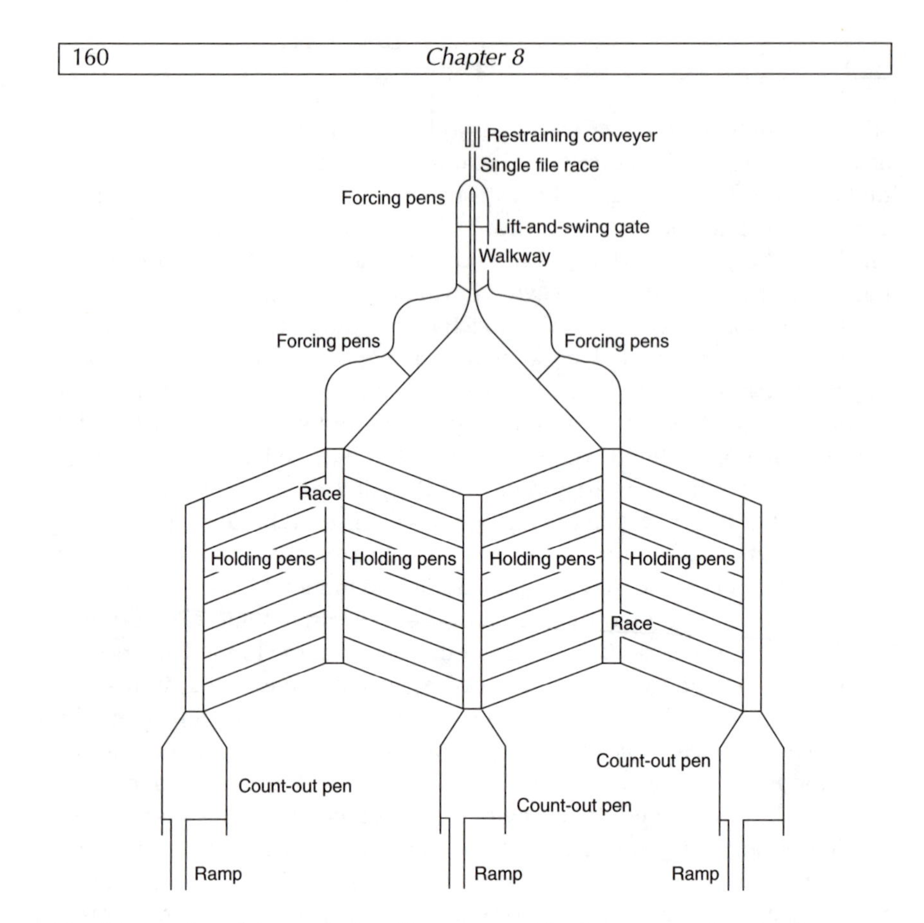

Fig. 8.3. Design of the yards, handling pens and lead-up to stunning at a sheep meatworks.

Meat quality

Meat buyers and consumers seem to be less sensitive about meat quality issues in lamb and sheepmeat than they are for other meats. This may be partly because lamb is often çooked before the appearance of the cut surface of the meat is inspected. Dark lamb in association with high pH_{ult} meat is not a complaint one often hears about, and yet the defect exists in 8% of lamb and 12% of mutton that is produced in New Zealand (Graafhuis and Devine, 1994). In that country, excessive exercise before slaughter is thought to be the main cause of high pH_{ult} lamb and mutton (Fig. 8.4) (Devine and Chrystall, 1988). Over-forcing the sheep during mustering can almost completely deplete muscle glycogen levels, and in that situation recovery takes too long (over 17 hours) for most meatworks throughputs. The carcasses go into rigor sooner after slaughter. When meat from such severely exhausted lambs was cooked and presented to a taste panel, it was found to be more tender than meat from unexercised controls (Chrystall *et al.*, 1982).

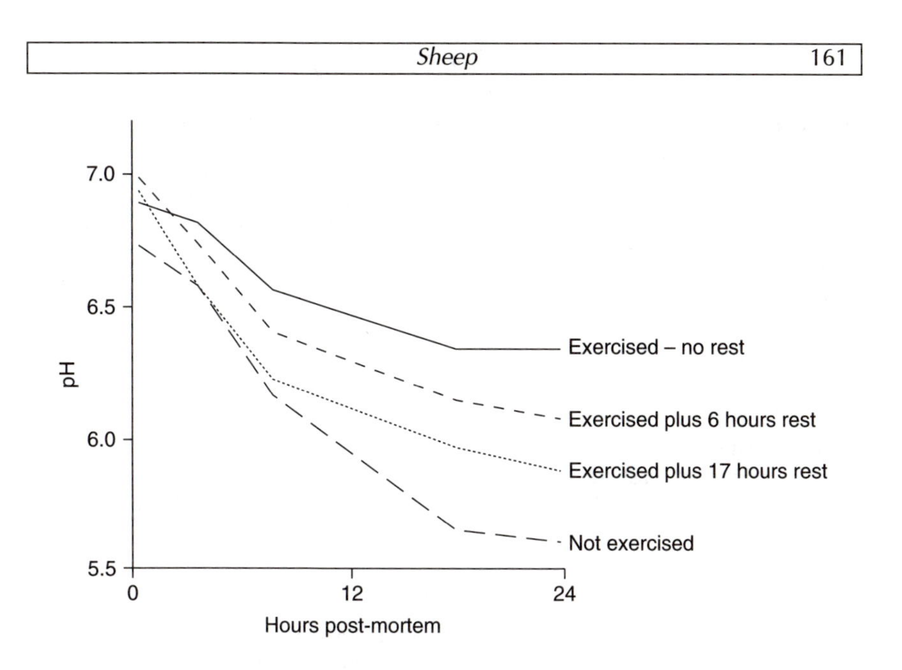

Fig. 8.4. Effect of preslaughter exercise on meat pH_{ult} in lambs.

The more stresses that a lamb has to go through before slaughter, the more likely it is to produce high pH_{ult} meat. When lambs are crutched or shorn before slaughter, and when they are fasted and swimwashed, these *multiple stresses* have additive effects in depleting muscle glycogen and causing high pH_{ult} meat (Table 8.4). The single most provocative of these stresses is swimwashing (Bray *et al.*, 1989). It is demanding on the strength of a lamb to pull itself through a waterbath race when its fleece is loaded with water.

Another provocative way that has been used experimentally for inducing high pH_{ult} meat is to inject a sheep with adrenaline before it is slaughtered. This also produces a very dark meat, the colour of burnt umber. The amounts of adrenaline needed to produce these conditions are greater than would normally be produced by the animal's own adrenal medulla. This raises the question whether *adrenaline stresses* such as fear, anxiety and hyperthermia are sufficient on their own to produce high pH_{ult} meat. One study approached this question by blocking physical activity in muscles in the hindquarters by applying a local anaesthetic to the spinal cord (Apple *et al.*, 1995). The sheep were then stressed emotionally by restraining them in isolation. Plasma adrenaline levels were high, and the pH_{ult} in both forequarter and hindquarter muscles was elevated (6.40). This showed that the adrenaline that can be produced by a lamb in response to stress and in the absence of physical exercise (in the hindquarters) was sufficient to produce high pH_{ult} meat.

Table 8.4. Effect of preslaughter management procedures on high pH_{ult} meat in lambs. (From Bray *et al.*, 1989).

Live sheep treatment	% Carcasses with l. dorsi $pH_{ult} > 6.0$
Control	12
Shorn	12
Underfed	12
Shorn + underfed	36
Washed	40
Underfed + washed	44
Shorn + washed	56
Shorn + underfed + washed	80

Not all muscles in the sheep's body respond to stress in the same way. This was shown by Monin (1981) when he compared pH_{ult} values in transported and non-transported lambs (Table 8.5). Muscles such as the triceps brachii, supraspinatus, semitendinosus and pectoralis profundus were prone to developing a high pH_{ult}. Under normal circumstances these muscles are continually active, and the additional activity imposed by the transport stress led to rapid depletion in their glycogen levels. Other muscles are only occasionally used, such as the psoas major, which helps to perform leg kicking, and the longissimus dorsi, which brings about back arching. These muscles are not particularly taxed during transport stress and so they are not prone to developing a high pH_{ult}. By contrast, the rectus abdominis is involved with breathing movements; it is continually active, and even in the unstressed state it has a high pH_{ult}.

High pH_{ult} lamb has a more bland *flavour and odour*, it can be tougher and less juicy and have a low overall acceptability rating (Devine *et al.*, 1993). The poorer flavour and odour occur in both ewe lambs and entire males, and it is associated with smaller amounts of 28 different compounds, including the aldehyde decadienal, the alcohols octenol and pentenol, and heptanoic acid, which are evolved from meat in the broth and fat that is produced during cooking (Braggins, 1996). Which of these compounds is most important in influencing overall flavour and odour is not yet known, but some of them have distinctive odours. For example, hexanal and decadienal have green, grassy odours.

There are other preslaughter factors besides stress that can influence lamb flavour. Lambs that have been grazing white clover or lucerne before slaughter have a distinctive flavour in their fat and lean which some people consider an off-flavour. Trying to eliminate these flavours by fasting the animals before slaughter does not work (Czochanska *et al.*, 1970; Park *et al.*, 1972).

Table 8.5. Effect of preslaughter transport on the pH_{ult} of different muscles in lambs. (From Monin, 1981).

Muscle	pH_{ult}	
	Transported lambs	Unstressed lambs
Triceps brachii	6.39	5.69
Supraspinatus	6.35	5.79
Semitendinosus	6.32	5.83
Pectoralis profundus	6.31	5.85
Infraspinatus	6.25	5.76
Rectus abdominis	6.18	6.11
Biceps femoris	5.95	5.66
Semimembranosus	5.90	5.71
Psoas major	5.78	5.71
Adductor	5.73	5.62
Longissimus dorsi	5.61	5.64

High pH_{ult} meat that has not been aged is likely to be tender. The relationship between *toughness* and pH_{ult} for lamb is shown in Fig. 8.5. The risk that the meat will be tough is greatest when its pH_{ult} is between 5.7 and 6.1, but this curvilinear relationship disappears as the meat ages. Meat of intermediate pH_{ult} is the only type of meat that is likely to tenderize with ageing, and this is most likely to occur if it is kept warm. High pH_{ult} and low pH_{ult}

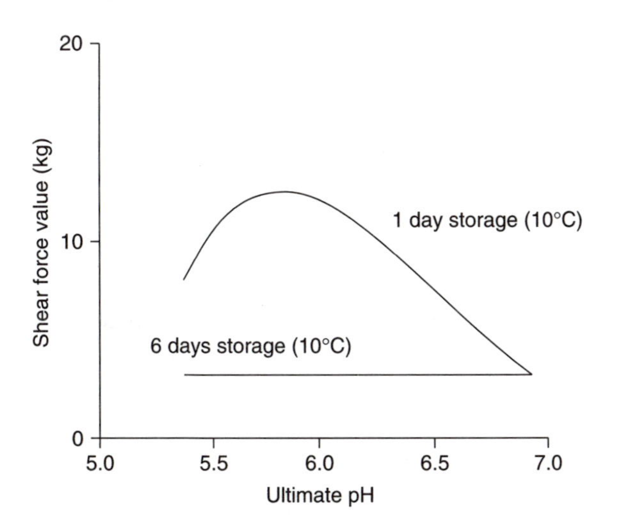

Fig. 8.5. Relationship between pH_{ult} and meat toughness in lamb longissimus dorsi.

meats do not become more tender with ageing. During ageing there is enzymatic degradation of the Z-line, titin and nebulin. The likely reason why extremely high pH meat is tender soon after slaughter is that the activity of one of the calpain enzymes responsible for breakdown of these structures is increased, whilst pH and temperature are elevated. Calpain activity is very sensitive to pH, and as the pH increases to 7.5 its activity in breaking down the structural components in muscle increases substantially (Fig. 8.6) (Cena *et al.*, 1992).

A high pH_{ult} in lamb can favour the growth of certain *food-borne pathogens.* An example is *Aeromonas hydrophila,* which is assuming greater recognition as a human pathogen. This bacteria is a facultative psychrotrophic anaerobe; in other words it tolerates low temperatures and low oxygen conditions. As such it is a threat to the chilled modified atmosphere packaged (MAP) lamb trade. Like *Listeria monocytogenes* and *Yersinia enterolytica,* it is capable of multiplying at normal refrigeration temperatures. If there is likely to be some high pH_{ult} cuts in a consignment of MAP lamb, the best way of controlling the growth of *Aeromonas hydrophila* is to use either 100% CO_2 or 50% CO_2/50% N_2 in the gas atmosphere. Vacuum packaging is not as effective in controlling this particular microorganism.

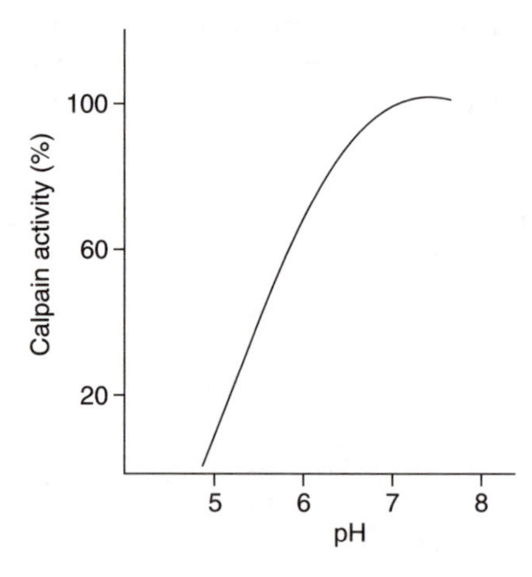

Fig. 8.6. Effect if pH on calpain activity in lamb longissimus dorsi.

Chapter 9

Pigs

The main welfare issues that confront the pig industry include:

- handling in abattoirs;
- stunning;
- confinement (e.g. farrowing crates, stalls and tethers);
- piglet mortality (e.g. crushing);
- aggression (e.g. at mixing or feeding);
- disease (e.g. pneumonia, osteochondrosis);
- barren environments (e.g. conditions leading to stereotypies);
- mutilations (e.g. castration, tail docking, teeth clipping).

Not all of these influence meat or carcass quality, but the features that can be affected are: dark, firm, dry (DFD) meat; pale, soft, exudative (PSE) meat; meat tenderness; rindside damage; skin colour; bruising; broken bones at stunning; boar taint; and reduced browning during cooking.

Some people consider that outdoor-reared pigs produce the best quality meat. *Free range pork* has an image of being more 'savoury' and 'pleasant' and less 'dry' than intensively reared pork (Oude Ophuis, 1994). It can also have the image of being 'fresher' with a higher nutritional value. The majority of studies, however, have indicated that the differences in eating quality between outdoor- and indoor-reared pigs are small. Two studies have in fact shown that free-range pork is marginally tougher than standard pork.

The most consistent differences are that outdoor pigs are slightly slower growing and leaner (Enfalt *et al*., 1997). They are also easier to handle during the preslaughter period. They are more calm, they show less exploratory behaviour and they tend to fight less than intensively reared indoor pigs. Their reduced activity when confronted with novel situations can lead to a lower prevalence of DFD pork. They settle sooner after arriving at the abattoir and so they are likely to have higher muscle glycogen levels at the time of slaughter and hence a normal pH_{ult} in their meat. This, however, will also depend on how they are handled; if they are exercised through rough handling, the advantage in terms of less DFD meat can be lost.

In recent years there has been a lot of focus on the environmental effects of intensive pig farming. This does not mean that there are no welfare problems. High levels of NH_3 in the atmosphere in indoor piggeries can be irritating and they suppress appetite and growth in the pigs. Dust can also be a nuisance in intensive piggeries, especially where the pigs are floor-fed with a mash or where dusty straw is used as bedding. Vacuum cleaners are recommended instead of brooms, and the addition of fat to the meal will also help to control dust. Intensive fattening piggeries which are poorly ventilated and have slatted floors over slurry tanks can develop odour problems. These are not normally a severe problem for the pigs, but occasionally pigs which have been in close proximity to an anaerobic slurry have died from H_2S poisoning as the slurry was being mixed before being pumped out of the building. In some countries the slurry must be stored in tanks that are separated from the piggery by a stench trap. Noise levels in piggeries are also an environmental hazard: Levels of 98 dB(A) have been recorded during meal feeding and levels of 110 dB(A) during castration. Noise levels exceeding 90 dB(A) for 4 hours are damaging to human hearing, and staff need to wear ear defenders.

Pigs kept indoors in hot climates have few ways of keeping cool. Normally they would wallow or move to the shade. Keeping pigs in hot conditions (32°C) has resulted in a slower rate of post-mortem muscle glycolysis compared with rearing at 21°C (Aberle *et al.*, 1969), and high humidities have resulted in meat that is more tender.

The systems used for breeding herds vary considerably. In some situations the sows farrow in arks outdoors. At weaning, the piglets are usually transferred to an indoor piggery where they are grown to the appropriate market weight. In intensive pig breeding units the sows have less opportunity to forage, build nests, take exercise, wallow, groom themselves by rubbing and to interact socially with other sows or their own litter. For example, in some countries sows are housed indoors the whole time: they are put into farrowing crates from just before farrowing until the litter is weaned at about 5 weeks; they are then held in dry-sow stalls during pregnancy. In other countries the sow only stays in the farrowing crate for 10–13 days; she is transferred with her litter to a nursery pen until weaning, when she may be held in a dry-sow stall; and once it is established that she is pregnant she is then moved to a large pen holding other sows. There are many variations on these approaches. Some of the advantages and disadvantages of using farrowing crates and of farrowing outdoors are summarized in Table 9.1.

Prolonged confinement in dry-sow stalls or with tethers is considered stressful for sows for several reasons: exercise is limited; there can be more leg and feet problems; there is reduced social interaction between sows; the sows are confined in less comfortable conditions; and behavioural oppor-

Table 9.1. Advantages and disadvantages of different pig breeding systems.

Advantages	Disadvantages
Using farrowing crates (in comparison with pens)	
Less space required	Absence of nesting behaviour
Less labour required	No exercise and limited movement
Ease of observation	Unable to turn around
Ease of supervision	Confinement leading to restlessness, fighting the crate and repetitive rooting behaviour
Can reduce piglet crushing (evidence is contradictory)	Bruising or skin blemishes in some sows
Keeping dry sows outdoors (in comparison with indoors)	
Enriched environment	Risk of sunburn and heat stress
Greater space allowance and opportunity for exercise	Individual feeding is difficult
	Risk of gut diseases
Potentially more comfortable	Individual sow inspection and care are more difficult
Less risk of prolapses	
Lower capital cost	Risk of bullying and fighting
No stereotypies	

tunities are restricted. Two methods have been used experimentally to assess this stress. One has been to examine the sows' stereotypies, such as bar chewing. The other has been to measure the plasma cortisol response to ACTH injection in the confined pigs and to compare this with pigs kept under other conditions. Tethered pigs have higher plasma cortisol responses to ACTH than loose-housed pigs (Janssens *et al.*, 1994). In particular, the increased cortisol response in tethered pigs was greater when there was no snout or visual contact between adjacent sows. This emphasizes that opportunity for social contact should be included in sow housing systems. Problems with aggression should be managed in a way that does not involve completely isolating the pig.

Several painful surgical procedures are performed on piglets without any anaesthetic, and in some parts of the world there is public pressure to stop their use. *Teeth clipping* is done to reduce facial scarring in piglets, and to control udder damage in the sow. If the sharp canine teeth are left untrimmed, the piglets can damage each other when competing at the udder. It is important not to trim the teeth too close to the gums, otherwise the teeth splinter and a tooth pulp infection could set in. Only the tips of the teeth should be clipped. Some piglets also have their tails docked to prevent *tail biting* later in life. Tail biting can lead to infections that result in carcass condemnation from abscesses and pyaemia. When tail biting is not corrected it can, in extreme cases, lead to cannibalism. The causes of tail biting vary from farm to farm, but predisposing factors include: hunger; lack of facilities, such as bedding, which encourage normal oral-based behaviours; early weaning; high stocking densities; insufficient trough space leading to frustration at not being able to feed whilst other pigs are feeding; high temperatures; insufficient ventilation; very bright light; and observing other pigs tail biting. There are a number of alternatives to tail docking, and these usually include providing rooting areas or bedding material and isolating culprit or victim pigs.

Castration is another painful procedure which is performed without anaesthetic on piglets. One study showed that in terms of the heart rate response, incising the scrotum and severing the spermatic cord were particularly stressful parts of the procedure. Removing the testicle from the cut scrotum was less stressful (White *et al.*, 1995). Castration without anaesthetic was more stressful once the piglets reached 8 days of age.

Castration is done in those countries where pigs are grown to high slaughter weights. If male pigs are left entire, the meat will have undesirable odours and flavours known as *boar taint*. These usually develop once the pigs have reached puberty, and so they are most noticeable in heavyweight pigs. Castration is not practised in every country. In Australia, Eire, New Zealand, Spain and the UK male pigs are usually left entire. The advantages of not castrating are that entire males grow faster, convert feed into liveweight more efficiently and produce leaner carcasses. The disadvantages, besides boar taint, are that boars are more aggressive; when fighting they acquire rindside damage and carcass bruises, and can exhaust themselves to the extent that they produce DFD pork. In addition, the fat in boar carcasses contains more water and it is softer. This makes the carcass and meat cuts more floppy and so butchery is more difficult. The subcutaneous fat is apt to separate from the lean and the softer less saturated fat is prone to rancidity if stored for long periods. These, however, are minor disadvantages in comparison with boar taint.

Boar taint is most noticeable when the meat is being cooked. Only a proportion of the human population can detect boar taint and women are more sensitive to the smell than men. It is usually described as an unpleasant male urine-like odour. Sometimes the smell has undertones of sweat, pig faeces, onions or camphor. Three compounds have been implicated in this combination of smells: androstenone, indole and skatole (Fig. 9.1). Androstenone imparts a urinous odour; it is a male sex hormone, which explains why the taint is less common in meat from gilts and castrates. Skatole is formed by bacteria in the hindgut of pigs from the amino acid, tryptophan. Along with indole, it is thought to be responsible for the pig-faeces and camphor-like odours sometimes found in the cooked meat. These two compounds are not necessarily specific to boars but their concentration can be higher in boar fat than in that of gilts because the boar's liver does not always break down the skatole effectively. Skatole levels in fat are also higher if the pigs are fed a dry feed instead of wet feed and if they are tightly stocked on the farm or lie in their own faeces and urine to

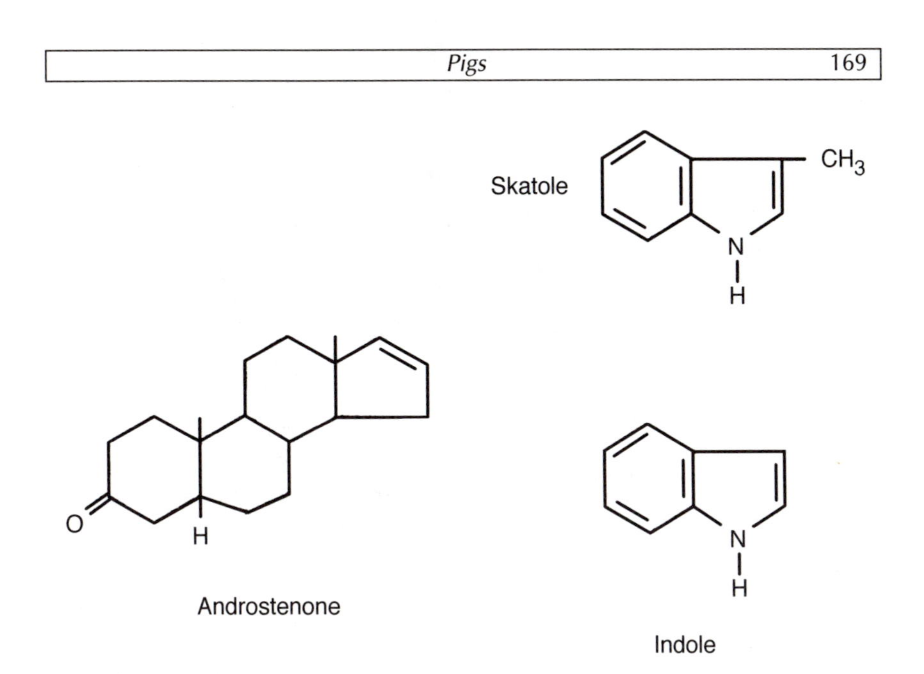

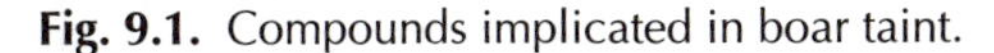
Fig. 9.1. Compounds implicated in boar taint.

keep cool. Holding pigs on slatted floors helps to reduce contact with faeces and urine, and so the levels of indole and skatole in the subcutaneous fat are reduced. It has been suggested that there could be a genetic factor that influences the skatole content of subcutaneous fat.

Osteochondrosis is a painful and debilitating leg disorder that causes lameness in breeding pigs. It is linked to high growth rates and to insufficient attention to genetically selecting against the condition. It is due to cracks and crevices forming in the cartilage layer of the bones at the hock, elbow, shoulder and hip joints. The cracks spread and cartilage flaps form which eventually detach and lie loose inside the joint (Reiland, 1975). Besides causing painful lameness, the condition may be linked to broken bones at stunning. Animals with osteochondrosis sometimes have cracks in the cartilage layer that lines the glenoid process of the shoulderblade bone (i.e. the cup of the shoulderblade which joins with the humerus bone). It is thought that, at stunning, these cracks break apart along with the underlying bone and a haemorrhage forms, which spoils the shoulder joint. The bloody meat has to be trimmed during jointing and this leads to loss of yield. In addition, the fractures also make it difficult to remove the shoulderblade automatically. During deboning, a claw grasps the neck of the shoulderblade and pulls the bone out of the shoulder joint. This is ineffective when the neck or glenoid process of the bone is broken (Fig. 9.2). Lameness can be due to other causes, including arthritis and abscesses, and these contribute to condemnation of parts of the carcass.

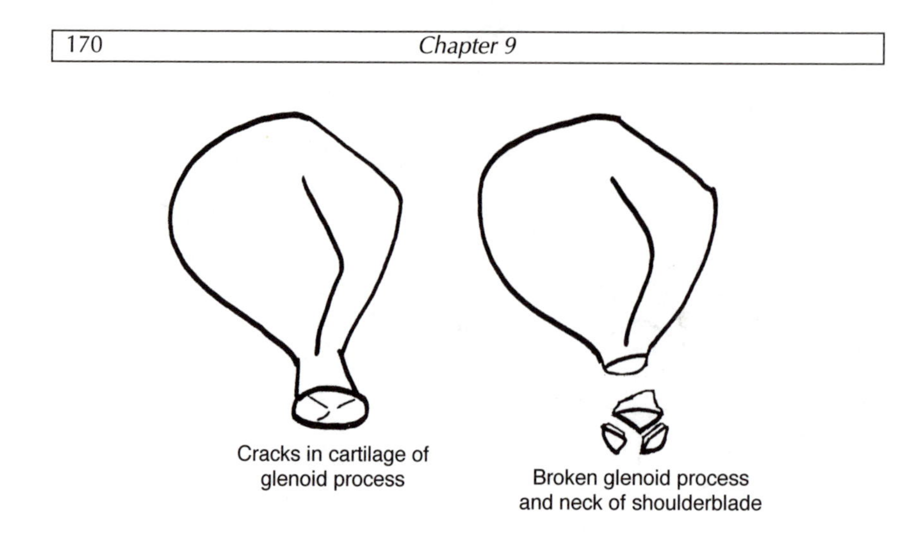

Fig. 9.2. Shoulderblade fractures in pigs.

It has been estimated that about two-thirds of all the pig farms in The Netherlands are infected with species of *Salmonella* bacteria. The salmonellas are present in the pigs' digestive tract and lymph nodes. The most important factors that determine whether a pig is infected are farm hygiene, particularly manure management. Preslaughter stress can have an effect, though it is of lesser importance, and it can occur in the following way. Pigs are normally fasted for at least 12 hours before slaughter, by which time their stomachs do not contain any solid digesta. The absence of solids in the stomach leads to a rise in pH of the stomach contents, through reduced gastric acid secretion. Gastric acid secretion is also inhibited by the acute stress of loading and transport, through the release of catecholamines. Stress also increases intestinal motility. Together, the increased pH and gut motility favour the survival, proliferation and excretion of salmonellas. Up to 20% of salmonella-free pigs are thought to become infected during transport and lairage through environmental contamination created by those pigs which are excreting the bacteria.

If instead the pigs are fed before they are sent to slaughter, there can be:

- higher mortality during transport;
- harder work involved in eviscerating the carcasses;
- spillage of gut contents during evisceration;
- greater waste disposal volume (gut contents) at the abattoir.

Feed is usually withheld overnight before despatch from the farm. When pigs are fasted overnight, their liver glycogen is converted to glucose which enters the bloodstream and is used as a source of energy by the rest of the body. The rate of decline of liver glycogen during fasting follows the pattern shown in Fig. 9.3 (Warriss, 1982). By measuring the liver glycogen content in a freshly slaughtered pig and relating this value to Fig. 9.3, one can estimate the time the animal was fasted. This approach was used at four abattoirs in the UK and it was found that half the pigs had been fasted for more than 19 hours and one-quarter for over 31 hours before slaughter (Warriss and Bevis, 1987).

From about 16 hours of fasting the pig relies on free fatty acids released from its body fat (instead of glucose from the liver) as the main source of energy. From this time onwards body fat is mobilized and there is a loss of carcass weight. Liveweight loss starts earlier than this because of loss of gut contents and reduction in liver weight. Much of the emptying of the stomach occurs wthin the first 5 hours and so the optimum period for fasting pigs before transport is not less than 5 hours. The optimum period of fasting before slaughter is not more than 18 hours.

Preslaughter fasting has only small effects on meat quality (Tarrant, 1989a). Long fasting periods will tend to decrease the prevalence of PSE meat and increase the prevalence of DFD meat. The effect on DFD meat is more noticeable in those muscles that are most active. Muscles such as the longissimus dorsi which are not continuously active tend to maintain their glycogen concentration during fasting, whereas those that support the animal's posture and weight are more prone to glycogen depletion and showing DFD characteristics following a long fast. Liver quality is also affected by the length of fasting. Longer fasts lead to a smaller, darker liver which is less tender and juicy when fried.

Death during transport to the abattoir is most common during the hotter months of the year. In Europe, when the mean daily temperature

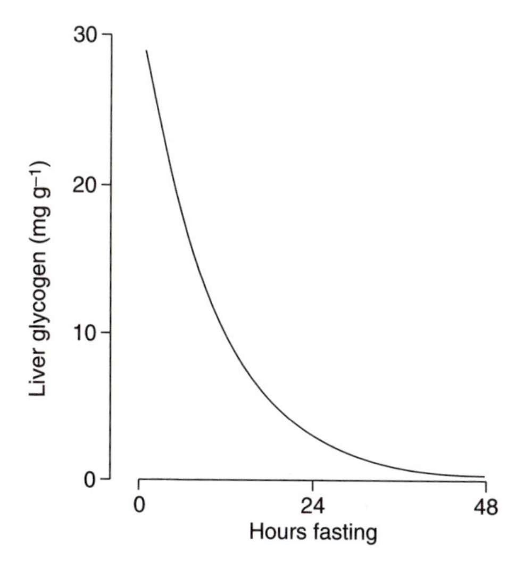

Fig. 9.3. Effect of witholding feed on liver glycogen concentration in pigs (Warriss, 1987).

exceeds 16°C, pig mortality during transport starts to rise. Under these conditions it is advisable to:

- transport pigs at night or during the cooler parts of the day;
- reduce the stocking density in the truck by carrying fewer pigs;
- park the truck in the shade or keep it moving to ensure adequate ventilation;
- give the pigs a cold shower on arrival at the abattoir.

In several field trials it has been found that increasing the ventilation in the trucks by enlarging the ventilation slots has reduced mortality substantially. Pigs which do die during transport usually die from stress-induced heart failure. The heart muscle has pale necrotic areas, which are a sign of poor blood supply, and this is also a feature of death from excessive levels of catecholamines in the bloodstream. Blocking catecholamine receptors in the heart muscle, or ablating the amygdalas in the brain, has been used experimentally to prevent stress-induced myocardial necrosis in pigs, which shows that the heart failure is closely linked to the stress response (Johansson *et al.*, 1982).

Stress-induced deaths usually occur in particular breeds or genetic strains of pig. These are often referred to as stress-sensitive (SS) genotypes or as halothane positive (*nn*) pigs. SS pigs also have an unusually responsive sympatho-adrenomedullary nervous system. The cardiovascular responses that are mediated through this nervous pathway are exaggerated, and so the hearts of these pigs are thought to be more prone to catecholamine overloading (Gregory and Wotton, 1981). Enhanced activity of the sympathoadrenomedullary nervous system may also contribute to the growth of a leaner carcass (Gregory, 1981).

Our understanding of what happens to an SS pig as it dies from a stress crisis during the preslaughter period has stemmed from work on *malignant hyperthermia* (MH). MH is a lethal condition which is metabolically similar but it is initiated with drugs (halothane or suxamethonium) instead of exercise. During MH the SS pig metabolizes energy in its muscle at an exceptionally fast rate. This leads to a rise in body temperature. The ability to supply oxygen, to keep up with the high rate of muscle metabolism, begins to fail and the muscle produces lactic acid instead. Large quantities of CO_2 are produced by the excessive muscle metabolism and this makes the animal breathless and cyanotic (blue). Adrenaline and noradrenaline levels in the blood rise and potassium is released from the liver. From a welfare perspective, it is an unpleasant death. The excessive muscle metabolism causes the animal to go into rigor whilst it is still alive. It is unable to move properly because of the rigor; it gets very hot, and the breathlessness can be extreme. The usual prevalence of deaths during transport is about 0.1%, but levels of 1% have been reported in some countries where SS breeds are common, such as Germany and Belgium.

In Belgium it is normal practice to inject SS pigs with a tranquillizer to minimize stress-induced deaths during transport and death from fighting in the lairage (Geverink *et al.*, 1996). In many other countries tranquillizers would be unacceptable because of the presence of drug residues in the meat.

Loading on to the truck at the farm can be stressful, especially with pigs that have not experienced loading before. It can be made easier if the following criteria are met.

- The loading platform is at the same level as the truck deck, or the angle of the ramp is less than 20°. Pigs manage to climb slopes of up to 20° relatively easily. Above 20° they are slower, but this effect can be reduced by providing close cleats on the ramp. The cleats should be 20 cm apart.
- The loading ramp is stable and has stairsteps.
- The inside of the truck has a light. Pigs move more readily towards light.
- A hydraulic tailgate lift is used, particularly with multi-deck trucks.
- There is continuity in the floor surface material between the loading platform and the truck. This can be created by spreading straw over the platform and the truck floor.

It is particularly important not to overstock the truck if there is going to be a long journey (longer than 24 hours). After such journeys there will be a high prevalence of DFD meat, and overstocking will make this worse as it reduces the amount of time the pigs will be lying down and resting.

Transit erythema is a skin blemish which is not common but is linked to transport conditions. It appears as red patches on skin that has been in contact with the floor. This is usually on the belly and hams. It may occur in response to cooling or to urine on the floor. It usually fades once the carcass is chilled, but at some abattoirs it has been trimmed. Skin bruising on the ham occurs when pigs slide down the unloading ramp, or if the floor of the transport truck is stippled to provide grip and the pigs slide whilst in a dog-sitting position.

Prolapses occur during transport when intra-abdominal pressure is too high and this occurs when pigs climb ramps, exert themselves during exercise and get squeezed together in the truck.

Electric goads are widely used for getting pigs out of trucks and for driving them along races leading to the restraining conveyor. Applying an electric goad increases the animal's heart rate and is inevitably stressful. Flexible slappers are less stressful. It has been claimed that excessive use of electric goads increases blood splash in the meat.

Pigs are not easy animals to handle in abattoirs. Common *handling problems* include the following.

- Pigs often respond to forced or hurried movement by fighting against it, instead of moving with it.
- In unfamiliar situations they are inclined to return to where they came from, and are prepared to fight to get back to the familiar site.

- They have poor short-range vision and show a preference for gradually exploring new situations. This makes them slow to move. Ensuring that the ground is well lit, but not dazzling, allows the pigs to move faster, and with less hesitation.
- They do not always show strong following behaviour; instead, they may split off to escape or to explore the surroundings.
- They do not necessarily respond to pressure from other pigs which are pushing from behind. When driving pigs from the holding pens to the stunning point they should be moved in small groups (up to 15 pigs per group) as this usually allows the operator to influence the behaviour of the leading pig.
- They do not respond well to 'stop–go' situations that commonly exist in the race leading to the restraining conveyor.
- When alarmed and stressed they pack together and sorting or handling becomes chaotic.

The following features should be considered when designing a pig lairage:

- horizontal unloading ramps, or ramps with less than 20° slope;
- non-slip floors;
- no discontinuities in floor material or texture;
- adequate lighting along the route the pigs have to pass;
- gates which swing both ways;
- solid sides to fences and pen walls;
- narrow pens instead of square pens;
- through-flow pens;
- wide corridors with few bends.

Pigs that are flighty or nervous of humans at the farm are also flighty and difficult to handle at the abattoir. Handling pigs at the farm from 4 weeks to 7 weeks of age helps to familiarize them with humans, makes them less fearful and makes subsequent handling easier. In addition, pigs that are aggressive to each other at the farm also tend to be more aggressive at the abattoir.

When pigs fight each other in the lairage, they inflict skin damage which shows up in the carcass as *rindside damage*. When severe this can cause downgrading of the whole carcass. Several factors lead to increased fighting, such as mixing unfamiliar pigs and the presence of entire male pigs. Rindside damage is usually worst when pigs are held at the abattoir overnight instead of being slaughtered on the day of arrival. They fight for longer and inflict more damage to each other. When they fight they try to bite or gash each other with their lower incisors and canines. Typically they strike the shoulder, jowl and chest of the opponent, but sometimes they will bite an ear or strike the flank. The red wheals in the skin persist in the carcass, creating an unsightly blemish on a joint or bacon due to be sold with skin attached. The most effective way of controlling this problem is avoiding mixing unfamiliar pigs. One of the cues that initiates fighting is the smell of an unfamiliar pig. Attempts at masking these smells by applying stronger-smelling compounds from an aerosol have not been particularly effective. Where it is inevitable that pigs will have to be mixed, this is best done as they are loaded on to the truck; pigs fight less on a moving truck and the journey gives them time to get used to each other. Fasted pigs tend to fight more aggressively than fed pigs. Fed pigs take rest periods between bouts, whereas fasted pigs keep fighting for longer. Linked to this, submissive behaviour is more obvious amongst fasted pigs.

The tendency to be aggressive in the lairage can also be influenced by the way the pig was reared. If piglets fight a lot whilst they are in the farrowing shed, they will continue to be aggressive after weaning. Presumably they learn at an early age to fight for what they want and the habit persists. In fattening units, aggression is also influenced by stocking density and the relationship is curvilinear (Fig. 9.4).

When pigs fight in the lairage they use their muscle glycogen and this can lead to exhaustion and *DFD meat*. The degree of glycogen depletion is controlled by three processes:

- glycogenolysis, which is activated by adrenaline from the adrenal medulla;
- ATP utilization, which occurs during exercise (glycogenolysis would occur as a secondary response to help replete the ATP);
- resynthesis of glycogen during rest periods after the fighting.

The extent of glycogen depletion also varies between muscles. When pigs fight, the muscles in the neck and shoulder are used to butt and strike the

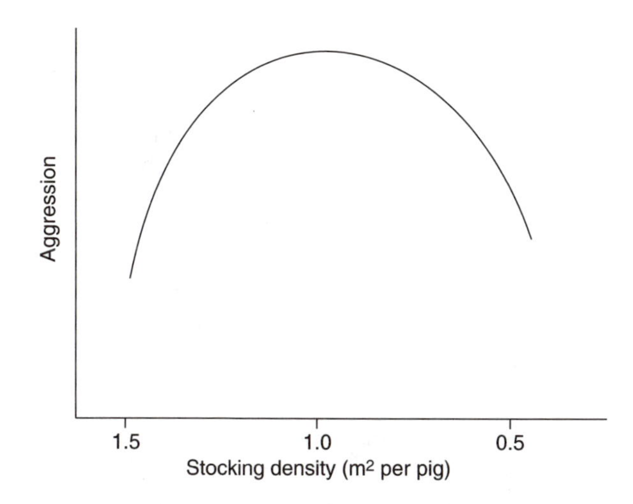

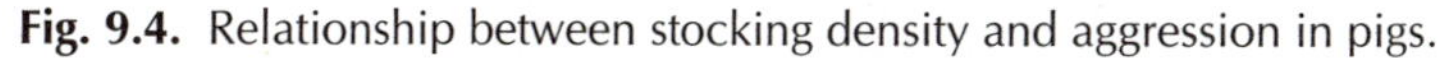
Fig. 9.4. Relationship between stocking density and aggression in pigs.

opponent, and so these muscles are particularly prone to becoming exhausted. The longissimus dorsi, on the other hand, is less active and there is only limited glycogen depletion (Fernandez *et al.*, 1995). Some muscles in the ham may become glycogen depleted, but it would be unusual to see DFD in the semitendinosus. Within a muscle, glycogen depletion tends to occur first in the fast twitch fibres; when these are exhausted, slow twitch fibres lose their glycogen.

Several situations can lead to DFD meat in practice. In one study it was found that 18% of pigs transported in a truck had DFD in the quadriceps femoris muscle. The truck had a slippery floor, it was not sectioned off and there was no mechanical ventilation. In contrast, only 10% of pigs were DFD after transport in a truck fitted with a non-skid floor, partitions and mechanical ventilation (Nielsen, 1977). The difference in DFD between the truck types was greatest for the muscles in the neck and shoulder, and presumably this was linked to the difficulty the animals experienced in maintaining their posture.

Sometimes it is found that pigs squabble as soon as they are placed in a holding pen at the abattoir. If they are slaughtered within 2 hours there will be a high risk of DFD meat. If instead they are left for 4 hours they will settle down, muscle glycogen will be recovering and there will be less risk of DFD meat. It is generally recommended that gilts and castrates should be given at least 3 hours in lairage to rest and recover their muscle glycogen. There is insufficient information to give a recommendation for boars.

If pigs are held overnight in the lairage it is important to encourage them to settle and not to waste energy interfering with each other. A restful night can be achieved by not stocking the pens heavily (e.g. provide 0.8 m^2 or more per pig) and by switching off the lights.

Glycogen repletion depends on the availability of substrates in the bloodstream. When energy substrates are available, muscle glycogen can be repleted quickly (e.g. within 3.5 hours of fighting). Feeding the pigs a sugar solution after mixing stress will help to restore muscle glycogen, and this strategy has been used at some abattoirs in the past.

Showering pigs with water whilst they are in the lairage is often used to clean the pigs, to reduce odour emission from the abattoir, and to reduce the pigs' activity. If the water is so cold that it reduces the pigs' muscle temperature, it can reduce the severity of PSE meat by controlling sarcoplasmic protein denaturation. In one study, severe chilling caused a reduction in muscle glycogen and this led to a darker meat (Sayre *et al.*, 1961).

In summary, the situations which can lead to muscle glycogen depletion and DFD meat are:

- fighting;
- difficulty in maintaining balance during transport;
- witholding feed in combination with exercise;
- long transport and holding times;

- lack of familiarity with being handled;
- selling through live auction markets before slaughter;
- insufficient resting time in the lairage.

The way pigs are treated before slaughter can also influence the extent to which meat will brown as it is being cooked. Normally, *browning of meat* occurs as amino sugars are formed during the Maillard reaction, but some browning is also due to caramelization. In the Maillard reaction, amino sugars join with reducing sugars which are present in meat as intermediates in the glycolytic pathway (e.g. glucose-1-phosphate, glucose-6-phosphate and fructose-6-phosphate). Feeding with sugar before slaughter raises the level of reducing sugars in the meat, and this increases the extent of browning that occurs when it is cooked. Meat from unexercised, unstressed pigs contains more reducing sugars than meat from exercise-stressed pigs, and so meat from the unstressed pigs is more likely to develop brown colours when cooked. DFD pork is less likely to brown than normal meat because it contains less glycolytic intermediate sugars. The browning reaction also contributes some flavour components to cooked meat, but there is no consistent evidence which shows that meat from stressed pigs has less flavour. In fact there is evidence that meat from stressed pigs has slightly stronger aroma when cooked, but the reason was not demonstrated (Lewis *et al.*, 1962).

According to one estimate, 22% of pig carcasses in the UK are DFD (Warriss *et al.*, 1989). It is unwise to give a general estimate of the

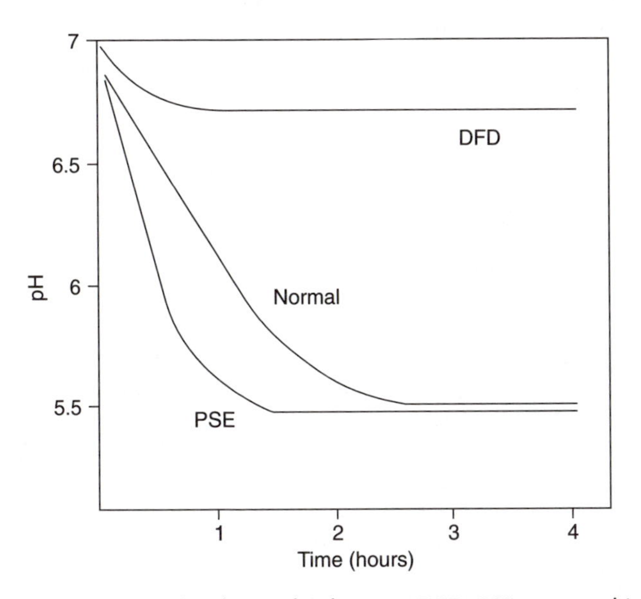

Fig. 9.5. Fall in pH in muscles destined to become DFD, PSE or normal in appearance.

prevalence of PSE meat as it is variable and depends on the genotype of the pigs. Like DFD, *PSE meat* formation is linked to stress before slaughter, but the mechanism is quite different. DFD is caused by depletion of muscle glycogen before slaughter. The shortage of glycogen limits post-mortem muscle acidification (Fig. 9.5). In PSE meat formation there is no shortage of glycogen. Instead, the animal is physiologically stressed by the stunning and slaughter process and this causes the muscles to acidify at a rapid rate whilst the carcass is still hot. The combination of a low post-mortem muscle pH and high muscle temperature is the critical situation which leads to PSE meat formation. The tendency to develop rapid acidification is largely influenced by the genotype of the pig. Preslaughter handling is less important, but it can contribute to PSE meat in two ways. Firstly, if the stress causes acid to build up in the muscle before the animal is slaughtered then this will exacerbate the situation. The muscle pH starts at a low level from the time of slaughter. Secondly, if the stress makes the pig hot just before it is slaughtered, the rate of carcass cooling can be reduced and so PSE meat may be produced through acidification at high temperatures.

The genotypes that are prone to producing PSE meat are the same as those that are stress-sensitive (SS) or halothane-positive (*nn* for the halothane gene). The different pig breeds are ranked according to SS in Table 9.2. Mildly SS pigs (*Nn* for the halothane gene) are less likely to produce PSE meat, and PSE meat is uncommon in stress-resistant (SR) pigs (*NN* for the halothane gene). In SS pigs, the muscle activation at stunning is sufficient to induce PSE meat formation. Handling these pigs more quietly and gently before slaughter has little effect on their meat quality, whereas in the mildly SS pigs reducing preslaughter stress is more effective. Exercise or heat stress during the hour before slaughter can cause these pigs to produce PSE meat, especially if they are acidotic at the time they are slaughtered.

Table 9.2. Stress sensitivity and proneness to producing PSE meat in different pig breeds.

Stress sensitive	Mildly stress sensitive	Stress resistant
Piétrain	Dutch Landrace	Irish Large White
Belgian Landrace	French Landrace	Australian Large White
Poland China	Swedish Landrace	French Large White
German Landrace	Swiss Landrace	American Yorkshire
	British Landrace	British Large White
	Danish Landrace	Duroc
	Norwegian Landrace	
	Australian Landrace	
	Irish Landrace	
	Dutch Yorkshire	
	American Hampshire	

The acidosis inhibits the uptake of sarcoplasmic Ca^{2+} by the sarcoplasmic reticulum (Greaser *et al.*, 1969), and the elevated Ca^{2+} activates myosin ATPase and hence the rate of ATP hydrolysis. Only extreme muscle activity, such as that produced by electrically stimulating the hot carcass, will produce PSE meat in an otherwise SR pig.

The mechanism that leads to PSE meat formation in SS genotypes is similar to the one just described for exercise and heat stress. The muscle in SS genotypes has a reduced ability to regulate the Ca^{2+} concentration in its sarcoplasm. The sarcoplasmic reticulum and the mitochondria in their muscle are unable to sequester the high levels of Ca^{2+} that are released during post-mortem muscle metabolism. The Ca^{2+} activates ATP breakdown by increasing the activity of myosin ATPase (Quass and Briskey, 1968), and this causes muscle contraction and an early onset of rigor. A characteristic feature of these carcasses is the development of early rigor, which can be seen as early stiffening of the forelegs in the suspended carcass.

At worst, PSE meat looks like a piece of soggy, light-grey blotting paper. Its physical properties are listed in Table 9.3. Its pale colour is caused by the denaturation of soluble muscle proteins when they are subjected to a low pH at high muscle temperatures. If, for any reason, the muscle fails to cool sufficiently before it reaches the critical pH at which the proteins are denatured, then the soluble proteins start to flocculate and they precipitate on to the structural proteins of the muscle. This creates a film of precipitated proteins which are pale in colour and increases the opacity of the meat. Together, these cause the meat to be pale in colour. The critical pH–temperature combinations are shown in Fig. 9.6. PSE meat is also less tender and less juicy and has a less desirable (sour) flavour than normal pork (Jones *et al.*, 1991).

Table 9.3. Properties of PSE (pale soft exudative) and DFD (dark firm dry) meat.

PSE meat		DFD meat	
Properties	Effect	Properties	Effect
Fresh meat		Fresh meat	
Abnormally pale	Customer resistance	Abnormally dark	Customer resistance
High drip loss	Weight loss	Rapid spoilage	Customer rejection
	Poor appearance		
Discoloration during retail display	Customer resistance		
Cooked meat		Cooked meat	
Reduced juiciness	Consumer dissatisfaction	Less weight loss on cooking	Less visible shrinkage
Slightly more chewy or tougher	Consumer dissatisfaction	Tender	Consumer approval

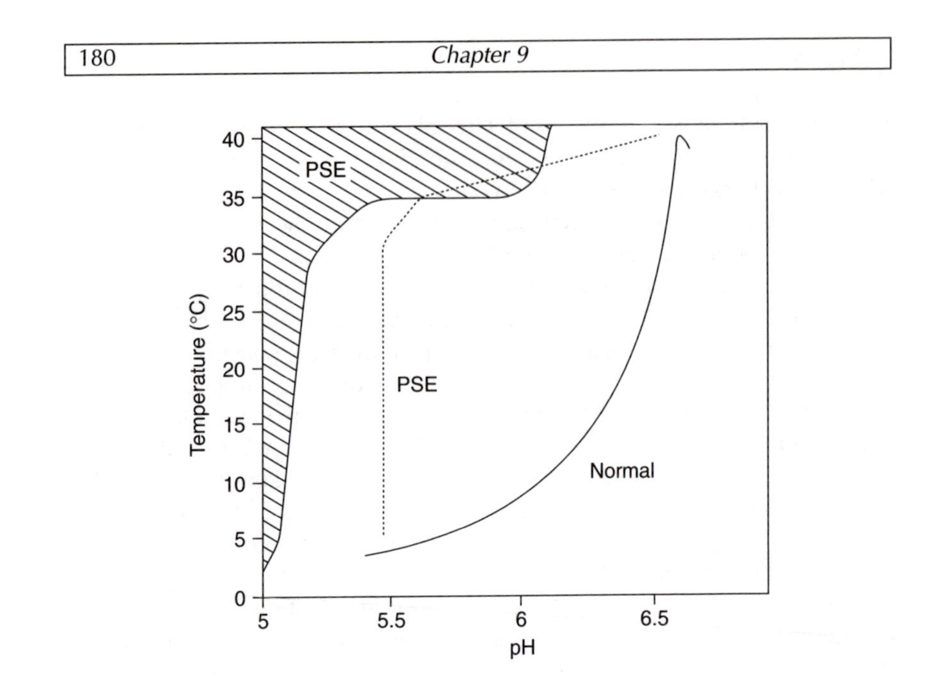

Fig. 9.6. Relationship between pH and temperature in normal (solid line) and PSE (dotted line) meat. If a muscle enters the hatched area during its post-mortem metabolism, it will develop PSE characteristics.

In the past, pig-breeding companies have inadvertently increased the prevalence of PSE meat through an inappropriate breeding policy. They selected pigs for leanness and superior ham conformation and sold them as meat sire lines for crossing with sows to produce a lean slaughter generation. The meat sire lines were developed by including SS breeds such as the Piétrain and Belgian Landrace, which have improved leanness and meaty hams. The aim was to produce lean slaughter pigs as offspring from these sires. The disadvantage with this approach was that it relied on all the offspring being slaughtered. If any offspring were retained for breeding, the semi-lethal SS gene would be distributed in the breeding herds instead of being limited to the sire line and slaughter stock. Stress sensitivity is inherited as a double recessive trait (*nn*). The heterozygote (*Nn*) is less prone to stress-induced deaths and to developing PSE meat after slaughter (Table 9.4) (de Smet *et al.*, 1996). If an *nn* boar from the sire line is crossed with an *Nn* sow, about half the offspring would be expected to produce PSE meat. In this way problems with PSE meat and stress-induced deaths increased.

Another strategy that was used by the pig-breeding companies was to select within the boar line for the halothane reaction. The halothane test picks out pigs that are *nn*. By selecting for this trait, leanness was rapidly improved. The halothane test is based on exposing the pig to the anaesthetic agent, halothane, which is delivered through a face mask. If the

Table 9.4. Effect of genotype and lairage duration on PSE meat characteristics. (From de Smet *et al.*, 1996.)

Genotype	Lairage time (h)	$pH_{40\ min}$ in loin	Colour, L value	Drip loss g kg^{-1}
NN	< 1	6.25 ± 0.04	50.7 ± 0.6	42 ± 4[b]
	2–3	6.27 ± 0.04	50.5 ± 0.5	37 ± 4[bc]
	4–5	6.23 ± 0.04	51.0 ± 0.5	34 ± 4[c]
Nn	< 1	6.03 ± 0.03[b]	51.2 ± 0.4	48 ± 3
	2–3	6.11 ± 0.03[bc]	50.7 ± 0.4	46 ± 3
	4–5	6.15 ± 0.03[c]	51.0 ± 0.4	44 ± 3
nn	< 1	5.69 ± 0.06[b]	56.8 ± 0.8[b]	70 ± 6[b]
	2–3	5.72 ± 0.06[b]	54.7 ± 0.8[c]	60 ± 6[bc]
	4–5	5.88 ± 0.06[c]	53.0 ± 0.8[d]	55 ± 5[c]

[a–d] Means in a column without a common superscript letter were significantly different at $P = 0.05$.

muscles of the pig become stiff and it starts to show rigor, the halothane is quickly removed to prevent the pig from dying; the animal is classified as halothane positive (*nn*), and it could be included in the meat sire line.

Experience showed that the heterozygote (*Nn*) was more prone to developing PSE meat and to death during transport than had originally been suspected. Once this was realized, the selection for *nn* was reversed. Lines that were halothane positive (*nn*) were removed from the sire lines, and leanness was selected by other means. In retrospect, selection for *nn* as a quick way of improving leanness was an irresponsible decision, as it was known beforehand that *nn* is a semi-lethal gene with adverse effects on meat quality.

If SS pigs (*nn*) are mixed in lairage there is a risk that some will die from a stress crisis. Those that survive the mixing stress and are slaughtered in the normal manner can have slightly better meat quality than unmixed SS pigs (Murray and Jones, 1994). This is because muscle glycogen levels are reduced by the exercise during mixing stress and this limits the rate of muscle pH fall. In effect, PSE-prone muscle is turned into DFD. The combinations of genotype and meat quality that can occur in the same animal are shown in Table 9.5.

Feeding pigs in the morning on the day of slaughter can increase the prevalence of PSE meat, especially if they are slaughtered as soon as they arrive at the abattoir (Nielsen, 1981). Giving pigs a rest period of 2–3 hours in the lairage before slaughter helps to reduce PSE meat, and prolonged starvation will also reduce it but at the risk of producing more DFD meat. A provocative way of inducing PSE meat is to subject the pigs to heat stress before slaughter. So, the cardinal rules in overcoming a PSE meat problem are, firstly, to change the breeding in order to eliminate those genotypes that produce the condition. Secondly, avoid heat stress from the sun and

Table 9.5. Links between pig genotype, muscle glycogen and meat quality.

Genotype	Muscle glycogen at slaughter	Meat quality
Stress sensitive[a]	High	PSE
(e.g. Piétrain)	Medium	PSE or normal
	Low	DFD
Stress resistant[b]	High	Normal
(e.g. Large White)	Medium	normal
	Low	DFD

[a] Stress-sensitive pigs are also halothane positive, *nn* for the halothane gene, susceptible to malignant hyperthermia, PSE-prone and susceptible to stress-induced deaths.
[b] Stress-resistant pigs are resistant to these complications and are *NN* for the halothane gene.

from excessive exertion before slaughter. Giving the pigs a cold shower in the lairage can help to reduce PSE meat, provided the shower is cold enough to lower muscle temperature (Long and Tarrant, 1990). In SR pigs it could make the meat darker (Sayre *et al.*, 1961).

In summary, three conditions must exist for a pig to develop PSE meat:

- a genetic predisposition (i.e. SS genotype);
- a triggering factor (e.g. electrical stunning);
- sufficient glycogen in the muscle at the time of slaughter.

It is important to note that PSE meat is not entirely due to ante-mortem factors, as it can be influenced by the way the carcasses are treated after slaughter. The following post-mortem situations can increase the level of PSE meat:

- overscalding;
- electrical stimulation;
- slow chilling.

Chapter 10

Poultry

The main welfare problems in the broiler, turkey and duck industries are:

- leg disorders;
- overstocking;
- breeder stock management;
    - underfeeding;
    - cannibalism;
- inadequate lighting;
- inadequate bird inspection;
- catching and transport;
- stunning and slaughter.

Leg disorders are one of the most common and the most serious welfare problems in poultry (Kestin *et al.*, 1992). In varying degrees they cause pain for the birds, and in some cases they cause wasting, dehydration and death. In the worst cases of lameness the birds have a *Staphylococcus aureus* infection, which they probably acquire through the navel when they are chicks. This results in structural changes in the femur, which becomes weakened, and often the bird is debilitated and growth is reduced. The condition is sometimes called femoral head necrosis, but a more accurate term would be osteomyelitis. In severe forms the bird cannot walk, or it can only walk to the feeders and drinkers by taking a few paces at a time. Typically, between 1 and 5% of a flock may be affected when the birds reach slaughter age. Affected birds should be culled when the flock is inspected each day. In birds that are not culled and survive to slaughter, the weakened femur can affect the quality of the thigh portions that are produced in the portioning line. If the femur breaks during automatic thigh bone removal in the portioning line, part of the femur is left in the meat as a contaminant.

In milder cases of leg disorders, birds may have angulated joints or swollen joints due to accumulation of undifferentiated cartilage at the growth plate of a bone. One of these disorders is tibial dyschondroplasia.

Collectively, these conditions can cause lameness in about 20% of the flock. The birds are often reluctant to walk for long and they have an unsteady, strutting gait. In a proportion of these birds walking is a painful experience, but their growth is not necessarily affected. The angulation of the leg creates problems at the processing plant. Firstly, it makes it difficult to insert the bird properly into the shackle without causing it pain. Secondly, birds are often suspended part of the way down the shackle, and the joints counteract one another to give an inflexible carcass. This makes the carcass more prone to machine damage when it is mechanically plucked.

One way of controlling the development of non-infectious leg disorders is to slow the birds' growth during the second week of life (Classen, 1992). This can be done by giving the birds less feed or by reducing the nutrient density of the feed. This helps to limit weight-bearing during a critical period in their leg growth. Overall efficiency of feed utilization is not necessarily affected as the birds show compensatory growth when the restriction is lifted. Another way of limiting feed intake during this early period is to control the lighting pattern. When the lighting is switched on, birds usually stand up and have a feed. By controlling the frequency with which the lighting comes on and off, feed intake and leg disorders can be reduced.

Another way of controlling leg disorders is to encourage the birds to exercise. This can be done through making them work to get feed and by providing adequate space. Keeping older birds at high stocking densities restricts their movement, and if they take limited exercise they are more prone to developing a poor gait.

Very few broilers are farmed in extensive alternative systems such as the free-range system. Extensive systems provide plenty of space for exercise and they usually allow more opportunity for expressing a wider variety of behaviour patterns. They help to reduce, but not eliminate, leg disorders. When meat quality has been assessed in free-range broilers and standard broilers, there has been no difference in their meat texture or the loss of weight during cooking.

The stocking density used on broiler farms is important in determining flock profitability. Profitability per square metre of floor space reaches a maximum at 40–42 kg m^{-2} (Puron *et al.*, 1995). At these high densities the birds are less active and they are more prone to skin as well as leg disorders. In terms of their behaviour, they walk less but there is more interference between birds. When a bird walks to a feeder or drinker in an overcrowded shed, it is likely to bump into other birds that are squatting on the floor. The squatting birds either stand up and move away, or just move their heads away from the interference whilst they remain sitting (Martrenchar *et al.*, 1997). At high densities the birds that are moving may scratch the squatting birds with their claws. This results in *scabby hips* which form unsightly blemishes in the carcasses and lead to carcass downgrading. As stocking density rises and the birds compete more, feed intake per bird starts to decline (Bolton *et al.*, 1972; Shanawany, 1988). This in turn leads to reduced growth rate per bird. Much of the evidence suggests that growth suppression starts to occur within the stocking density range of 20–29 kg m^{-2}.

Keeping broilers in dim lighting reduces their activity, but it does not necessarily compromise their walking ability. It is often used as a way of limiting the amount of energy they use in taking exercise. Dim lighting is apt to make the birds more flighty when they are taken out of the sheds and experience bright daylight for the first time. Flightiness causes red wingtips and bruising through wing flapping and this leads to downgrading of the carcasses.

As the birds grow, they fill the available space in the shed. As they get taller, they knock against the drinkers which are suspended from the roof. This causes spillage of water on to the litter, making it sticky and the birds dirty, and the moisture encourages bacteria in the litter to produce ammonia, which fouls the atmosphere in the shed. These problems are managed by raising the drinkers as the birds grow, increasing the clearance above the floor. This in turn creates a risk for lame birds and undersized birds, which are unable to reach the drinkers, and some of them may die from dehydration. Those that survive to slaughter and are killed whilst dehydrated have a tough skin and a dry, sticky meat.

Undersized birds should not be presented for slaughter. Their carcasses are of little commercial value and are usually rejected for being too small. In addition, small birds are usually slaughtered without being stunned because they do not reach the water level of the waterbath electric stunner.

The litter in the rearing shed has to be managed as it has some important effects on bird quality. Litter moisture content is mainly controlled by regulating the rate of air flow through the shed. This becomes more difficult at high stocking densities, as the birds form a windproof layer over the litter, which fails to dry. If the birds sit on wet litter they are prone to developing *hock burn* (scab on the hock). In the past, hock burn has been a source of embarrassment for supermarkets in countries where animal welfare pressure groups have complained to the company that by selling carcasses with hock burn it is fostering poor farming standards. The supermarkets have passed complaints on to the processing firm, which in turn has put pressure on the farmers to stop the problem. Hock burn is now less common than it used to be.

Lame birds are more likely to develop hock burn because they spend more time squatting on the litter. Similarly, large lame birds are more likely to develop *breast blisters*, especially on hard floor surfaces. When a bird squats on the floor, 59% of its weight is borne by its keel; if the surface is hard, watery cysts can develop where the keel presses against the floor. They are a cause of carcass downgrading, because they are unsightly. Breast blisters occur below the skin, whereas *breast burns* occur in the skin. These are patches of dead skin tissue over the keel where it has been in contact with wet or badly compacted litter. The corrosive effect of the faeces and urine causes localized burning of the skin, which may become infected through prolonged exposure to wetness. It is more common in males than females and in birds kept at high stocking densities. Less commonly, the follicles in the breast feather tracts become infected, resulting in an unsightly *folliculitis*, which is also a cause of carcass downgrading. All these carcass quality problems are avoided by not overstocking, by managing the broiler shed litter correctly and by avoiding situations that lead to diarrhoea in the birds.

A particularly unpleasant (and no doubt painful) condition in broilers is rupture of the gastrocnemius tendon at the base of the drumstick. This rupture occurs if there is weakening of the tendon and it happens as the bird gets up from a sitting position. A haemorrhage is produced at the site of the rupture. If this is formed several days before the bird goes for slaughter, it changes colour and gives rise to the so-called *greenleg condition.* Affected carcasses are either rejected or downgraded.

Turkeys, broiler breeders and broilers can have an unsightly defect called *green muscle disease* or Oregon disease. It affects the pectoralis minor, sometimes on both sides of the keel. In its early stages the muscle is white or salmon pink but gradually turns green as the muscle atrophies and forms fibrous scar tissue. It is due to ischaemia which leads to necrosis of the whole muscle. The ischaemia develops after an episode of vigorous wing flapping, and heavily muscled breeds are more prone to the condition than lighter breeds. The condition is analogous to human 'march gangrene' seen in the leg muscles of unfit soldiers who go on a forced march.

Modern broiler strains have been bred for growth rate and breast conformation. Compared with broilers of the 1950s, they are faster growing and they convert feed into liveweight more efficiently, but they are more prone to dying early in life as well as developing leg disorders (Havenstein *et al.*, 1994). Some of these strains produce more fat in the carcass, which is not wanted by consumers. *Sudden Death Syndrome* (SDS) is one of the more common causes of early death in these birds after the first week of life. It is due to a ventricular fibrillation in the heart, and high prevalences can be avoided by limiting the birds' feed intake. It is thought that overcrowding of the abdomen with digesta and with a large abdominal fat pad are predisposing causes for the deaths, through a raised intra-abdominal pressure acting on venous return to the heart and on the pumping action of the heart.

Feed should be withheld before the birds are slaughtered, to allow the gut to empty. This should help to reduce the likelihood of gut contents leaking or spilling on to the carcass, but on the down-side it will assist the establishment of *Salmonella* within the caeca (Moran and Bilgili, 1990). A *fasting time* of 16 hours will reduce the overall burden of gut contents in broilers (Papa, 1991). Beyond 16 hours, the rate of loss of intestinal contents is very slow.

The period of feed deprivation should not lead to unnecessary loss of carcass weight. When broilers are fasted their liver glycogen levels can be depleted within 6 hours (Warriss *et al.*, 1988) and from that time onwards they are likely to lose carcass weight. By 24 hours there may be as much as 10% loss in liveweight and a 6% loss of carcass weight. The overall optimum fasting period that allows adequate gut emptying without excessive loss of carcass weight is 10 hours. Where the aim is just to ensure that the birds have empty crops, withholding feed for four hours should be adequate (Summers and Leeson, 1979). When 43-day-old broilers are transported under cool conditions, a liveweight loss of 5 g per hour can be expected (Jensen, 1976). In terms of meat quality, the evidence is somewhat contradictory. When birds are transported for 6 hours or longer, the pH_{ult} of the thigh meat can be raised (Warriss *et al.*, 1993), but other work has shown that the pH_{ult} is normal and, instead, the $pH_{15\ min}$ is lower (Ehinger and Gschwindt, 1981). If the $pH_{15\ min}$ of breast meat is ever 6.5 or higher, the meat is more prone to bacterial growth (Stawicki *et al.*, 1976). Fasting birds for 12 hours or longer can adversely affect tenderness (Scholtyssek *et al.*, 1977).

There is little doubt that birds are stressed when they are caught and loaded into transport crates before slaughter. This has been shown by measuring the plasma corticosterone concentrations in plasma (Fig. 10.1) (Knowles and Broom, 1990). When birds were caught and carried in the normal manner whilst held upside down by the legs, the stress response was greater than that in birds caught and carried gently in an upright position. Catching teams are expected to load birds at a rate of 1000 to 1500

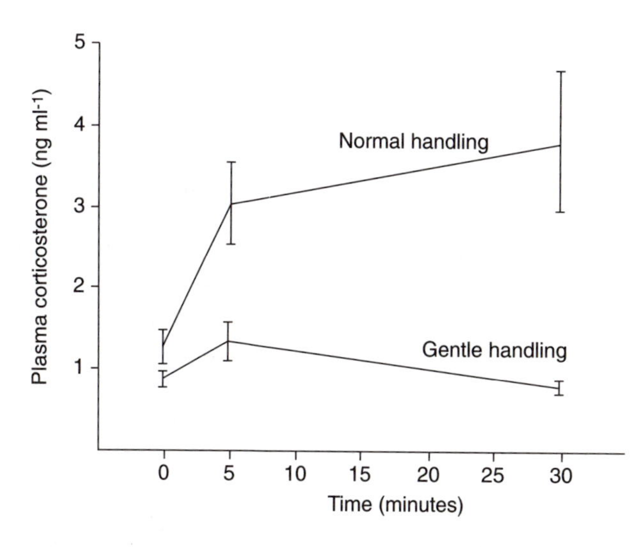

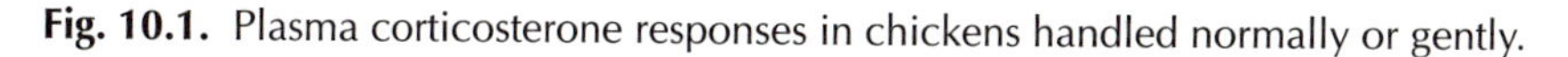
Fig. 10.1. Plasma corticosterone responses in chickens handled normally or gently.

birds per person per hour, and it is inevitable that at these rates there will be some emotional stress in the birds.

During the catching procedure there is also a risk that the birds will damage each other. If the flock gets alarmed the birds migrate towards one end of the shed, where they may pile up on each other and cause backscratching and death from smothering. In the past this has been a problem with ducks and turkeys. It has been controlled by not alarming the birds. The lighting is turned off or kept to a low level and noise is controlled.

The prevalence of *deaths during transport* is low when expressed as a percentage of the birds in a flock (e.g. 0.2%), but high when considered on an absolute basis (e.g 120 birds per processing plant per day). The longer the journey between the farm and the plant, the higher the number of deaths. The number of deaths accelerates with time rather than being constant, which indicates that the condition of the birds deteriorates as the journey progresses.

Some of the causes of death can be identified from post-mortem dissections. In one survey it was found that 47% of deaths were linked to congestive heart failure (CHF) (Gregory and Austin, 1992). It appeared that the stress associated with loading and transport precipitated a heart attack in broilers that had CHF. In its severe form, CHF leads to ascites (waterbelly). Ascitic birds produce carcasses that are not fit for human consumption, but in its milder form the carcasses are edible if the birds arrive at the processing plant alive. Death also occurs from trauma, which accounts for about 35% of the total deaths. In the Gregory and Austin (1992) survey, the main causes of trauma were:

- dislocated or broken hip 76%
- haemorrhage from the liver 11%
- head trauma 8%
- internal haemorrhage (not from the liver) 3%
- other 2%

Hip dislocation occurs as birds are carried in the broiler sheds and loaded into the transport crates. Normally the birds are held by one leg as a bunch of birds in each hand. If one or more birds start flapping they twist at the hip, the femur detaches, and a subcutaneous haemorrhage is produced which kills the bird. This is more common in larger birds and quite often the detached femur is forced into the abdominal cavity, where it ruptures an air sac, allowing blood to enter the lungs. Dead birds that have a dislocated hip often have blood in the mouth, which has been coughed up from the respiratory tract. Sometimes this damage is caused by too much haste on the part of the catchers. For example, one company had a problem with dislocated hips which it stopped by changing to an hourly staff payment system instead of a job completion basis. The incentive to work fast was removed, and hip damage declined.

There are two important forms of ante-mortem *bruising* in poultry; breast bruising and red wingtips. Breast bruising can occur during transport on rough roads and in trucks with inadequate suspension. This would not be a common situation in most countries. It can also occur when heavy birds, especially turkeys, are loaded into the transport crates. If they are thrown in and the breast hits the edge of the transport crate, a breast bruise can develop. Red wingtips can be due to violent flapping when the birds are hung on the line at the processing plant. The location of the bruising is shown in Fig. 10.2, along with other common sites for carcass bruising. Most of the carcass bruising seen in poultry carcasses occurs post-mortem as the birds are being plucked, and the ways in which this occurs are described in more detail in Chapter 14. Wing flapping in the hanging-on area at the processing plant can be controlled by:

- using breast comforters (these are plastic strips that are hung parallel to the line which the birds rub against as they are conveyed to the stunner);
- ensuring that the line runs smoothly and evenly (for example, there should not be any jolts at the joints in the overhead rail);
- dimming the lights and ensuring that there are no sharp contrasts in lighting.

When bruising occurs before slaughter there is a risk that the bruise will carry *Staphylococcus aureus* bacteria. The way in which the contamination occurs is not fully understood. One theory is that proteolytic enzymes in the bruised tissue increase the permeability of the chicken skin and bruised tissue, and this allows entry and penetration of bacteria.

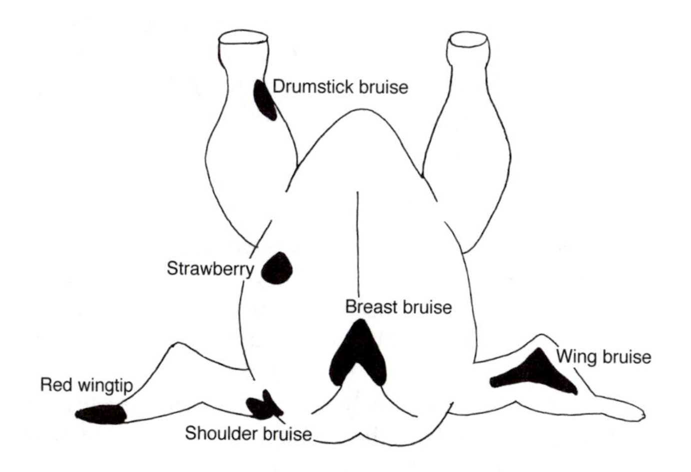

Fig. 10.2. Common sites of bruising in poultry carcasses.

Birds also acquire *broken bones* during preslaughter handling (Gregory and Wilkins, 1992). Crushed skulls can occur when plastic drawers in modules are used as containers for transporting the birds. If a bird's head is sticking up when the drawer is being closed, it gets caught. Other damage can occur in the trunk of the body. In one study the prevalence of broken bones in broilers that arrived live at the processing plant and had been hung on to the shackles of the killing line was 3%. From the processor's perspective this is a loss, because of the haemorrhaging associated with the fractures. In terms of bone fragments contaminating the final product, this cause is trivial in comparison with the fractures that develop during processing. By the time the carcasses reach the end of the processing line, 96% have broken bones with on average three broken bones per carcass.

Broken bones in the live bird is a serious welfare problem in end-of-lay battery hens when they are sent for slaughter. The hens' bones are particularly fragile because of the long period they spend without exercise and because of the high demands on bone calcium for eggshell formation.

Emotional and *temperature stress* are not easy to recognize in crated birds on a truck, and so it is useful to consider the environmental conditions as well as the state and behaviour of the birds. From a welfare point of view the optimum temperature for slaughterweight chickens that are reared in temperate climates is 22–24°C. Prolonged temperatures above 38°C are dangerous. Normally the rectal temperature is 41°C but when it exceeds 42.5°C the birds begin to pant. Beyond 45°C panting declines and may cease altogether, so as to conserve body water. Besides panting, the other means of losing heat are vasodilation in the shanks and comb, increasing the body surface area to encourage convective heat loss and drinking large amounts of water. By taking cold water into the crop, the base of the neck is cooled and this helps to lower the temperature of the blood in the carotid arteries which supply the brain. As birds do not have access to any water once they leave the farm, they no longer have this means of keeping their heads cool. Panting and vasodilation are the only cooling mechanisms available to crated birds, but the heat exchange through panting can be compromised if the humidity is high (greater than 70% relative humidity). In tropical climates it is advisable to transport the birds during the cooler periods of the day, and tall crates should be used which allow air movement over the birds' heads. If the crates are stacked on top of each other they should be spaced on the truck in rows with wide aisles. The object is to allow adequate airflow over and around the birds (in particular around their heads) to encourage convective and evaporative cooling. There is bound to be some sacrifice in the weight of birds that can be carried when wide crate spacing is used, but this will be offset by a lower mortality.

At the other extreme, the lower critical temperature for chickens is about 16°C. This corresponds to the ambient temperature at which a bird will increase its rate of heat production in order to maintain body temperature. The lower lethal body temperature, at which 50% of a truck load would be expected to die, is between 19°C and 24°C. The only obvious sign of cold stress in crated birds is feather erection. In countries with a cold climate such as Finland, birds are transported during the winter in insulated, mechanically ventilated vehicles. Whatever the climate, whether it be hot, temperate or cold, it is advisable to alter the stocking density in the crates according to the anticipated weather conditions. A more common approach is to raise or lower curtains which hang from the sides of the truck, according to the weather. These help to control air movement, and in general when they are lowered the lower modules are likely to be warmest, and when they are raised the upper modules are warmest.

In some countries it is a legal requirement that the birds are protected from all adverse weather. Cold stress is aggravated considerably if the birds are wet, because additional heat is lost through evaporation of the water. Besides protecting the birds from rain, it can be important to ensure that the crates are reasonably dry and in particular that they are free of ice before the birds are loaded.

In most situations birds are removed from the transport crates by hand when they are hung on to the shackles at the processing plant. Automatic *unloading* is used at some plants: the module is tipped and the birds slide out, on to a conveyor which takes them to a turntable where staff pick them up and place them in the shackles. When the birds are tipped out of the modules they all start flapping. This is a natural response in a bird which is either losing its balance or falling. Wing flapping causes bruising and carcass downgrading from red wingtips. In other systems the transport crates are withdrawn from the module and conveyed to the hanging-on area. Some crates have perforated floors. This assists cooling but it also means that some birds (about 3%) have their claws or toes sheared off as the drawers are pulled out of the modules. Their toes protrude through the holes in the perforated floor and are sheared at the rim of the module.

In broilers there is considerable variation in the thickness of the birds' shanks, particularly between males and females. The size of the gap in the shackle where the bird's leg is held also varies (range between plants is about 0.95–1.4 cm), but in general there is greater variation in the birds. This means that birds with thick shanks require more force when inserting their legs into the shackles. Compression of the periosteum of the bone in this situation is potentially painful for the birds. Evidence which supports this is as follows. The average force applied on the chicken's leg during *shackling* is about 90 N. A force of 75 N applied to the shank is sufficient to cause a rise in heart rate in a chicken, and that response is prevented if a local anaesthetic is applied to the legs. Evidently 75 N is painful, and this is less than the normal shackling force. The tightness of the shackle is important in two other respects. Firstly, the fit should be sufficiently tight to ensure good electrical contact between the shackle and the bird (when using constant voltage stunners), otherwise there is a risk of inadequate current flow. Secondly, the grip must ensure that the bird does not become dislodged from the shackle during plucking. Clearly, there is a compromise between the need to provide a low electrical resistance at the shackle electrode, thus ensuring an adequate stun, and not hurting the bird through compression of the shank. Some broiler plants and many turkey plants use shackles which have a choice of gap widths for birds of different shank thicknesses. At bigger plants it may be possible to provide different shackles for the males if they are killed on a separate line from the females.

Besides being potentially painful, it is likely that suspending a bird upside down from a shackle causes it some distress. For this reason it is advisable to minimize the time between shackling and stunning. However, it is also important that the wing flapping that occurs at shackling has subsided by the time the birds reach the waterbath. Survey work has shown that the minumum hang-on period which allows activity to subside is 12 seconds for broilers and 25 seconds for turkeys.

If the birds are stressed before slaughter and this causes depletion of their muscle glycogen, the meat is likely to be more tender. The greater tenderization is probably due to the high pH of the meat allowing greater enzymatic breakdown of the myofibrillar proteins in the meat fibres (Etherington *et al.*, 1990). If, on the other hand, the birds struggle and flap their wings excessively just before they are killed, this will cause a build-up of lactic acid in the breast muscle and the meat is likely to be tough. In this situation the muscle is not glycogen depleted. Instead, it becomes acidic whilst it is still hot. The relationship which reflects this effect is shown in Fig. 10.3 (Khan and Nakamura, 1970). As the lactic acid content in the muscle at the time of slaughter increases, so also does meat toughness 24 hours later. The increased toughness is due to more extensive muscle contraction during rigor development, and this effect is temperature dependent. The higher the temperature as the muscle goes into rigor, the stronger will be the contraction. This is known as *heat shortening*. The relationship between muscle temperature and the degree of shortening in breast and thigh meat is shown in Fig. 10.4. Two incidental points arise from this figure. Firstly, breast meat is more prone to heat shortening than thigh meat; and secondly, broiler meat is not prone to cold shortening. Cold shortening has been induced experimentally in chicken but it is not common in practice.

Meat toughness due to heat shortening has also been observed in broilers that have been heat stressed before slaughter, and in birds that convulsed violently as they died because they were not stunned before neck cutting. Breast meat from heat-stressed broilers is also prone to producing more drip after filleting (Northcutt *et al.*, 1994). In turkeys, it is likely to be paler as well as having a lower water-holding capacity. The paleness is due to a higher reflectance, and the meat is less red probably because the haem pigments are denatured by the high temperature–acid conditions. This type of turkey meat is similar to PSE meat in pork. In general, toughness in heat-shortened poultry meat does not resolve when the meat is left to age for 48 hours.

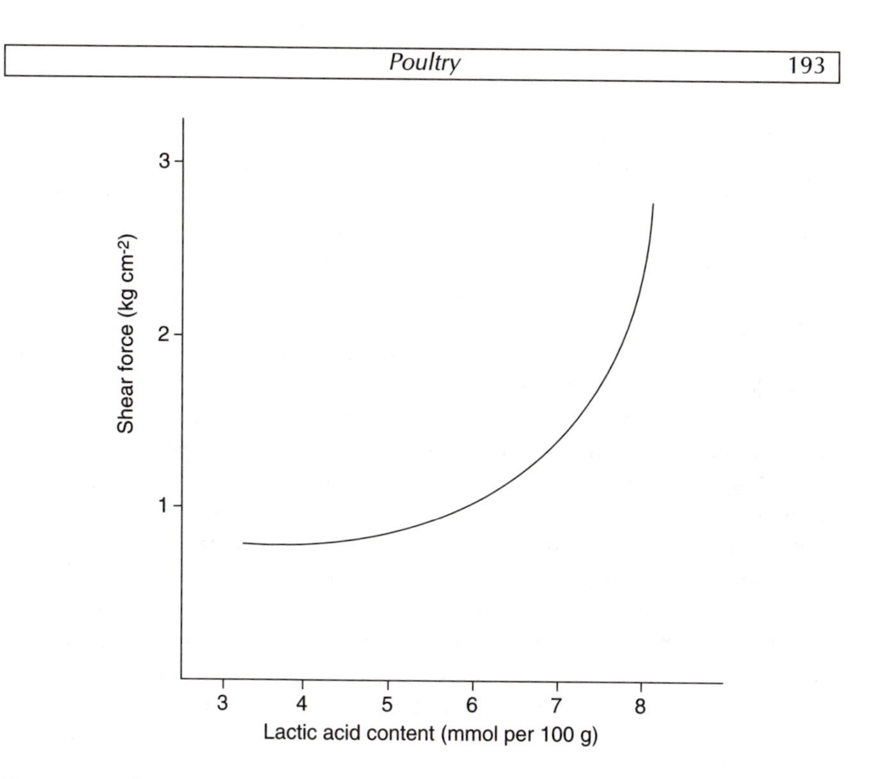

Fig. 10.3. Relationship between lactic acid content of chicken breast muscle immediately after death and shear force after 24 h ageing.

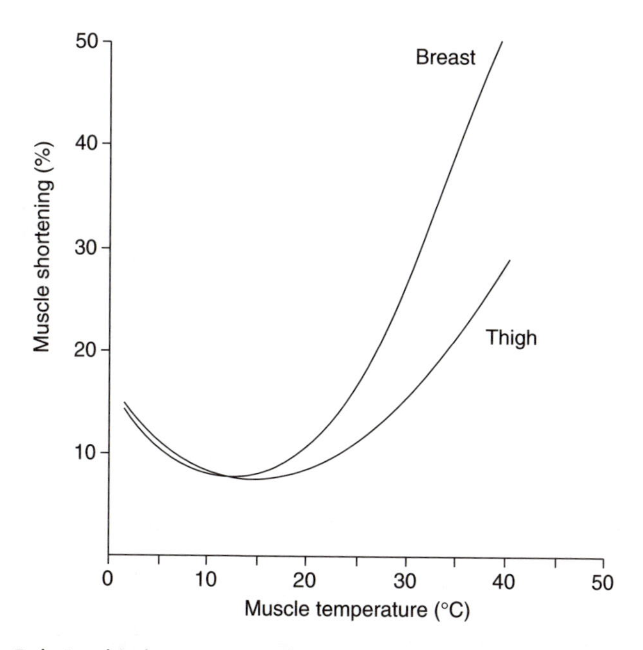

Fig. 10.4. Relationship between muscle temperature and muscle shortening in chicken breast and thigh.

The way birds are treated before slaughter can also influence the force required to pluck their carcasses. Normally, efficient *plucking* is achieved by scalding the carcass, which reduces the force required to remove the feathers, and by ensuring that the presentation of the plucking machine to the carcass allows good coverage and contact between the plucker fingers and the feathers. It is widely accepted in the poultry processing industry that the birds will be more difficult to pluck if they experience cold weather before they are slaughtered. Part of this effect could be due to cold birds entering the scalder and lowering the temperature of the water, and part of it could be due to residual activity in the sympathetic nervous system, which would cause tightening of the smooth muscle in the skin that grips the feather shaft. The role of the sympathetic nervous system was demonstrated by pretreating chickens with reserpine, which causes depletion of noradrenaline in the sympathetic nerve endings, and this allowed the feathers to be removed from the live bird with less force (Knapp and Newell, 1961). In practice, increasing the force of the plucker or raising the temperature of the scaldwater are the most appropriate options, provided they do not damage the carcass or cook the breast meat. Excessive exercise stress before slaughter can also make feather removal harder, as can fasting the birds for longer than 8 hours.

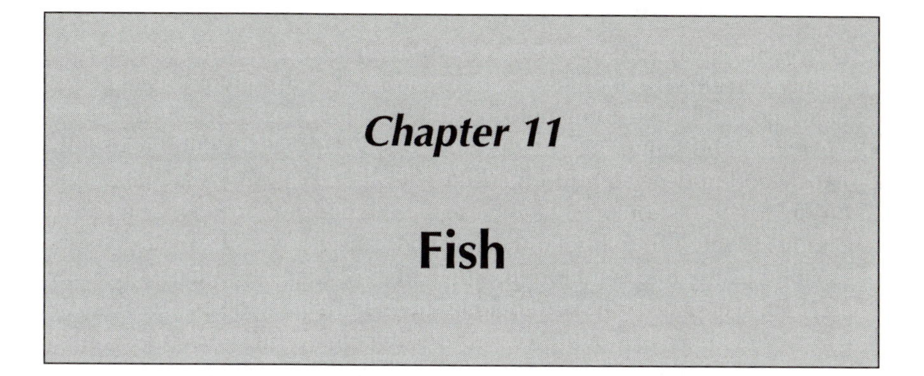

Chapter 11

Fish

MARINE FISH

The methods used for catching and killing fish affect their scales, skin and the quality of the meat. Fish are capable of experiencing pain and so any damage that occurs during fishing is important to welfare as well as causing food wastage. With some methods there is also wastage from harvesting by-catch (unwanted and underutilized species), and in some sectors of the fishing industry, such as shrimp fishing in the tropics, only a small proportion of the catch (10–30%) may be used. The discarding of unwanted by-catch is an ethical dilemma which will be confronting the fishing industry more in the future.

The fishing methods that will be considered in this chapter have been described by Sainsbury (1971) and are grouped as: trawling; purse seining; gillnetting; longlining; trolling; pole-and-line fishing; harpooning; jigging lines; angling.

- In bottom otter *trawling* a large bag-shaped net is drawn along the seabed to scoop up fish on or near the bottom. The net has a wide open mouth and tapers to a quick-release closed end (cod-end). Wings extend from the mouth, increasing the area swept by the net, and they guide the fish towards the mouth. The wings are held outwards by otter boards, and opposing floats and weights keep the mouth of the bag open.
- In *purse seining* a long net is set around a school of fish, the top of the net usually being at the water's surface. When the school is encircled, the bottom is pulled together to create an artificial enclosure which holds the catch. By drawing in the top lines the purse is made smaller until the fish are gathered alongside the vessel. The catch is removed from the net either with a fish pump or with a net winch, or by brailing with a scoop net.
- The *gillnet* relies on fish swimming into a stationary net and becoming

trapped by the gills and operculum as they try to swim through. In some versions there are several layers of net with different mesh sizes and the fish become entangled (tangle nets).

- *Longline* and gillnet fishing are done with static gear which is usually anchored underwater and marked with buoys. With longlines, a line (often up to 60 km long) fitted with short lengths of line carrying baited hooks is set. The fish take the bait, become hooked and are brought aboard as the line is taken up. The length of time that a fish is held by a hook depends on how frequently the gear is hauled up.
- In *trolling* a slow-moving vessel tows weighted lines, each bearing a number of lures or baited hooks. The fish snap at the lures and after hooking themselves they are hauled in. The hooking of a fish is detected by a jerk at the outrigger. In some systems the fish are gaffed to bring them aboard.
- *Pole-and-line fishing* is arguably one of the most humane methods of catching a fish. When a school of fish is located they are brought to a feeding frenzy by scattering bait over the side of the vessel. A gang of pole fishermen, or mechanical poles, cast their lines and the fish snap at the splash of the hooks. On striking, the fisherman swings a fish on to the deck behind, and as the hook is barbless the fish disengages at the end of the swing and slides to a collecting area.
- *Harpooning* has been used for large species such as swordfish. When the fish is struck and the harpoon takes hold, the fish is allowed to run until it tires itself out. It is then snubbed, secured in a sling and hoisted aboard.
- *Jigging lines* are used in squid fisheries in Asia. Incandescent lamps are hung over the side of the vessel to attract the squid. The vessel is stabilized to dampen pitching, thus minimizing fouling of the fishing lines. The lines are weighted; they have coloured plastic lures with hooks and they are wound on to elliptical reels, so that when a line is wound in automatically it has a jerking or jigging motion. The squid attack the lures and hook themselves. With multiple jigging lines and strategically placed hand jigging lines, the squid can be brought into a feeding frenzy which greatly increases the catch.
- In *angling* the fish are caught individually with a rod and line. The fish may be played whilst reeling in as part of a sporting contest for the enjoyment of the fisherman.

Catching fish in a trawl net depends on guiding them to the mouth of the net, and then exhausting and overrunning them as the net is towed forwards. The fish are guided towards the mouth of the net in two ways. The bridle wires which stretch between the wings and the otter boards guide the fish towards the centre path of the net, and the wings of the net act as a funnel (Fig. 11.1). The bridle wires are set at an angle to the towing path. As they move they create the illusion for the fish positioned on the nearside

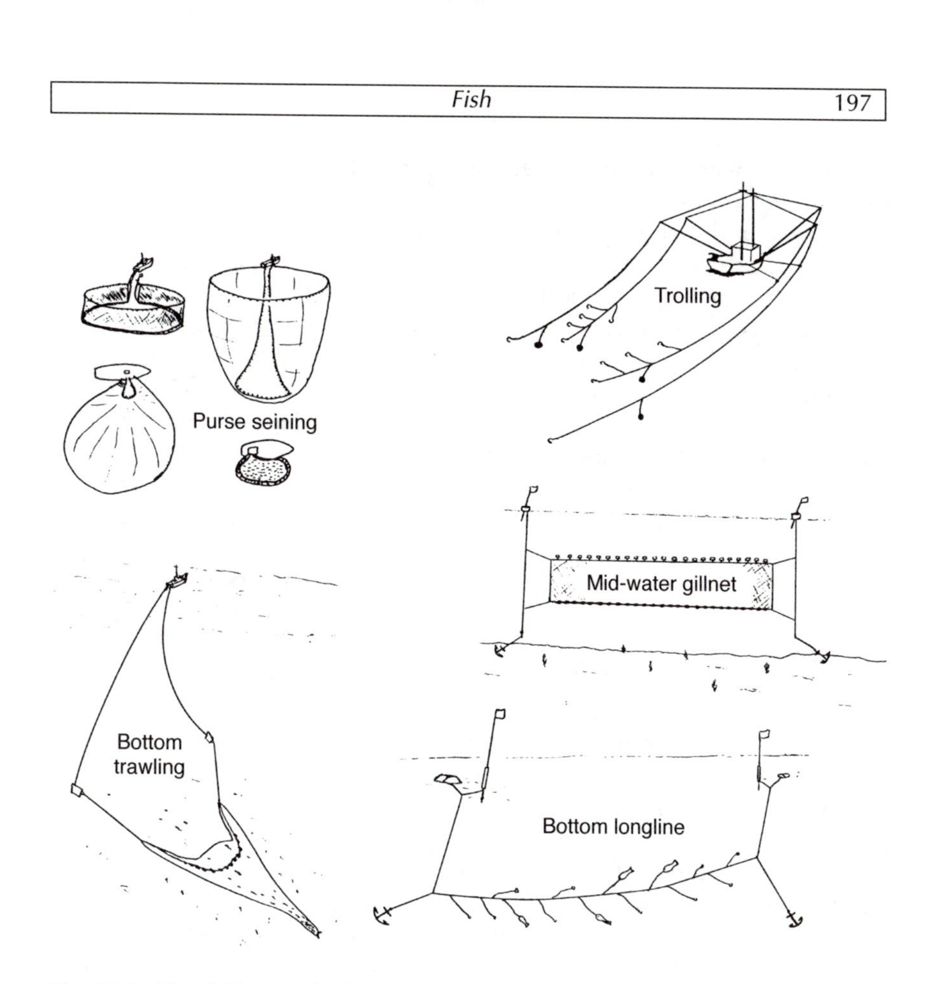

Fig. 11.1. Five fishing methods.

of a bridle that the wire is moving towards them. This makes the fish manoeuvre away from the wire and towards the central axis of the net.

Underwater filming of bottom *trawling* has shown that the fish swim in front of the mouth of the trawl net; as they tire they slow down, rise up from the seabed and enter the body of the net. Overrunning the fish depends on outlasting its stamina. Normally cod and haddock can swim for long periods, relying mainly on their dark muscle, when swimming at speeds which are up to twice their own body length per second. For a 50 cm fish this is up to 2 knots. Above that speed, the staying power or endurance is quite short. The 50 cm fish can sustain a speed greater than 2 knots for a distance equal to only about 500 body lengths (250 m). At these faster speeds a fish relies on its anaerobic muscle system, which is powered by a limited reserve of glycogen. Endurance is limited by the supply of glycogen, and the time taken before a fish tires varies considerably with species. When the towing speed is 3 knots, haddock swim for no more than

2.5 minutes, whereas pollack keep going for about 15 minutes. Mackerel often speed up and swim out of the net. Larger fish can sustain faster speeds and at the end of a tow those at the front of the mouth of the net swim away as the net slows down. A burst of faster towing speed towards the end of a tow helps to put these fish into the cod-end.

As the fish pass down the trawl net they come to a position where the net tapers to a funnel. At this point they become constricted and they start to panic. They swim with fast tail beating, and an erratic flick–glide action, often striking the net and colliding with each other whilst trying to maintain a position ahead of the funnel. Eventually the net overtakes them and they pass down to the cod-end whilst scraping and bumping against the net. By the time they reach the cod-end they have acquired skin and scale damage. As the cod-end fills with more fish there is an increase in turbulence within the net. This can cause the cod-end to twist on itself. After two or three such revolutions in the same direction, the entrance of the cod-end is sealed off and the fish become compressed. The compression causes additional skin and scale damage. After a time the net will untwist itself and return to its normal position.

Some of the fish die within the cod-end from compression. Death presumably occurs from compression of the opercula (gill covers) against the net and from adjacent fish preventing breathing movements of the gills. The fish asphyxiate. Another possible cause of death in a minority of fish is failure in venous return to the heart due to pressure on the body at particular points. This would lead to reduced cardiac output and perfusion of the brain. The proportion of fish that are dead by the time they are hoisted on board varies considerably, according to the size of the catch and the duration of the tow. The longer the towing period, the more likely it is that they will be dead; for example, in one study a 2-hour trawl was associated with 29% mortality on raising the net whereas a 4-hour trawl resulted in 61% mortality (Hattula *et al.*, 1995). High pressures are exerted on the fish when the nets are hoisted out of the water and this can cause intestinal contents to be expelled. These need to be washed off before the fish are packed and stowed.

Regulations govern the mesh size of the cod-ends of the trawl nets. These aim at allowing undersized fish to escape and hopefully survive. Smaller fish usually escape through the upper part of the cod-end, immediately in front of the bulk of the catch, but not all of them survive. Mortality amongst escapees from a herring trawl during the first 7 days following escape has varied between 30% and 72%. Small fish are more prone to dying after escape (Suuronen *et al.*, 1996), and herring are probably more prone to dying than other species such as snapper. Death is thought to develop from skin injuries inflicted when the fish are in the net and from exhaustion.

In *seine netting* the fish are encircled and herded by ropes and a net at a relatively slow speed so as not to alarm the fish. The vessel then speeds up to 2–3 knots to outpace the fish as the circle is completed. In seine fishing the towing speeds are slower and so seine-caught fish often have less skin and scale damage than trawled fish. Monofilament *gillnets* cause considerable damage to skin and scales. As the fish struggle, the net material cuts through the skin and the net scuffs the surface of the skin. When the gillnet and fish are hauled in, the weight of the net does additional damage to the snared fish as they pass over a roller guide. As the fish and net land on the deck the fish are unmeshed and, in the case of shark, the fish may be bled by cutting the throat. In some shark species delayed bleeding after death affects their quality through the accumulation of urea and ammonia in the flesh. Using nets with knotless mesh, and retrieving the nets at short intervals, helps to minimize skin and scale damage during gillnet fishing. On some vessels a crew member may stand alongside the net roller to make sure that any fish that are not properly meshed do not escape. The loosely attached fish are gaffed with a handheld hook, and this causes additional damage to the product.

Net fishing causes more *skin and scale damage* than line fishing. This affects quality in two ways. Fish skin is normally covered with a layer of mucus which acts as a water-repellent and as a barrier to bacteria and other pathogens. Skin and scale damage allows easier entry of bacteria into the flesh, which increases the risk of spoilage and off-odours, and it detracts from the appearance of the fish, spoiling its marketability. During *troll fishing* some species tend to roll and become entangled in the troll lines whilst they are towed by the hook and line. This is not particularly common, but when it occurs it causes skin and scale damage.

Depending on how the fish is hooked, trolling can be very stressful for the fish. Table 11.1 shows the results from three vessels which were trolling for chinook salmon off Alaska in 1987 (Wertheimer *et al.*, 1989). The

Table 11.1. Parts of the fish that were hooked, and the hooking mortality, in 913 trolled salmon.

Parts hooked	Proportion of catch (%)	Proportion dying immediately (%)	Proportion dying within 4–6 days (%)
Corner of mouth	23	1	6
Eye	23	3	18
Lower jaw	15	2	10
Isthmus	12	4	31
Cheek	9	4	12
Upper jaw	8	1	7
Snout	6	0	5
Gills	4	30	55

majority of the fish were hooked in or around their mouths, and a further 23% were hooked through an eye. Only 3% of the fish were dead when they were unhooked on the vessel, and most of these were hooked by the gills. In this study the fish that were alive were unhooked and held live in sea pens; 16% of them died within 4–6 days. Those that had been hooked by the gills, isthmus or eye had a reduced chance of survival. These results are important for two reasons. Firstly, they show which parts of the fish are particularly sensitive to hook trauma in terms of fish survival, and they indicate the likely *capture mortality* in fish that are released instead of being used for meat consumption. In fish, blood passes from the heart to the brain via the gills. If a fish is hooked by the gills and this interferes with blood flow to the brain, unconsciousness and death could be rapid. However, entanglement or hooking in the gills could be irritating as this region is sensitive to physical stimulation by even fine foreign objects such as weed.

The world's marine fish reserves have fallen dramatically during the 20th century. This is now being addressed by limiting the by-catch, by defining the size of target fish that can be taken and by setting quotas for particular species. These are prescribed either as legal requirements or as voluntary undertakings by the fisheries. In purse seine fishing, part or all of the catch may be slipped (released) if the average size in a catch is too small or if the total catch is too large for what is required. In some fisheries there are regulations that limit either the number and tonnage of fish that can be landed, or the length of the fishing season, or the size of each fish that can be marketed. Fish smaller than the legal size have to be returned to the ocean. These regulations and recommendations are based on the assumption that most fish that are returned will survive. In salmon troll fisheries, mortality during the first 4–6 days after being fished is 18% in undersized fish that are returned to the water, and most of these deaths occur within 24 hours. Where trials have been done on the survival of fish that were caught by trolling or angling, mortality has been related to the severity of the exercise stress. Those fish that died during the recuperation period were the ones which developed the highest lactate levels. When muskellunge were caught by angling and then released, 30% died after release. Those that died within 6 hours developed a severe acidosis and rises in plasma potassium levels. When salmon were caught by angling, the pH in the white muscle fell from 7.46 to 6.80. The struggle associated with playing the fish caused near depletion of muscle creatine phosphate and glycogen, and a marked reduction in ATP. Muscle lactate levels rose from about 1 $\mu mol\ g^{-1}$ to 37 $\mu mol\ g^{-1}$, but plasma lactate showed only a small rise.

During angling, carp show the following behaviours once they are hooked: rapid darting movements; coughing and spitting; head shaking; fleeing; belching gas from the swim bladder; sinking; and lying on the bed of the tank. If, after hooking, the line is payed out and there is no line tension, the fish do not show escape behaviour. Instead, the main behaviours are coughing or spitting and head shaking, and they resume feeding within a few minutes. This implies that playing the fish is more aversive than hooking the mouth.

Two types of *livebaiting* are used in commercial hook-and-line fishing. Chumming is used for pelagic (near-surface) species which need to be brought together or set into a feeding frenzy. The livebait is thrown into the water, usually alongside the vessel. Typically the livebait remains motionless for several seconds upon hitting the water, and then it swims underneath the hull for protection. This brings the predatory fish nearer to the vessel, where they are taken with hook and lure. After the initial catch the vessel is eased forward to flush out the livebait from under the hull and a second catch follows. The choice of livebait species is important. In pole-and-line fishing a species that jumps when attacked is better than one that dives. The other type of livebaiting is attaching a live fish to a hook to draw the target species. This method is commonly used in longline fishing and it has been condemned by some welfare protagonists. In the past the chief practical disadvantage has been the time involved in attaching the livebait to the hooks. This has been overcome with a semi-automatic machine which attaches the live fish as the line is payed out.

Bruising and mechanical damage occur in fish when they are pumped automatically from seine nets or from tanks, cages or ponds. Three types of *fish pump* are used: vacuum (and venturi), centrifugal (and turbine), and Archimedean screw pumps. Transferring fish by turbine pump or brailing with a lift net causes more skin abrasions than using a vacuum pump (Grizzle *et al.*, 1992). Vacuum and turbine pumps cause more broken dorsal and pectoral fins than lift nets.

Most fishing methods impose physiological and physical *stress* on the fish. When marine fish are caught by net or line they often show pronounced increases in plasma catecholamines, p_aCO_2, lactate, K^+, Na^+, creatine phosphokinase and cortisol. For example, adrenaline, which is released from chromaffin tissue near the kidney, increases from less than 0.15 nM to 36 nM in the plasma when ludderick are gillnetted, and it can exceed 300 nM in blue mao mao which are caught and played on a line for about 10 minutes (Lowe and Wells, 1996). Adrenaline and physical activity both promote glycogen breakdown and the formation of acid as H^+ in muscle. Much of the acid is produced in a fish's white muscle, and fish are capable of producing high levels of lactate in this muscle when exercise stressed. The protons that accompany lactate production in muscle are potentially harmful, and fish need to protect themselves with a buffering mechanism. This is provided by the imidazole group of L-hisitidine. Histidine, and its related derivative anserine, buffers the muscle by absorbing the protons. Anserine acts as a store of histidine which is made available during periods of activity. Athletic species such as tuna and marlin have large quantities of anserine in their white muscle.

Fish also have to protect themselves against the osmotic forces of their environment. The osmolarity of fish plasma is typically 300–400 mOsm per litre, whereas seawater has an osmolarity of 1000 mOsm. Marine fish expend energy in maintaining their body fluids in a hypotonic condition relative to the environment. This energy expenditure accounts for 15–20% of the fish's basal metabolic rate. When energy substrates are chanelled towards other functions, as occurs when fish are stressed, osmotic homeostasis may be lost; the fish lose body water and hence weight. Several mechanisms are involved in this weight loss. Normally, marine fish counteract the diffusion of water from body fluids to the hypertonic seawater medium by swallowing seawater and extracting the water component through the gut. Monovalent ions, principally Na^+ and Cl^-, are absorbed with the water. Excess chloride is excreted by the gills and sodium is exchanged across the gills in return for potassium. When fish are stressed, the release of adrenaline leads to constriction of intestinal sphincters, causing a prompt decrease in water uptake by the gut. At the same time adrenergic receptors in the gills are activated which inhibit chloride excretion and Na^+–K^+ exchange at the gills. Water loss occurs across the gills through osmosis and, as this is not adequately replaced by water absorption through the gut, weight loss follows. Freshwater fish experience similar problems but the osmotic gradient is in the opposite direction. The osmoregulatory disturbance created by hooking stress in freshwater rainbow trout is greatest at about 2–4 hours after the fish has been hooked and played, and it is exaggerated at high water temperatures. In marine fish which are caught and sold live, these osmotic stresses can be countered by lowering the salinity of the water in the holding tanks. In freshwater fish the salinity should be raised slightly. Adjusting the osmolarity of the water may help to reduce mortality in some species.

The loss of osmotic homeostasis during exercise stress can be lethal. Exercise to exhaustion for as little as 6 minutes has been known to kill 40% of trout (Wood *et al.*, 1983). Death is not necessarily immediate. Typically, the fish lose balance 1–2 hours prior to death by rolling on to their backs, and their ventilation becomes rapid and shallow. Ventilation ceases before they develop a cardiac arrest. Another situation where stress is associated with suppressed respiration is tonic immobility. Some species go into an inactive catatonic state with subdued breathing movements when they are captured and restrained (Davie *et al.*, 1993). In practice this reaction makes them easy to restrain and handle, especially for livebaiting.

Successful capture by trawling, harpooning and angling depends on exhausting the fish as they are caught. Gillnetting, longlining, trolling and some types of pole-and-line fishing also cause exhaustion through the high levels of activity and excitement. With all these methods the white muscle in the fish is almost depleted of glycogen by the time the fish is captured. The muscle may not be particularly acid, but it has high lactate levels. In fish, most of the lactate that is produced from glycogen is retained in the muscle during a stressful episode, and it is eventually metabolized to CO_2

or back to glycogen. The H^+ produced with the lactate is released into the blood for excretion by the gills. For these reasons, in some species blood pH is more likely to reflect exercise stress than blood lactate.

Fish that are stressed during trawling develop high levels of glucose-6-phosphate and fructose-1,6-diphosphate in their meat in comparison with unstressed fish. This can influence the *colour* of the meat. Brown colours form as a result of Maillard reactions between these compounds and amino groups during cooking. Dehydrated and dry-salted fish are particularly prone to these reactions, which can be prevented either by the addition of sodium bisulphite or by soaking the meat in water before cooking.

If fish continuously exercise for several weeks before they are caught and killed, the haem pigments in the dark muscle are likely to be enriched. In particular the myoglobin levels are higher and the meat is darker in colour. This may detract from the fishes' value if the market expects a white meat.

The normal pH_{ult} of fishmeat is higher than in other meat species, and its exact value varies with species. In haddock it is between 6.3 and 6.6, whereas in cod it varies according to season, from 5.9 to 6.9. The pH is lowest in summer, when the cod are feeding well, and it is highest in winter. One of the reasons the pH_{ult} is high in fish is that muscle glycogen is broken down by amylolysis besides producing lactic acid, and in some species lactic acid production is lower. In amylolysis, glycogen is broken down to maltose and then glucose. The intermediate and final products in amylolysis are sweeter than those in the glycogenolytic pathway, and so fishmeat tends to taste sweeter than other meats (Tarr, 1966).

Fish flavour can be influenced by the metabolism of nucleotides in the meat. During the early stages of storage, AMP is deaminated to inosinic acid (IMP), which has the beneficial effect of intensifying the flavour of other compounds. As the fish ages further, IMP is converted to inosine, which is flavourless and has no flavour-enhancing properties. Later still, inosine is broken down to ribose and hypoxanthine, and hypoxanthine has a bitter flavour. The production of hypoxanthine is probably the reason for the bitterness that occurs in cod that is held for long periods after death. There is no reason to suppose that the levels of IMP are influenced by catching stress; there were no differences when IMP levels were compared in herring caught by trawling, gillnetting and trapnetting.

Gaping is one of the most common quality problems with filleted fish (Love, 1988). It occurs when adjacent myotomes (muscle blocks) separate from each other. Gaps are created within the meat and the fillet is likely to fall to pieces. Gaping makes it difficult to skin the fish without breaking it, especially when using skinning machines. It also makes thin slicing of cured meats such as smoked salmon more difficult. The most effective ways of countering gaping and disintegration of a fish during cooking are either to cook it with the skin on or to coat it with a binder (e.g. batter) which holds the fillet together.

Several factors cause fish fillets to gape. One is weakening of the binding between the mycommata (connective tissue) and muscle fibres; the mycommata help to hold adjacent myotomes together. The other is excessive tension during rigor, which causes adjacent myotomes to shrink and the muscle tears itself to pieces. The likelihood of gaping is increased if the freshly caught fish is allowed to warm up in the sun whilst on the deck. In the case of cod, the muscle temperature has to increase above 17°C, and for trout 26°C, before gaping is more likely to occur. The higher temperatures have two effects: they increase muscle contraction as rigor sets in, and they reduce the strength of the mycommata. Heat-treated fishmeat that develops gaping also tends to be tough and it loses fluid. An important practical recommendation is to chill fish rapidly in order to avoid gaping.

Gaping is not likely to occur in meat from stressed fish. Fish that are severely stressed during catching have low levels of muscle glycogen and ATP and so they will have insufficient energy to permit the vigorous contraction that causes the myotomes to tear apart. Only fishmeat that is destined to have a low or intermediate pH_{ult} has sufficient energy to experience this severe form of contraction, and because of this there is a negative relationship between gaping and pH_{ult} (Fig. 11.2). Part of this relationship is also due to a direct effect of pH on the strength of the mycommata. Under acid conditions the connective tissue in the mycommata is physically weaker and the meat is more prone to developing gaping (Love *et al.*, 1974).

In cod and farmed salmon the prevalence of gaping varies with season. It is more common in the warmer months. This can be due to inadequate chilling of the meat, but more frequently it is because the fish are eating more and their muscle glycogen and ATP levels are higher. This allows a stronger contraction during rigor and creates the acid conditions that cause weakening of the mycommata.

The seasonal variation in pH in cod also explains the seasonal variation in its *mushiness.* During early winter and spring, when the fish are starving

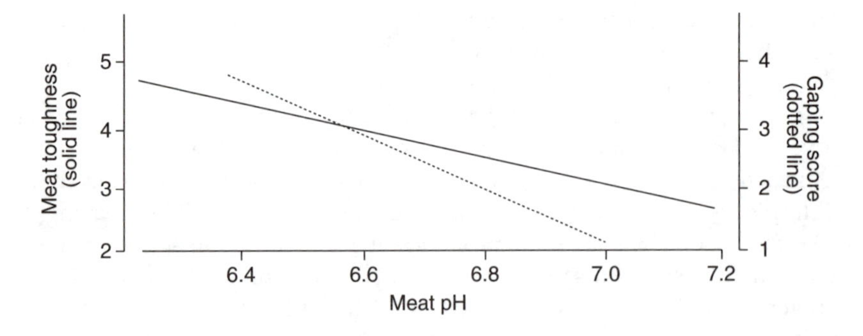

Fig. 11.2. Relationships between meat pH, toughness and gaping.

and the pH is high, the meat has a higher water-holding capacity and moisture content and it tends to be mushy. Such fish spoils more quickly when stored in an unfrozen state. Freezing helps to improve its texture by making it firmer. At the end of spring the fish pass abruptly from a period of semi-starvation to full feeding as they enter the summer feeding grounds. This allows supercompensation of glycogen, and glycogen storage capacity increases. The meat not only has a low pH but also contains more glycolytic intermediate compounds, which help to make it sweeter.

The reason that freezing makes fishmeat firmer can be explained as follows. The water in fishmeat exists in two states: water that is bound to proteins in the meat, and water that is unbound or 'free'. During freezing, water is forced from the proteins to join the column of ice that has been formed from free water. Once the protein-bound water has joined the free water, it will not return to its former place on the protein molecules when it is thawed. The protein fibres in thawed meat are less hydrated; they feel more fibrous and chewy and dry to the palate, and the meat is sometimes described as 'raggy'. In this way, short-term freezing can be used to firm up mushy high pH fishmeat. Freezing may have a detrimental toughening effect in low pH meat, which is likely to be firm anyway. The mechanisms that cause firmness in low pH fish are different from the toughening effect created by freezing, and the two are additive. Large cod are more likely to have a lower pH than small cod, especially when feed is available, and so where part of the catch is to be frozen and part iced, it is logical to freeze the smaller fish to reduce mushiness and avoid overall toughening. The toughening effect of freezing is species-dependent; species such as cod and whiting are more likely to develop toughness than sole and halibut.

Burnt tuna is an interesting example of how exercise during catching affects meat quality. It shares many similarities to the PSE condition that occurs in pork (Watson *et al.*, 1992). High quality tuna should be translucent, red and firm. Burnt tuna is soft, with a pale muddy brown colour and a slightly sour taste. Although burnt tuna is edible, it is unacceptable for the sashimi trade (raw fish consumption). It is only evident when the fish are cut up, and it is customary for fishermen in Hawaii to give a rebate to wholesalers who discover the condition during butchery. It occurs in about 25% of tuna caught by commercial pole-and-line fishing, and it is common in sport-caught tuna. Longline tuna are less affected.

Tuna have remarkable athletic and line-fighting abilities. When alarmed they have been known to sustain speeds of 35 knots for over 5 minutes, and this produces large amounts of lactate in their white muscle. Some of the highest muscle lactate concentrations that have ever been recorded have been in tuna. Their unusually active muscle leads to muscle temperatures that can be more than 10°C higher than other parts of the body. During line fishing, the longer the fish fights the line and the longer it takes to bring the fish in, the worse will the burnt tuna condition be (Cramer *et al.*, 1981). Fish that fight the longest have particularly high muscle lactate levels and low muscle pH at death. The combination of low pH and high temperature induces opacity and fluid leakage through denaturation of the sarcoplasmic and myofibrillar proteins, respectively. Prompt chilling when the fish are caught may help to reduce but not eliminate the problem.

Highly active marine species also produce high levels of trimethylamine oxide in their meat, especially fish living in cold waters. Trimethylamine oxide is an excretory product formed during detoxification of ammonia. It does not impart any flavour to the meat, but on storage bacteria reduce it to trimethylamine, which produces the characteristic fishy off-odours of spoiled fish.

Slime secretion continues for a number of days after slaughter, and this results in some *weight loss*. If the skin is removed and the fillets are stored in saltwater, the meat gains weight by an osmotic effect created by Na^+ uptake. Na^+ uptake is inhibited for as long as the muscle ATP levels remain elevated. In exhausted fish the ATP level is reduced and Na^+ uptake starts sooner during the post-mortem period. Muscle from exhausted fish that are skinned post-mortem is likely to gain more weight by this process than muscle from unexhausted fish.

In some longline and trolling fisheries the fish have their brains spiked as soon as they are landed. A narrow-bladed knife is pushed through the top of the head into the brain and the blade is twisted. This reduces physical activity and hence the rate of ATP degradation in the muscle, and it delays the onset of rigor. Of commercial significance, it helps to extend the period of *translucency* of the chilled meat and delays the onset of opaqueness, but it is ineffective if the fish is severely stressed during capture.

Fish are not usually bled when they are slaughtered. However, trials with trout and catfish have shown that bleeding at slaughter reduces redness in the meat and the development of rancid odours in frozen fish. The iron in haem *blood* pigments acts as a pro-oxidant, accelerating the production of oxidative rancidity. The yield of blood during slaughter has been greatest when the tail is cut off at the caudal peduncle. Cutting the ventral aorta at the isthmus provides a satisfactory bleed-out, whereas severing the spinal cord and dorsal aorta at the nape results in a poor bleed-out. Some fisheries which specialize in smoked fish production routinely bleed the fish as soon as they are caught. Blood spots can be a problem in frozen tuna and carp. The severity of the spotting can be reduced (but not eliminated) by storing the fish in a chilled state for 2 days or more before freezing.

Several species of fish are prone to bursting their bellies after catching. These include capelin, herring and sprat. *Burst bellies* are more important in summer, when the fish are feeding well, than in winter. This is partly because fish in the summer have a larger gut fill and the stomach wall is weakened through stretching, and also because the stomach has a larger concentration of digestive enzymes than at other times of the year. The digestive enzymes cause autolysis if the belly does burst. They diffuse into the edible tissues over a period of days if the fish is sold uneviscerated.

In benthic species (fish that live at low depths) which are physoclistous (have a closed swim bladder) there is a risk that the rapid change in pressure experienced as the fish are brought to the surface results in overinflation of the swim bladder. This is common in fish that are raised from depths of 30 m or more and it is important in catch-and-release fishing as the chances of survival are greatly reduced. In extreme cases the build-up in pressure within the abdomen causes a *prolapse*; parts of the gut are forced out of the mouth and anus, the eyes may be forced from the orbits and there can be distortion of the scales and flesh.

CRUSTACEANS AND SQUID

Lobsters and crabs are caught in trap pots, by spearing, by handheld scoop nets or by gloved hand and lantern. Spearing can result in a short storage life unless processing facilities are very close to the fishery. When lobsters and crabs are not processed immediately, they are often stored alive in tanks which are irrigated with seawater. When crabs are sold alive, freshness is assessed from their vitality. This is determined as follows.

- *Lively* – quite active when held by the carapace (back) with legs extended out horizontally.
- *Weak* – active only when pressure is applied to the apron. Periodic slight movement of the legs and mandibles when held by carapace.
- *Critically weak* – very heavy drooping of legs, mandibles and apron. No physical movement. Life only detectable by observing heart action (after removing carapace).
- *Dead* – distinguishable from critically weak crab by absence of heart action (after removing carapace).

Vitality provides the buyer with an indication of how well the live crab has been stored. In warm climates the crabs have to be stored in iced, insulated containers to maintain a lively condition and freedom from bacterial proliferation.

Healthy crabs do not have a sterile haemolymph; they harbour low levels of bacterial infection (about 14 cfu ml^{-1} haemolymph). Crabs caught in pots and confined to the pots for as long as 24 hours have similar bacterial counts in their haemolymph, but crabs subjected to the stresses of commercial capture, handling and transport are likely to be more heavily infected. This may be due to the injuries that occur during commercial handling. It has been suggested that the bacterial contamination may contribute to the risk of *Vibrio* poisoning amongst crabmeat consumers.

Claw loss is quite common in lobsters caught in traps. In one study in Canada, 19% of the lobsters had a missing claw. Up to 11% of the lobsters were also wounded in another part of the body. Not all of this damage occurred during handling; some occurred in lobster grounds where Irish moss had been harvested from the seabed using drag rakes. Needless to say, the damage reduced the marketability of the lobsters.

Crabs and lobsters may be killed by pegging (pithing), boiling, freezing or during evisceration and dressing. The stage at which an animal loses sentience during these killing procedures has not been examined in any detail. On some vessels crabs are killed on the deck. In Asian fisheries the pegged crab is often cut along the ventral midline and meat is cut out from each half. In other fisheries, the carapace is removed by striking the anterior projection against the edge of the processing table, prising the body in half, removing the gut and gills with a rotating nylon brush and then packing the two halves which still contain the meat into a basket net which is subsequently lowered into a cooking vat. The method used for killing lobsters can affect the flavour of its meat. When lobsters are killed by pegging (slicing through the carapace just behind the eyes) without being boiled, IMP will form in the tailmeat from AMP after about 2 days when stored at 0°C. Inosine starts to form between 3 and 7 days post-mortem, and hypoxanthine at 7–9 days. If, instead, the lobsters are boiled alive, the enzymes responsible for these conversions are denatured. This results in lower levels of the flavour-enhancing IMP as well as lower levels of the bitter compound, hypoxanthine.

Some species of prawn and shrimp are thin-shelled and fragile (e.g. Royal red prawns) and require careful handling to avoid stress-induced discolorations. Melanosis (blackspot) quickly develops when they are removed from the sea. This is caused by the enzyme dopa oxidase which produces the black pigment melanin, particularly at high temperatures. In warm conditions, the prawns need to be sorted and chilled quickly. Sodium bisulphite is sometimes used for delaying blackspot formation in ice-stored shrimps and prawns.

Eyestalk ablation is practised in breeding stock in farmed crustacea (especially prawns and shrimps). The eyestalks are essential for vision, and they secrete a number of hormones, one of which inhibits reproduction. By cutting off the eyestalks the inhibitor is removed and the females will mate repeatedly, and lay successive batches of eggs until they die. In males, ablation induces precocious moulting and reproduction. Male prawns (*Macrobrachium rosenbergii*) die within 48 days of bilateral eyestalk ablation, but if only one eyestalk is removed they survive considerably longer. Although the animals are blinded they are able to feed, and in fact their appetite and growth rate are increased following eyestalk removal. Removing a single eyestalk is more difficult and takes longer than cutting off both together.

Squid are caught by trawling, basnig nets (stick-held dipnet or a bagnet operated by dugout boats called basnigans), purse seining, round haul seining, scoopnets and jigging lines. Trawling takes most of the catch, but jigging is more common in municipal fisheries. The main edible parts in a squid are its mantle and tentacles. The tentacles in particular are damaged when jigging lines are used. Normally, the squid strikes its prey with its tentacles in a rapid lunging motion which draws the prey to its arms. Squid meat is mainly cream coloured and any bruising caused by the hooks strongly discolours the meat, even when it is processed by blanching and retorting.

FISH FARMING

Fish that are farmed in coastal floating cages or freshwater ponds experience a variety of different stresses. These include:

- overcrowding;
- predation;
- increased prevalence of disease;
- failure to migrate in mature stock;
- cage noise;
- inability to swim to deeper water during storms;
- abrasion against the cage walls;
- handling stresses;
- cannibalism.

Overcrowding in cages or ponds can lead to elevated plasma cortisol and catecholamine levels, greater scale loss and entry of pathogens, and decreased sodium possibly resulting from damage to the gills. At high stocking densities it is the subordinate fish that are likely to become most stressed. Recommended stocking rates have been 15 kg m^{-3} for salmon and less than 30 kg m^{-3} for trout (Farm Animal Welfare Council, 1996). In some salmon farms the stocking density is as high as 40 kg m^{-3}. Controlling disease outbreaks can be difficult at the higher stocking rates.

A major expense in farming fish is the cost of the feed. Two strategies are used for minimizing this cost: ensuring that feed is not wasted, and maximizing feed conversion efficiency (growth per unit weight of feed consumed). In salmon and trout farming, wastage is controlled by giving the fish a pelleted feed which is slow to sink. This is done by impregnating the pellet with air when it is manufactured in the mill. The fish have more time to eat the pellets if they sink slowly and so less is wasted on the estuary or pond bed. Growth rate and feed conversion efficiency are maximized by including high levels of fat in the pelleted feed. This acts as a concentrated source of energy and it helps to slow the sink rate, and hence the bottom wastage, of the feed. Over the years the fat content of salmon and trout feeds has increased from 10 to 30%, whilst the more expensive protein content has been kept constant at about 45%. The faster growth rates benefit the fish farmer, but this is offset by adverse effects on the appearance and eating quality of the product. Fish reared on high-fat pellets have more oily flesh. This is thought to create a fatty mouth feel when the meat is eaten; it is associated with more gaping on storing; there can be poorer uniformity in the colour of smoked salmon and there may be oil separation in vacuum-packaged product. The flavour of the meat is not necessarily affected. In trout farms these quality problems are managed by forcing the fish to metabolize surplus fat in the muscle before they are slaughtered. This is done in two ways; firstly, by fasting the trout for 1–4 weeks before catching; in addition to this they may be penned in a fast-flowing current to provoke muscular exercise. Fish such as trout are adapted to short bursts of activity rather than sustained continuous activity. In this respect these treatments are severe, but they need to be severe in order to achieve the aim of reducing fat levels in the muscle. During fasting the level of monounsaturated fatty acids decreases more than the polyunsaturated fatty acids, and there are reductions in flavour and juiciness. Some salmon farms use a low-fat finishing ration which, from a welfare perspective, is a more acceptable option.

At feeding time the fish compete for feed, and the smaller fish may be intimidated by the larger ones. Over time the sizes diverge and there is a risk of cannibalism if they are not periodically graded and sorted into cages or ponds according to size. The smaller fish are attacked by the larger fish, and the early signs of cannibalism are loss of tail fins in the smaller stock. To reduce aggression and competition at feeding time, the feed should be distributed evenly and widely.

The following risks occur when fish are handled:

- inadequate oxygenation when removed from the water
- inadequate oxygenation when crowded together
- death in association with exercise and stress
- mechanical damage from pumps, nets, vaccination tables and grading equipment
- infections developing from fin, skin and scale damage.

On the farms, considerable damage and losses occur from predation. In Europe the main predators on fish farms are seals, otters, mink, herons, and cormorants, shags and other seabirds. The primary control objectives should be physical exclusion or scaring. Destruction of a predator will not be effective if its place is taken by another of the same species.

In caged salmon, injuries to the snout and fins are common. They can be controlled to some extent by using cage nets with a small mesh size or nets that have been treated to reduce abrasiveness, but small mesh sizes have the disadvantage of reduced water flow and the need for more frequent cleaning.

If fish are severely stressed during the handling that precedes stunning, they develop rigor more rapidly and the rigor is stronger. The rapid, strong contractions result in disruption of the muscle structure and produce a softer meat (Sigholt *et al.*, 1997). It can also have a lower water-holding capacity.

The main killing methods used for farmed fish are:

- concussion with a priest (small club)
- CO_2 stunning followed by exsanguination
- overdosing with iso-eugenol
- emersion
- exsanguination without prior stunning
- electrical stunning/electrocution.

Concussion is not widely used on fish farms but it is highly effective in producing unconsciousness and it is usually effective in reducing physical activity. The low levels of physical activity are associated with reduced levels of lactic acid during the early post-mortem period (Azam *et al.*, 1989). The blow should be aimed at the head in a restrained fish. Striking a freely moving fish is likely to bruise the edible parts as well as cause suffering. Restraint is sometimes achieved by holding the fish by the tail with the fingers pressing on the lateral line and the fish resting on a sheepskin. Salmon killed by concussion take longer to enter rigor than fish stunned with CO_2 saturated water and then killed by bleeding. Carbon dioxide causes more physical activity and so muscle ATP is depleted sooner, allowing rigor to occur earlier. The increased physical activity with carbon dioxide is thought to be a sign of irritation in the fish. They jump and swim actively, presumably in an attempt to escape, before losing consciousness at 30 and 60 seconds after tipping them into the CO_2-enriched water. There is concern that carbon dioxide is not an acceptable method from the welfare perspective, and some farms have stopped using it because the increased activity causes too much skin damage. The gills in uncooked salmon that have been stunned with carbon dioxide are prone to premature browning, and this can give a false impression that the fish have been stored for a long period. If salmon are kept in stagnant water in a holding pen for 10 minutes before CO_2 stunning, the additional stress of overcrowding provokes vigorous muscular activity and accelerated rigor once they are dead. The muscle structure becomes disrupted and meat texture can be unacceptably soft (Sigholt *et al.*, 1997). In eels, CO_2 stunning can be associated with a lower water-holding capacity in the meat, and in carp there can be a more intense rigor, in comparison with electrical stunning, concussion stunning or severing the spinal cord (Marx *et al.*, 1997). In Australasia, AQIS (iso-eugenol) is used on some fish farms for anaesthetizing the fish before slaughter. Exsanguination without prior stunning is used in some countries. It is done by tearing or cutting one or more gill arches or the isthmus and returning the fish to water to bleed out. Damaging the gill arch is likely to be irritating, if not painful, for the fish. Electrical stunning is not widely used for fish because it can lead to haemorrhages, especially when the spinal column breaks during the electrically induced muscle contraction.

Eel farms are often stocked with wild elvers which are grown on in tanks or ponds. When they reach a marketable size they may be sold live or processed, depending on the market being served. Live eels are reasonably resilient to emersion because they can absorb oxygen through their slime layer, and they are sometimes transported and sold live without paying much attention to the condition of the water. They are awkward animals to kill. The combination of a slippery layer of slime and their ability to wriggle makes them difficult to restrain. Some processors de-slime the eels before slaughter by placing them in a deep container with dry salt. The eels thrash around together for up to 2 hours, gradually absorbing salt before they die. Failure to remove the slime results in white discoloration of the skin in the smoked product, and it is claimed to affect the flavour of the meat. Part of the perceived off-flavour may, however, be due to the fact that non-deslimed eels are often sold whole with their viscera present. Muddy flavours can be transferred to the meat if evisceration is delayed. In some countries live eels are de-slimed using ammonium hydroxide. The eels are first weakened by holding them out of water for 12 hours. When placed in a tank of 6% ammonium hydroxide they take on average 16 minutes to die, and they show pronounced writhing in the intervening period. At this concentration the smoked meat contains small amounts of ammonia (about 25 mg per 100 g) and this is not usually sufficient to affect its taste or smell. Ammonium hydroxide is an irritant for fish. It is NH_3 rather than NH_4^+ which is toxic, and the equilibrium between the two depends on temperature and pH. From the welfare perspective there is a need to replace this and the salt de-sliming method with a post-mortem de-sliming system.

Eels killed at fish shops and public markets usually have their spinal cords severed at the third vertebra. This does not produce immediate death or immediate unconsciousness. They should be concussed beforehand (Flight and Verheijen, 1993). Eels that are killed for export are often frozen alive. During this process they intertwine with one another, and European buyers look for this condition when making sure that the eels were not dead before freezing. Some processors use an electric current to immobilize or stun the eels, whilst kabyaki manufacturers are said to skin the eels live. This is done by quickly pinning the head to a board, slitting down the side of the back and removing the guts and backbone.

Chapter 12

Processed Meats

This chapter examines some of the ways that animal welfare interacts with the quality of further processed meats. The welfare issues include stresses and insults which affect the pH of the meat, and cause broken bones, bruising and blood splash, heat stress, and physical contractions associated with stunning. The quality issues that are affected include water-holding capacity and weight loss, fat retention, myosin gel formation, heat-stable pinkness in meat, oxidative rancidity, the presence of contaminants such as bone or blood and poor binding of re-formed meats.

In practice, the most important relationships between welfare and processed meat quality are exerted through the effects of preslaughter stress on meat pH. Meat pH affects the following features in processed meats:

- water-holding capacity and weight loss;
- protein solubility and myosin gel formation;
- extent of myoglobin denaturation during cooking and hence pinkness of cooked meat.

The *water-holding capacity* of a meat is strongly influenced by the electrostatic charge of the proteins within the meat. These charges help to attract and hold water in its dissociated ionized form (H^+ and OH^-). If for any reason the proteins lose their charge, the bound water is released and will leak from the meat, and an unsightly drip forms in the packaging. In addition, when adjacent myofibrillar proteins have the same charge there is electrostatic repulsion between the myofibrils, and the meat has an expanded bulk. If the charge on the protein is lost, the repulsion is also lost and the structure shrinks, forcing fluid out as drip. The pH of the meat influences the extent to which the proteins are charged. Most of the proteins in meat lose their charge when the pH is between 5.1 and 5.5. The pH at which this occurs for an individual protein is known as the isoelectric point for that protein. To summarize, in the pH range 5.1–5.5 the proteins in meat fail to attract and hold water and the muscle releases drip. This range is close to the normal pH_{ult} for meat.

The relationship between pH_{ult} and water-holding capacity in ground beef is shown in Fig. 12.1 (Hamm, 1975). As meat acidifies post-mortem, the proteins reach an isoelectric point where there is little or no net charge. If the muscle fails to acidify and the pH does not reach the isoelectric point for its proteins, it is likely to have a higher water-holding capacity. There are two main causes for meat failing to acidify post-mortem. Firstly, preslaughter stress can lead to muscle glycogen depletion and this may limit post-mortem glycolysis and lactic acid formation. Secondly, not all muscles in the carcass acidify to the same extent. For example, neck muscle tends to have a high pH_{ult} (e.g. 5.8), which is well above the isoelectric point of its proteins. The relationship shown in Fig. 12.1 explains why some manufacturers of processed meat prefer to use high pH meat from stressed animals. It has high water-holding capacity and so it does not lose weight during processing. In addition, because of its dark colour it is unsuitable for the fresh meat trade and this makes it cheaper to buy. Adding acid to meat which has a normal pH_{ult} will enhance its water-holding capacity, and this is sometimes used during marinading. Alternatively, polyphosphates can be used to make the meat more alkaline and increase the water-holding capacity in the other direction (Fig. 12.1).

In many meat products, water-holding capacity and *fat retention* are closely linked. When water retention is good, fat retention can also be high. This is important in finely comminuted products, which in general have poor fat binding. If, for example, a batch of finely comminuted product was made from unusually high pH meat, water-holding capacity would be good;

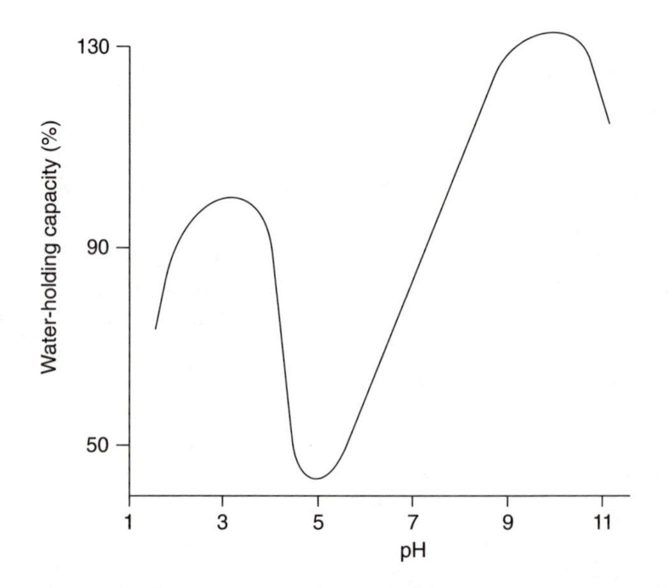

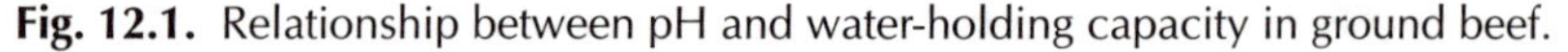
Fig. 12.1. Relationship between pH and water-holding capacity in ground beef.

there would be less risk of the product breaking up and falling apart, or of the fat coalescing and running together during cooking. The reason for the relationship between water-holding capacity and fat binding is as follows. The most important protein in muscle which influences fat and water retention in meat products is myosin. When salt is mixed with comminuted meat, part of the insoluble myosin passes into the liquid phase and dissolves; and, associated with this, the meat swells. In comparison with other meat proteins, myosin is relatively hydrophobic. The presence of a hydrophobic protein in the aqueous phase reduces the repulsion between fat droplets and water in the meat mix. It does this by encapsulating the fat droplets and holding them as an emulsion in the mixture. In this way, myosin helps to retain fat. Myosin improves water retention through the swelling effect that occurs when it is solubilized by the added salt. Part of this effect is due to retention of water by capillary forces between the myofibrils, which become more widely spaced as the myosin dissolves, and part is due to the more open structure being filled with free water.

PSE meat has an inferior water-holding capacity. This applies both to the fresh meat and to processed meats made from PSE meat. The poor water retention of PSE meat is particularly important in processed meat manufacture as it reduces yield. Poor yields are a serious burden for some meat processors, and it has been known for managers at some factories to suspect that there has been a theft, when in fact the loss has been due to water leaking or evaporating from the product during manufacture or storage. One of the reasons that PSE meat products have a poor water-holding capacity is because the myosin in PSE meat has a low solubility. When myosin dissolves during the manufacturing process, the meat swells and can hold more water. The myosin in PSE meat has a low solubility; the meat does not swell as much as normal meat, and so water retention is reduced.

Water-holding capacity in PSE meat can be improved to some extent by increasing the pH of the meat mix during the manufacturing process, using the relationship demonstrated for beef in Fig. 12.1. One way of doing this is to add polyphosphates to the PSE meat. Polyphosphates act synergistically with salt to improve water uptake and retention during curing and during sausage manufacture. Part of this effect is due to raising the pH, but chelation of divalent cations, increasing the ionic strength, disassociation of actomyosin and improved solubilization of myosin may also contribute. The addition of phosphates does not markedly affect other properties of PSE meat, but it can make cured hams slightly darker in colour (which is a benefit). When used in excess, phosphates can make the product mushy and slightly bitter (Merkel, 1971). In the case of frankfurter sausages, water retention can be improved by raising the pH of the blended pork, and this can give the sausages a softer, juicier texture.

PSE meat is more prone to evaporative moisture loss during cooking, and this could contribute to its slightly greater chewiness. As water-holding capacity decreases, there is also likely to be more drip on thawing the meat.

So, when frozen PSE meat is thawed it sheds more water in comparison with normal pigmeat. This also results in a fibrous texture in the PSE meat product which is less appealing. When a side of PSE pork is used for producing bacon by immersing it in a tank of curing solution, it often takes up more Na from the brine than normal pork. The absorbed salt creates an osmotic gradient which initially causes greater weight gain during curing in PSE sides. However, the meat still has a poor water-holding capacity and so the additional water may leak out again during storage, and the overall yield during curing will be poor (Smith and Lesser, 1982). The formation of the pink pigment, nitrosomyoglobin, during immersion curing does not necessarily mask the paleness of PSE meat. If, however, the product is cured and canned, and during the canning process the cans are heat sterilized at over 100°C, the unattractive paleness that is normally present in the fresh meat will be virtually undetectable. Dry-cured PSE meat is also indistinguishable in overall appearance from dry-cured normal pork. In other respects the eating quality of cured PSE meats is usually comparable to cured normal meat.

PSE meat is unsuitable for making processed meats which rely on myosin gel formation. The myosin in PSE meat has a low solubility and this results in poor binding of its products. Normally, when a meat is used for making a re-formed product, it is ground or diced with salt. The salt helps to solubilize and extract the myosin in the meat. The solubilized myosin is present within a liquid layer which coats the meat particles. When the meat is cooked the myosin forms a gel which binds to the meat and acts as a cohesive matrix throughout the product. The strength of the gel is important in determining whether the comminuted meat product will hold together or crumble and fall apart when it is sliced. The myosin in PSE meat has a low solubility because it is shielded from the salt which would normally help to dissolve and extract it during processing. The myosin is coated by a layer of sarcoplasmic proteins that denatured and precipitated on to the myosin during post-mortem metabolism. The salt has to get access to the myosin in order to solubilize it and the precipitated proteins prevent this. In extreme cases of PSE meat, the myosin itself may be denatured and this would also contribute to its reduced solubility during salt extraction (Briskey, 1964).

Another undesirable feature of using PSE meat in manufactured meats is that it can produce large volumes of jelly. This is because of the large amount of exudate that develops when the meat is cut and worked mechanically. Although myosin extraction is lower in PSE meat in comparison with normal meat when they are treated with salt, there is sufficient gelatin and solubilized myosin to allow gel formation.

PSE meat can be used to make acceptable dry-fermented sausages. Large quantities of these sausages are made every year, particularly in Central and Eastern Europe. There are many different recipes but typically pork and beef are blended together with pig fat, salt, sodium nitrite and a *Streptomyces* starter culture. The mix is stuffed into a casing and allowed to ferment at a high humidity for about a week. The sausages are then smoked slowly before allowing them to dry for a fortnight or longer. If PSE pork is used as a starting material, the sausage has a lower water-holding capacity and it dries more easily. Eating quality is not affected but visual appeal of the sliced fermented sausage can be improved by including PSE meat, as it appears less raw. The processing properties of PSE meat are summarized in Table 12.1.

DFD pork has a high water-holding capacity and so it loses less weight during curing. It tends to take up less salt during curing, and its translucency gives it a characteristic appearance which is known as glazy bacon. It also loses less weight during cooking (Lewis *et al.*, 1961). *Dark-cutting beef* also has a high water-holding capacity which means that it is less prone to losing water during processing and cooking. From a yield perspective, dark-cutting beef is well suited for grinding into meat patties. It is, however, prone to bacterial spoilage and so it should be frozen for much of the time that it is used in processed meat manufacture. It is more variable in its physical properties than normal meat, and is not tolerated for some manufactured products because of this. In emulsion-type products the meat is finely comminuted and so the presence of a small quantity of dark-cutting beef is of little consequence. As the size of the pieces of meat increases, the more difficult it is to overcome any adverse effects. Dark-cutting beef often affects the hindquarter muscles, whilst the forequarter muscles (which are normally preferred for manufactured meats, because of their cheaper price) are less affected.

The pH_{ult} of a meat influences the behaviour of myosin in the meat, which in turn can determine the quality of re-formed comminuted meat products. The solubilization of the myosin by salt and the formation of a myosin gel during cooking are critical steps in binding the myofibrils together and in forming a cohesive gel around the pieces of meat. Gel

Table 12.1. Processing properties of PSE pigmeat.

Property or process	Effect
Lower water-holding capacity	More drip from fresh meat
	Greater weight loss (as water) on cooking
	Greater release of gel (along with the water) during processing or cooking
	Lower yield when producing cooked ham
	Unsatisfactory rehydration of dried meat products
Curing	Increased salt uptake
	Cured meat may be paler in colour
Flavour	Acidic fresh meat flavour
	Saltier cured meat

formation depends on the ionic strength, pH, heating temperature and rate, the species and the muscle fibre type. The highest gel strengths occur at a pH of 6.0–6.5. So, meat from animals that have been stressed before slaughter is more likely to form stronger myosin gels which are less prone to falling apart. This could be important where there is no monitoring and control of the pH of the ground meat used in manufactured products.

The addition of salt to ground or diced meat usually improves its water-holding capacity. However, the extent of the increase in water-holding capacity depends on the pH of the meat. If the pH is greater than the isoelectric point, then the water-holding capacity will be increased by the salt. If the pH is close to or less than the isoelectric point, then salt has less effect on water-holding capacity.

The strength of a myosin gel helps to determine whether a re-formed meat product will hold together or fall apart when it is sliced. Myosin from *chicken* breast muscle has a greater gel strength than myosin from leg muscle. This is due to differences in the isoforms of myosin found in the two muscle types. If birds are losing weight before slaughter (for example, through feed restriction) leg muscle myosin gels are weakened further but breast meat gels are unaffected (Asghar *et al.*, 1984). A high pH favours the production of meat products that have a finer, more open gel structure.

Heat stress prior to slaughter has been found to cause toughening in turkey meat loaves and in cooked chicken breast meat, and this is probably due to slower cooling and more pronounced heat shortening in the carcass after slaughter (Lee *et al.*, 1976). It can also result in a PSE-like condition with greater drip loss from the breast meat.

Pinkness in cooked meat is a problem in the poultry meat industry. It can be due to one of two causes. The normal pigments in meat may have been converted to a heat-stable pink pigment; for example, myoglobin may have been converted to nitrosomyoglobin. Alternatively, the normal pigments have not been completely denatured during cooking. When chicken carcasses are cooked from chilled temperatures, the region in the carcass where heat penetration is slowest is the vertebral column. It is not uncommon to see, in supermarkets, cooked chicken halves with pink spines because of inadequate cooking. However, when product is cooked to the same internal temperature, high pH_{ult} meat can be redder than normal pH_{ult} meat, and this applies to beef and pork as well as poultry (Trout, 1989). Preslaughter stress and hence a high pH in the meat reduces the extent to which myoglobin is denatured during cooking. This effect is particularly noticeable at low cooking temperatures (70°C or less), but it can be reduced if the meat is salted. Other possible reasons for the link between stress and pinkness in cooked meat are that this meat could have higher levels of heat-stable cytochromes or nitric oxide, which binds to myoglobin, forming nitrosomyoglobin.

A common cause of nitrosomyoglobin formation in chicken at some plants is a high level of nitrate in the water supply to the plant. Nitrate in the spin chiller is taken up with water by the carcass. During storage it is converted to nitrite, which then combines with myoglobin to form the pink nitrosomyoglobin pigment that does not turn brown on cooking. To prevent excessive pinkness in precooked meat products, meat processors should avoid using meat with abnormally high pH_{ult}, and in poultry processing plants they should avoid using water containing high nitrate levels.

Fat quality is important in terms of its softness and colour, its susceptibility to becoming rancid and its separation from meat. Fats can become rancid during storage either by oxidative rancidity, or by hydrolytic rancidity if the appropriate enzymes are present. Oxidative rancidity is more common in meat products than hydrolytic rancidity. Factors that promote oxidative rancidity include high storage temperatures, presence of unsaturated fatty acids in the fat, exposure to light, irradiation of the product, perforation of the packaging, prolonged storage periods, and contamination of the fat with pro-oxidant cations (copper or iron) or with blood (which contains iron). Poor sticking can lead to poor bleeding and theoretically this could contribute to oxidative rancidity. More importantly, the inclusion of bruised meat which contains blood in minced meat or a processed product will increase the risk of spoilage from rancid flavours. At very low levels, rancidity can add 'character' to the flavour of a meat, but more commonly it produces off-flavours which taste soapy, fatty, stale or bitter. PSE meat is more prone to developing rancid off-flavours during frozen storage than normal pork (Merkel, 1971).

Sliced bacon produced from boars is prone to falling apart when a rasher is pulled away from its retail pack. The fat and lean are poorly bound to each other and they separate when under tension. This problem can be controlled by making thicker slices, but a more common remedy is to temper the bacon before it is sliced. This is done by chilling the bacon joint to close to its freezing point. Whilst frozen, the joint of bacon holds together and the fat–lean interface is less likely to be weakened during slicing. Unfortunately, tempering creates another problem. When the rasher is cooked, a puddle of protein solution leaks out of the meat and this forms a pool of white coagulated gel on the lean part of the bacon. This unsightly exudate is due to chilling or freezing the bacon.

In some situations inferior or downgraded meat is channelled into the processed meat market. This is particularly true for blood-splashed, bruised and high pH_{ult} meat. Bruising or colour problems are less evident if the meat is ground and diluted with other meats, or coated with a batter or breadcrumbs, or included with a gravy in a pie. Standards vary considerably between companies as to how they deal with this type of meat.

When *bruised meat* is used in processed meat production it can create unsightly bloody patches in the meat. This is important in pressed ham production, as a gel of dark blood can show up very strongly on the cut surface of a ham. Bruising within a bacon joint can create a smear of blood across the surface as the bacon is sliced. Blood is also thought to promote autolysis in the product if the enzymes in blood are not inactivated by heat treatment.

If *blood splash* or spots of blood are present in meat, they will turn brown when the meat is cooked. In the case of blood-splashed beef, the browning can be indistinguishable from the browning that occurs when the meat surface becomes charred during normal grilling. In the case of white poultry meats, the browning is more noticeable. Freezing before cooking causes the red blood cells to rupture and this may make the problem worse by allowing the haem pigment to spread over a large area. Short bleeding times at slaughter (less than 2 minutes) also make blood-spot browning worse in breast fillets (Lyon and Lyon, 1986).

Broken bones can be a problem in processed poultrymeat production. In many instances the fractures do not involve any pain to the animal, as they occur post-mortem and are often due to machine damage. However, the system under which the animal is kept on the farm can influence the likelihood of bone damage. Turkeys that are reared in cages are more prone to developing dislocated joints during catching and processing than are birds reared in deep litter. On account of this, turkeys are not reared in cages. Battery laying hens develop weaker bones than barn or free-range hens and this makes them more prone to bone fractures during catching and processing. By the time a battery hen carcass leaves the evisceration line at the processing plant, it has about six broken bones per carcass. Free-range hens have about four broken bones per carcass (Gregory and Wilkins, 1992). After the carcasses have been chilled, they are aged and then cooked. The cooking allows easier separation and hence a high recovery of the meat. However, it also allows bone fragments to come away with the meat and some end up in the final products, which include chicken pies, chicken soup and chicken meat pastes. Catching the live bird, plucking and mechanical offal withdrawal are the main causes of bone breakage that lead to contamination of hen meat products (Table 12.2).

Catching damage often occurs as the birds are removed from their cages. This is done by grasping a leg and pulling the bird out through the front entrance. The ischium (bone above the vent) and the keel tend to strike the entrance of the cage or the trough, and as these birds have weak skeletons by the time they reach the end of lay, the bones are easily broken. The bones are brittle because of the drain on body calcium reserves from egg production and because the birds do not take much exercise, which would otherwise strengthen their bones.

Wishbones commonly break during electrical stunning in broilers. They are a problem during further processing when the breast fillet is removed from the carcass. If the wishbone comes away with the breast meat and is not separated out it will be present as a contaminant, which can give rise to consumer complaints. Bone fragments such as this are particularly serious if they cause mouth damage in a consumer. Hen packers are particularly concerned about sharp bones such as the needle bone (fibula), wishbone and pieces of rib.

Table 12.2. Cummulative damage incurred by battery hens during handling and processing. (After Gregory and Wilkins, 1992.)

Sample point	*n*	% Birds with broken bones	Broken bones per bird
After removal from cages at farms	982	24	0.4
Before hanging on killing line at packing plant	207	31	0.6
After hanging on	375	39	0.7
After scalding	225	87	2.9
After plucking	65	95	6.1
After evisceration and spin chilling	167	98	5.9

In many East Asian countries the method used for slaughtering a pig is to tie its legs together, let it rest on the floor for up to 2 hours and then to cut its throat. The pigs fight initially, when they are tied, but they usually give up struggling if they are left alone. By the time they are bled, the muscle is usually in a rested and relaxed state. In contrast, with electrical stunning the activation of the nervous system by the current causes pronounced muscle contractions at the time of slaughter. Trials have been done which compare the two slaughter methods, and the traditional method of tying the legs, resting and sticking was preferred for producing semi-dried meats. This is because electrical stunning was associated with fracture and *fragmentation of muscle fibres* (Chang and Pearson, 1992). Pork products such as Zousoon (a semi-dry pork floss product) rely on long, uninterrupted muscle fibres, but the fragmentation caused by electrical stunning results instead in short-fibred dried pork, which is inappropriate for this particular meat product.

If *fish* are not severely stressed before they die, and if they are filleted and frozen pre-rigor, the meat contains ATP whilst it is still frozen. The ATP persists and, if the fillet is thawed gradually before it is cooked, provides energy for rigor development. On the other hand, if it is thawed rapidly it contracts violently, acquires a corrugated over-contracted appearance, exudes fluid and becomes very tough. Rapid thawing by putting a frozen fish into a deep fat fryer can produce a very rubbery texture. Long-term cold storage of fish causes it to release drip. This can be reduced by dipping the fillets into a solution of sodium polyphosphate prior to freezing. This helps to seal the surface of the fillet with a film of protein, but it does not necessarily improve the texture. If fishmeat develops gaping during processing, the fillets may be downgraded and used for manufactured products such as fishcakes.

Foie gras is used in processed gourmet products such as pâté de foie gras and terrine de foie gras. It is made from the livers of force-fed Barbary and Muscovy ducks and geese. Typically, the birds are reared to 12–14 weeks of age as a flock and then transferred to the cramming sheds, where they are housed in pens or cages. Whilst in the cramming sheds the birds are force-fed twice (ducks) or three to four times (geese) daily, using a funnel fitted with a piston which is inserted into the oesophagus. The birds have to be restrained during each feed, and after it they are torpid for 3–5 hours. The amount of feed that can be delivered increases substantially after the first week of force-feeding as the crop stretches. The aim is to produce a bird which at slaughter has a large liver containing a high level of fat. Geese produce a superior product, as the livers are heavier and lose less fat during cooking in comparison with duck livers. Before it is cooked the force-fed duck or goose liver consists of about 60% fat, and during cooking the duck liver may lose 40% of its fat and the goose liver about 20%. On account of this difference in yield, it is possible to sterilize goose foie gras using high temperatures without risking high losses of yield. Lower temperatures are used for duck foie gras and this can raise potential public health risks. Geese that are held in cages during the force-feeding period can produce heavier livers than birds held in pens. The potential welfare compromises with this system of liver production include:

- the frequent stress of handling and restraint;
- the forced introduction of a feeding tube into the oesophagus;
- cramming the birds with feed, producing abdominal discomfort and laboured breathing;
- aversion to and fear of repeated force-feeding.

Some birds die during or shortly after a feed. The counter-argument used in defending foie gras production is that it is used only in migratory species which, in their natural habitat, would cram themselves prior to flying long distances.

Chapter 13

Stunning and Slaughter

REDMEAT SPECIES

When animals are killed in slaughterhouses they are stunned and then they are slaughtered (Fig. 13.1). Stunning and slaughter should be regarded as two separate procedures, as they have quite different functions. The purposes of stunning are:

- to make the animal unconscious so that it can be stuck and bled without causing pain or distress;
- to immobilize the animal so that it can be bled conveniently and safely by the operator.

The usual stunning method is to pass an electric current through the animal's brain.

The usual slaughter method is sticking (bleeding the animal out), and the purposes of sticking are:

- to kill the animal before it regains consciousness;
- to remove blood from the carcass.

The most common combination of stunning and slaughter methods is electrical stunning followed by sticking. Other systems are shown in Table 13.1.

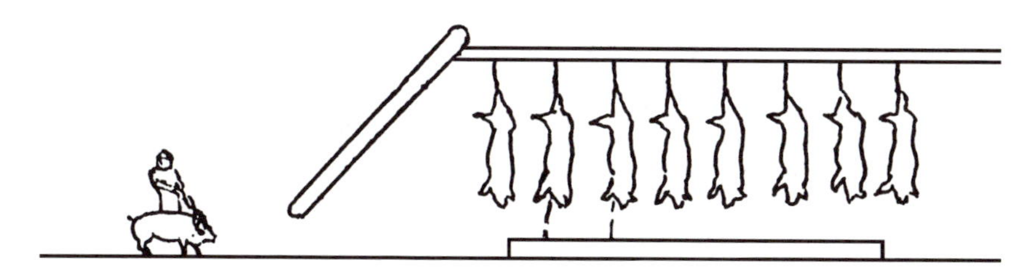

Fig. 13.1. Pig stunning and slaughter.

Table 13.1. Stunning and slaughter methods used internationally in abattoirs.

	Stunning methods					Slaughtering methods		
Species	Electrical stunning	Captive bolt	Percussion bolt	Carbon dioxide	Free bullet	Sticking after stunning	Cardiac arrest with bleeding	Sticking without stunning†
Cattle	*	***	*			***		*
Pigs	***			**	*	***		*
Sheep	***	*				***	*	*
Poultry	***			*		**	**	*

† Includes religious slaughter.
***, Main method; ** common method; * uncommon method used at some abattoirs or for certain types of stock.

Not all animals are stunned before they are slaughtered. In many countries it is still common practice to kill by the traditional method of cutting the neck with a knife without stunning the animal beforehand. Animals are killed without stunning by one of three religious slaughter methods. These are: *shechita*, which is used for producing kosher meat for people of the Jewish faith: *halal slaughter*, which is used in the Islamic faith; and *jhatka* (decapitation), which is used by Sikhs. In countries where these are minority faiths, most governments allow religious slaughter methods out of respect for the rights of the people who practise those religions. This has been a controversial issue and one where the debate has often focused on the question of whether the method used for killing an animal is a human right or an animal right. From the animal welfare perspective, the issues that concern us are the same as those that apply to non-religious slaughter:

- is the restraint that is required for killing the animal unduly or unnecessarily distressing?
- is the killing method painful?
- do the animals experience pain or distress whilst they are bleeding?

Stunning

Of the *stunning methods* listed in Table 13.1, the captive bolt, percussion bolt, carbon dioxide and free bullet usually (but not always) cause permanent insensibility. So from the humanitarian perspective there is less need to bleed the animal immediately. It is less likely to be able to regain consciousness when these methods are applied correctly.

With *captive-bolt* stunning the purpose is to concuss the animal by firing a bolt against its head (Gregory, 1988). It is called a captive bolt because the bolt is captive within the gun – as distinct from free-bolt guns, which are no longer used because of the difficulty of retrieving the bolt for reuse. The effectiveness of the concussive blow depends on the kinetic energy imparted to the head, and that in turn depends mainly on the velocity of the bolt. Three practical considerations determine bolt velocity:

- gun design and how the gun is applied to the head;
- choice of cartridge (the cartridges have different gunpowder grain strengths and particular grain strengths are appropriate for different classes of stock);
- bolt friction or jamming due to inadequate cleaning of the gun.

When the gun is fired, the explosive in the cartridge expands and it propels the bolt forwards. Carbon particles and gases are released during the explosion. Some of the carbon is vented out of the gun and some sublimes on the inside of the chamber, particularly if the gun is cold. With use, a crust of carbon is deposited in the chamber and if it is not removed by regular cleaning it slows the bolt down when it is next fired.

Most captive-bolt guns are fitted with compressible rings around the bolt. These are squeezed together when the gun is fired. They prevent the bolt from slamming into the muzzle, causing damage to the gun and bolt, and they return the bolt automatically to the primed position as they spring back to their normal shape. If there is a build-up of carbon inside the gun, the bolt fails to return fully to the primed position. This results in a larger-than-normal expansion chamber volume, which reduces the power of the next shot. It is important to ensure that the bolt is fully returned between each shot, and to clean the chamber when the bolt fails to return to its primed position.

Some guns have a bolt that protrudes from the muzzle when it is in the primed position; other designs have a bolt that is recessed within the muzzle (Fig. 13.2). The way these guns are held against the animal's head will influence the impact velocity. Normally, when a bolt is fired it requires a short distance to reach its maximum velocity. Guns with protruding bolts should be held slightly (up to 5 mm) away from the animal's head to allow for this, whereas guns with recessed bolts can be pressed against the head.

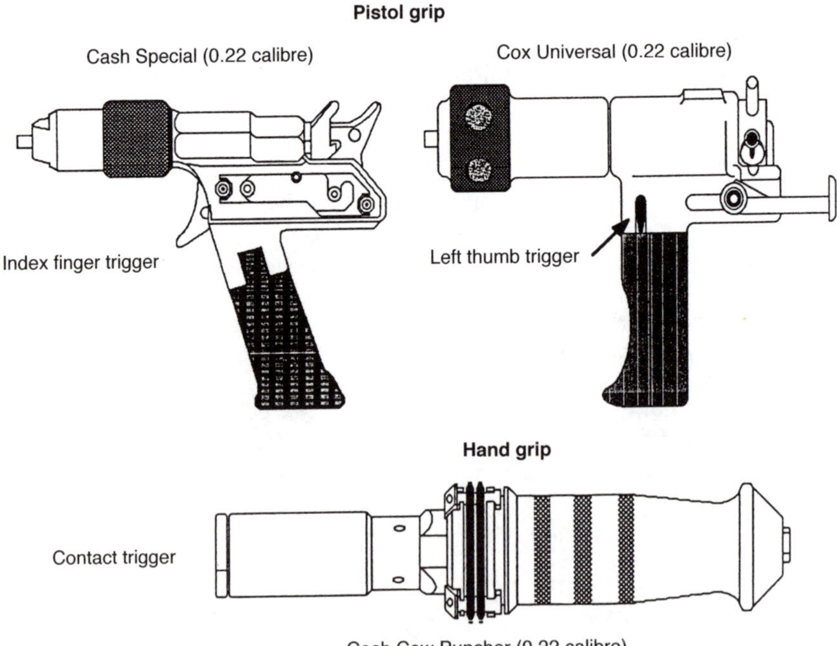

Fig. 13.2. Three types of captive-bolt gun. The Cash Cow Puncher has a recessed bolt, unlike the Cash Special and the Cox Universal.

Some guns with recessed bolts are triggered by contact firing (Fig. 13.2). Instead of having a trigger, the muzzle has to be struck against the animal's head to force the cartridge on to a non-moving firing pin. The advantage with this design is that the gun has to be in contact with the head to get it to fire, and this reduces the likelihood of an inadequate stun due to holding the gun too far away from the head.

Bolt diameter can affect the transfer of energy to the skull. If the diameter is too fine, the bolt would easily pierce the skull and much of the momentum would be taken up by the compressible rings. If the diameter was larger, more energy would be transferred to the skull as the bolt worked through the bone of the head. This can be visualized by comparing a bolt that is the diameter of a fine knitting needle with one that is 7 mm in diameter. For the same reason, a bolt that is blunt is preferable to one with a tip that is shaped to help penetration.

The ideal shooting position on the head is often considered to be at the cross-over point between imaginary lines drawn between the base of the horns and the opposite eyes (Fig. 13.3). Some authorities contend that the shot should be offset slightly to one side from this position, but this is a fine distinction which in reality is difficult to control and may not be that important. Deviation from the ideal position will be less important when high velocity guns are used. In other words, the size of the target area on the head can be increased when guns with high bolt velocities are used.

Much of the research into captive-bolt shooting has been based on an analysis of their effect on evoked responses in the brain. An evoked response is the electrical activity in the brain which occurs in response to

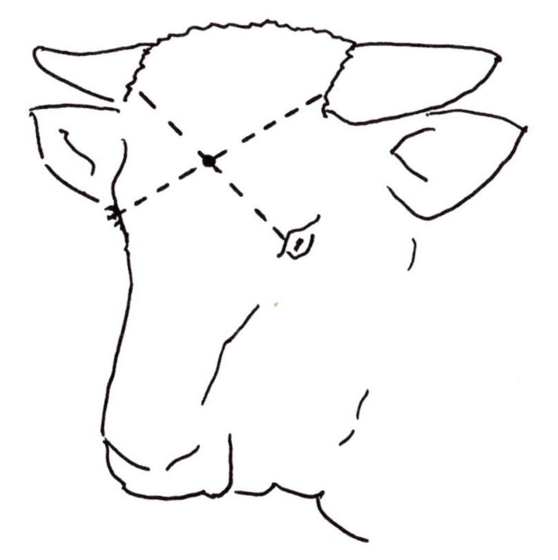

Fig. 13.3. Correct shooting position.

an external stimulus, such as a flash of light, a clicking noise or a mild electrical pulse applied to a limb. When recorded at the primary cortex of the brain, evoked responses are present when the animal is anaesthetized and when it is unanaesthetized. So, the presence of a response does not indicate consciousness. However, a response is essential for perception of that stimulus, and so the disappearance of a response demonstrates a loss of ability to perceive the stimulus. Recommendations on minimum bolt velocities have been based on the velocity that will obliterate the visual evoked responses in the brain. For steers, heifers and cows it is $55\ \mathrm{m\ s^{-1}}$ and for young bulls it is $72\ \mathrm{m\ s^{-1}}$. It is important to select guns and cartridges that are capable of delivering these velocities. Research using evoked responses has also produced the following list of signs that indicate an effective stun with a captive bolt.

- The animal must immediately collapse.
- Breathing must be absent.
- The muscles in the back and legs should go into spasm (Fig. 13.4). The forelegs and hindlegs should be flexed, and after about 5 seconds the forelegs will straighten and become extended. If the muscles are flaccid immediately after stunning, this is a sign that the stun is not as deep and there is a risk that the animal will regain consciousness.
- The eyes should not be rotated. A rotated eyeball indicates that a deep stun is not present and there is a risk that the animal will regain consciousness.

A common misunderstanding is that the bolt has to enter the brain to produce unconsciousness. This is not the case, otherwise the percussion-bolt gun would be totally ineffective. The *percussion-bolt* has a blunt end

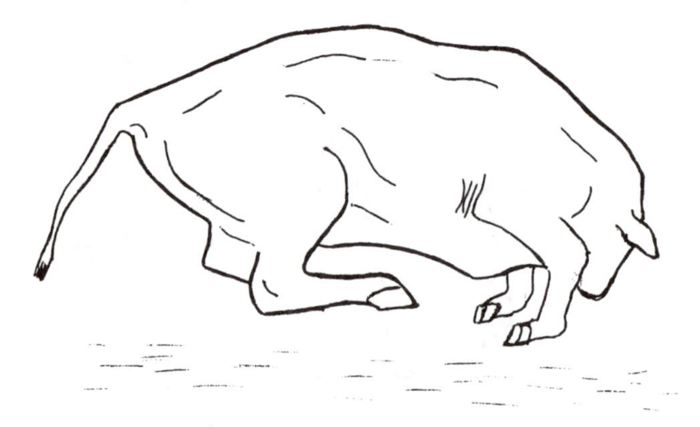

Fig. 13.4. When cattle are stunned with a captive bolt, the muscles in the body go into spasm and the animal collapses with the legs flexed.

which looks like a mushroom. It is designed to concuss without penetrating the brain and it is used mainly for stunning cattle before halal slaughter and (for worker health reasons) for stunning cattle that are thought to have bovine spongiform encephalopathy.

The *free bullet* also depends on concussion for stunning an animal. It is used in abattoirs when an animal runs amok, and at some abattoirs it is used on breeding pigs and horses. From a human safety perspective, it is advisable not to use an unnecessarily high velocity bullet, otherwise there is a risk of the bullet going through the animal's head and endangering personnel and equipment. On the other, hand the velocity must be sufficient to stun the animal. For bulls, a low velocity 0.44 bullet has been recommended; there should be less chance of it passing through the head than a high velocity 0.303 or 0.27. Alternatively, bullets which fragment inside the skull could be used.

During *electrical stunning* a current is passed through the brain. The intention is to induce epilepsy (Gregory, 1991a). The electroencephalogram (EEG) during epilepsy is shown in phase B of Fig. 13.5. In humans, there are no known instances where this type of epilepsy has been associated with consciousness. On this basis, it has been assumed that epileptiform activity (phase B) can be used experimentally to diagnose unconsciousness following electrical stunning. The electrical stunning current that is required to induce epilepsy varies with species. For pigs it is 1.25 amps, sheep 0.5 A and calves 1.0 A. If the stunning current is at these levels, 98% of the animals will be stunned, and so these values are used as the recommended minimum currents.

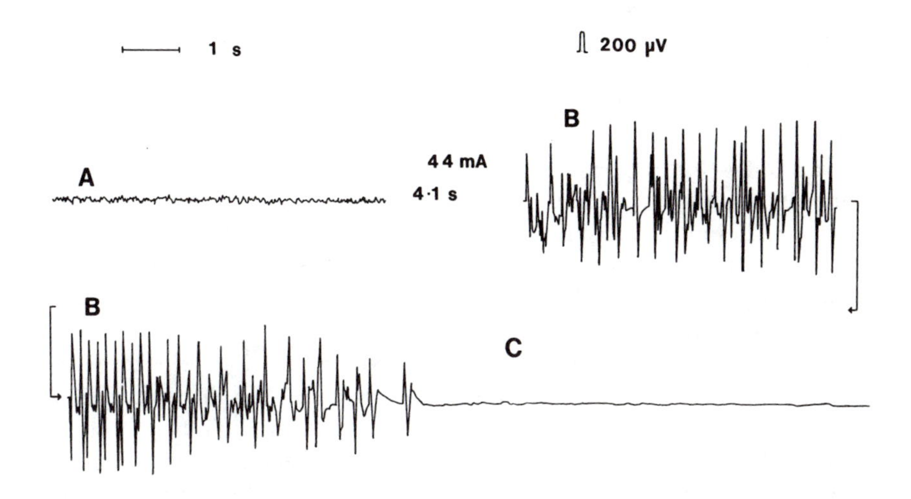

Fig. 13.5. Electroencephalogram (EEG) before (A) electrical stunning and during the (B) epileptiform and (C) quiet phases following application of the current.

Two methods are used for ensuring that the currents delivered do not fall below these levels. The first is to use high voltage stunning equipment. With constant voltage equipment, the actual current that is delivered depends on the resistance of the animal between the electrodes of the stunner. If it is assumed, for example, that the resistance for a pig's head is 160 ohms, the voltage required to achieve 1.25 A is 200 V (calculated from Ohm's law, $V = IR$). Some pigs, however, may have a resistance of 240 Ω, and for them the voltage required to deliver 1.25 A would be 300 V. In practice it is not possible to control all the variation in resistance. Instead, most equipment is designed to supply sufficiently high voltages to stun all animals. This approach has some drawbacks; in the above example, if 300 V was applied to a 160 Ω resistance pig, the animal would receive 1.9 A. Very high stunning currents such as this are thought to be an unnecessary safety hazard and to lead to carcass quality problems (discussed in Chapter 14). An alternative system is to use a constant voltage–current limiting stunner. The controlling voltage is set at a high level, but for each animal the excess current above a predetermined level is dissipated through a choke resistor in the control box. In this way the current delivered to each animal is regulated on an individual animal basis. It should be noted that this is not the same as a variable voltage–constant current stunner, which is more expensive; it has a sensing circuit and the output voltage is automatically adjusted according to each animal's resistance. In current-limiting systems, the voltage is kept constant and excess current is tapped off.

With most electrical stunning systems the aim should be to place the electrodes on or across the head, otherwise there is a risk that the current will not pass through the brain. With pigs, it is not always easy to place the electrodes across the head and instead it is common to put the electrodes across the neck. The 1.25 A recommendation for pigs is, however, based on neck application of the tongs. If, instead, the electrodes can be placed across the head in all pigs, a minimum current of 0.41 A should be sufficient (Anil, 1991).

Electrical stunning equipment requires routine maintenance. Where saline or water are not used, the electrodes often to develop a layer of charred material, which increases the electrical resistance. This can be removed with a powered wire brush situated alongside the operator. The operator should also be able to see from an ammeter the current that is delivered to each animal.

The way in which an animal is presented for stunning helps to determine the accuracy of placing the stunning device. Restraint in a conveyor or headbail assists accurate stunning but it may lead to additional stress in manoeuvring the animal into the restrained position and in holding it there. Stunning an unrestrained animal can be associated with misapplication of the tongs or gun and the animal may experience an electric shock or a non-concussive blow. Cattle are a particular problem when they are reluctant to lift their heads for a captive bolt shot when confined in a stunning pen, and this makes it difficult to get an accurate shot.

When head-only electrical stunning is used, it is important to stick the animal immediately. Sheep and pigs usually start regaining consciousness at about 60 seconds after applying the current, but in some animals it may be as soon as 40 seconds. As a general recommendation, it is advisable to stick within 20 seconds of head-only electrical stunning to avoid recovery of consciousness. In some countries there has been a legal requirement that animals should not be bled in sight of another conscious animal. This means that the stunned animal has to be conveyed away from any conscious animals before it can be stuck. This introduces an inevitable delay in the time to sticking. Research in pigs and sheep shows that heart rate and cortisol concentrations are not elevated when animals witness their penmates being slaughtered. In view of this it seems unreasonable to require 'out of sight' slaughter where this introduces a risk of recovery of consciousness because of a delay in sticking.

There are two approaches to assessing the effectiveness of electrical stunning (Gregory, 1985). The first is to inspect the equipment to make sure that it is delivering the recommended current for the species, to check that the electrodes are being applied in the appropriate position and to check that the animals are stuck within the prescribed time period. The second approach is to observe the behaviour of the animal. The physical signs of an epileptic fit can be checked as well as the absence of responsiveness to particular stimuli. Normally, when an animal is electrically stunned by the head-only method the hindlegs immediately go into flexion and the animal collapses if it is not supported in a restraining conveyor. The forelegs usually go into extension but in some situations they may be flexed for a brief period before straightening into rigid extension. During the epileptiform phase (phase B, Fig. 13.5) the body is tense and tonic (rigid), breathing is absent and the eyeballs may be obscured. In some animals there will be running or paddling movements with the legs. At the end of phase B the body relaxes and rhythmic breathing resumes. A quiet phase (C) follows, which is linked to exhaustion of the nervous system. Its duration is highly variable and sometimes it is virtually absent. It is followed by a clonic (kicking) phase, which can be either a galloping, cantering or erratic kicking action. This occurs during the high amplitude/low frequency phase in the EEG. Eventually the kicking subsides and the animal is alert and responsive. Recovery of consciousness occurs at some stage following resumption of rhythmic breathing. A common method used by inspectors at abattoirs for assessing the effectiveness of a stun is to check the corneal reflex, which indicates whether the brainstem is responsive. It does not distinguish accurately between consciousness and unconsciousness, but when the reflex is absent it is likely that the animal is unconscious. It is unwise to give precise times for the complete recovery of consciousness following electrical stunning because consciousness has many facets and there is a sequence in which different faculties recover. For example, sheep regain responsiveness to a smack on the snout before they regain responsiveness to a threatening gesture. Responsiveness to an ear pinch and other painful stimuli takes even longer to recover (Gregory and Wotton, 1988a).

The length of time that the current is applied to the head is not important from the welfare perspective when high currents are used. However, at currents that are below the recommendations given earlier, short current durations have been associated with quicker recovery of consciousness in sheep. High stunning currents are also more likely to act instantaneously. If the stun is not instantaneous, the animal will experience an electric shock before the stun is induced.

Several design features in electrical stunning affect the safety of personnel working near the equipment. The most important feature is whether the electrical potential of one of the electrodes is earthed. If this is the case, current can flow to earth from that electrode by any low-resistance pathway. Stray earthing of the current (e.g. through an operator) can be avoided by using a stunning current that passes through a transformer with a secondary winding that has both outputs isolated from earth.

Sticking

When an animal is bled the objective is to deflect blood flow away from the brain. In sheep, the carotid arteries on both sides of the neck supply the brain with blood, and they should be severed. When this is done the time to loss of consciousness, if the animal had not been stunned, would have been about 6 seconds, and the time to loss of visual evoked responses (VERs) is 14 seconds. If only one carotid artery is cut, the time to loss of VERs is five times longer (70 seconds); and if instead only the jugular veins in the neck are cut it takes about 5 minutes for the VERs to disappear (Gregory and Wotton, 1984a). When the venous return from the brain is cut (jugular veins) instead of the arterial supply, the animal dies slowly by venous haemorrhaging and circulatory collapse instead of quickly through deflection of blood away from the brain. Pigs are bled with a *chest stick* and the aim should be to sever the common brachiocephalic trunk which gives rise to the carotid arteries. Sometimes a subclavian artery is severed instead, and this should be satisfactory, provided the rate of bleeding from the artery is rapid. Problems with slow bleeding can occur in pigs if the size of the sticking wound in the skin is too small.

Cattle and calves should be bled by cutting the brachiocephalic trunk using a chest stick (Leigh and Delaney, 1987). The blade of the knife must be long enough to reach the brachiocephalic trunk. Cattle have an anastomosis in their blood vessels which allows blood to flow to the brain through the vertebral arteries if the carotid arteries are cut instead (Fig. 13.6). As a result, the time to loss of brain function can be quite long if only the carotid arteries are severed when using a gash stick (Newhook and Blackmore,

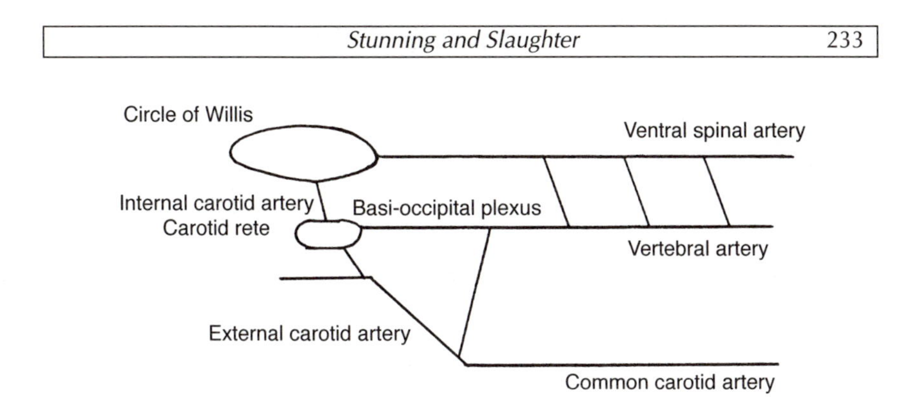

Fig. 13.6. Blood supply to the brain in cattle. The basi-occipital plexus is absent in sheep.

1982). In addition, when only the carotid arteries are cut, sometimes their cut ends develop aneurysms (ballooning), particularly when the sticking knife is blunt. This impedes blood flow and the animals take even longer to die. A chest stick is preferred from the welfare perspective for cattle and calves.

There are two neck-sticking methods used in sheep (Fig. 13.7). In *spear sticking*,the neck is pierced with a knife between the trachea and backbone, with the sharp edge of the blade pointing away from the backbone, and the knife is withdrawn along the path of entry. In *gash sticking* (ear-to-ear sticking), the knife is inserted as for spear sticking but all the soft tissues on the underside are cut as the knife is withdrawn. Alternatively, the blade is inserted into the neck and, using an overhand grasp of the knife handle, the blade is pulled through all the soft tissues of the underside of the neck. The back of the neck is facing the operator and may be pulled against a capstan block to extend the chin and expose the underside of the neck. With spear sticking, the best way of ensuring that both carotid arteries are cut is by inserting the knife correctly. If the muzzle or jaw is grasped with one hand and the chin is extended, the carotids are pulled taught against the backbone in the neck. This makes it difficult to cut the carotids as the knife either passes at too shallow a depth or there is a risk it will strike the backbone. Typically, the carotid artery on the side opposite to the point of entry will be missed. This can be avoided by rotating the knife after it has been inserted and withdrawing it with the sharp edge pressed against the backbone. Alternatively, a double-edged sticking knife can be used and the same pressing action applied without having to turn the knife.

Checking the effectiveness of sticking is best done by observing the animals on the bleeding line, and inspecting the sticking wound in animals which show physical activity that could indicate sustained brain function. It is worth checking these animals to make sure that both carotid arteries have been cut, or that they have not formed aneurysms. This will involve opening up the sticking wound, and the carcass may have to be removed from

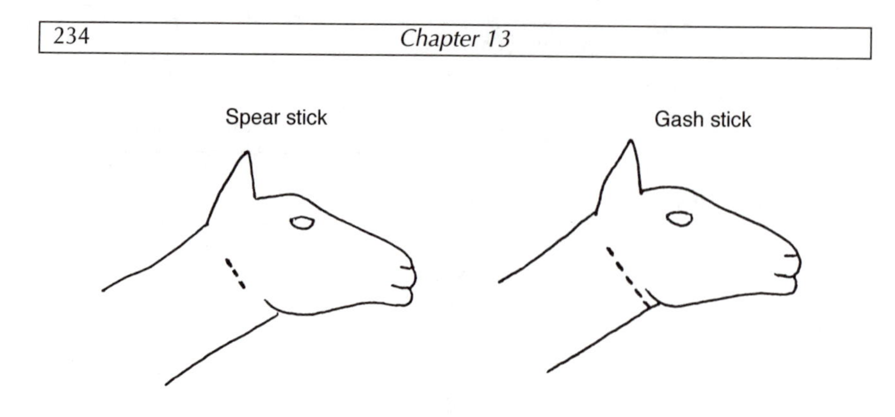

Fig. 13.7. Position of the neck-sticking wounds.

the slaughterline to do this. The carotid arteries can be identified from their close association with the vagus nerve.

Other methods

One way of avoiding all the welfare problems that can be encountered with sticking is to use a cardiac arrest stunning method instead (Gregory and Wotton, 1984b). By stopping the heart, perfusion of the brain comes to a halt and, in terms of brain function it is irrelevant as to when and which blood vessels are severed at sticking. In practice, this is done in sheep with *head-to-back stunning* (Fig. 13.8). The electrodes are designed to span both the brain and the heart. It is important that the electrodes are placed at the front of the brain rather than on the neck, otherwise the animal will be electrocuted. *Electrocution* is the induction of a cardiac arrest without simultaneous stunning. It is potentially painful for the animal and should never be used. A satisfactory current for inducing epilepsy in the sheep's brain plus a ventricular fibrillation in its heart is 1.0 A.

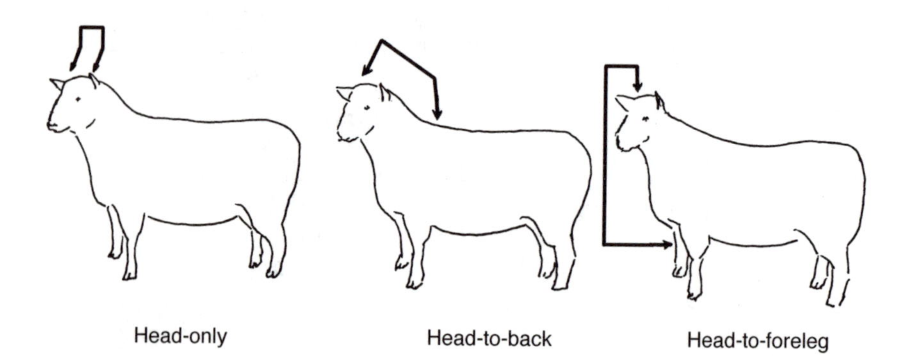

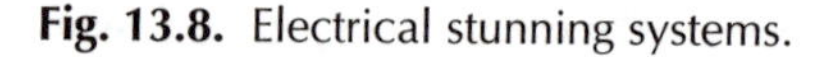

Fig. 13.8. Electrical stunning systems.

The advantages of inducing a cardiac arrest at stunning are as follows.

- There is less risk of the animal regaining consciousness after the stun.
- From the welfare perspective, it is not important to bleed the animal immediately.
- It is no longer essential to cut both carotid arteries, or the brachiocephalic trunk in the case of cattle and pigs, to ensure a humane slaughter.
- Physical convulsions are usually reduced.
- There is less risk of blood splash and bruising in the carcass.

In some countries electrical stunning is used as an alternative to no preslaughter stunning during halal slaughter of cattle. Some halal authorities accept electrical stunning before the halal cut is made, but they will not accept stunning methods that simultaneously induce a cardiac arrest.

The following summarizes the behavioural indicators which should be examined when checking the welfare of animals during head-only electrical stunning and sticking:

- checking that the animal shows the physical signs of an epileptic fit
- checking for absence of head turning or head righting behaviour and the absence of breathing movements
- after the convulsive phase, checking that jaw tension is relaxed. If it is relaxed, the animal is unconscious. If it reacts by chewing or biting when the jaws are prised apart, it is likely to be conscious.

With electrical stunning systems which induce a cardiac arrest, the animal may show a slow, shallow rhythmic breathing before it dies. If this occurs in an otherwise relaxed state, which is unresponsive to stimuli such as ear pinching and corneal stimulation, the animal is likely to be unconscious.

Carbon dioxide stunning is the preferred method for stunning pigs in Scandinavian countries. During the 1990s the most common system was the compact stunner. In this system the pigs were loaded individually into a chair, which was then lowered into a well that was prefilled with CO_2 (Fig. 13.9). The Combi system is a modification of this, where two or more pigs are loaded into each chair, and more recently a high throughput dip-lift system has been developed. Carbon dioxide has been criticised from a welfare outlook because it inevitably leads to a sense of breathlessness before the animal is unconscious. Behaviour studies have demonstrated that pigs show aversion to CO_2 and that they develop laboured breathing before they collapse.

WHITEMEAT SPECIES

Stunning before slaughter is not a legal requirement for poultry in every country, but it is common for the birds to be put through a waterbath electric stunner before they are bled with a neck cut (Fig. 13.10). The waterbath

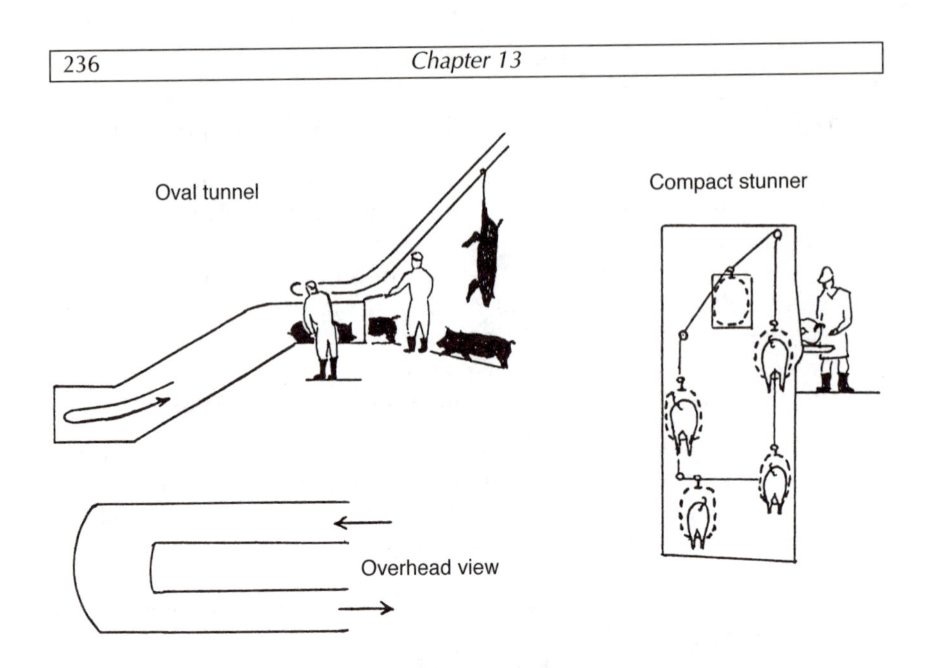

Fig. 13.9. The oval tunnel and compact carbon dioxide stunning systems.

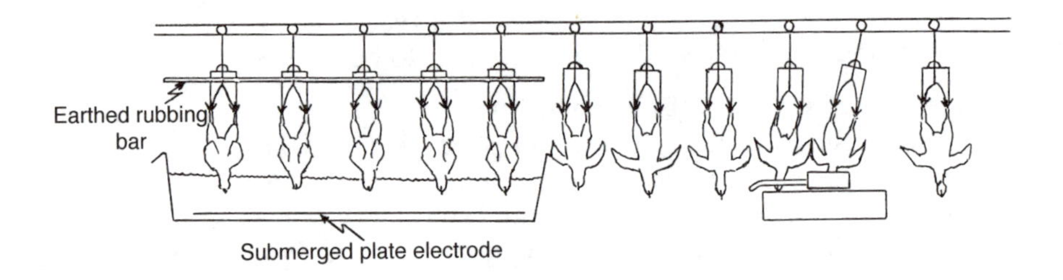

Fig. 13.10. Poultry waterbath electric stunner and neck cutter.

stunner is an open tank of water through which the birds are drawn as they are conveyed upside down by shackles along an overhead line. The water acts as the live electrode, and a metal bar which makes contact with the shackle usually acts as the earth electrode. Thus, current flows through the whole of the bird (except for its feet) when it is being stunned. In order to stun the bird, some of the current must pass through the brain. As many as 15 birds may be making contact with the water electrode at any time, but the exact number depends on the length of the waterbath.

Present stunners supply a current at a constant voltage. The voltage can be regulated with a dial or switch and the required average current per bird is titrated into the circuit using the current displayed on an ammeter.

Constant current stunners should not be used for poultry except where they supply current separately to each bird. Otherwise, current will take the route of least resistance and low-resistance birds will be overstunned while the high-resistance birds will be understunned.

Poultry do not usually produce the same type of epilepsy as the red-meat species when they are electrically stunned. Instead the EEG shows a *petit mal* epilepsy, and this is not necessarily diagnostic of unconsciousness. So, for bird species the recommended minimum currents have been based on other criteria (Gregory, 1992b). Two approaches have been used. One was to assess the minimum current which produced an acceptable period of overt behavioural unconsciousness. A current of 105 mA per bird was found to produce at least 52 seconds of apparent insensibility before broilers showed a return of head-righting behaviour and coordinated neck movement. Another approach was to examine responsiveness in the EEG to sensory stimuli. If the brain failed to show any somatosensory evoked responses, it lacked the neural integrity that is a prerequisite for perception of that stimulus. In other words, absence of the evoked response was an indicator of unequivocal unconsciousness in that sensory modality. The current necessary to induce loss of somatosensory evoked responses in broilers was over 120 mA per bird.

Some authorities take the view that, from the welfare standpoint, it is best to induce a cardiac arrest at stunning in at least 90% of the birds. Where this has been adopted as the standard for stunning poultry, the following average minimum currents (mA) per bird have been recommended:

- Chicken – 120
- Duck – 130
- Goose – 130
- Turkey – 150.

It so happens that the minimum current that guarantees an effective stun is approximately the same as that which induces a ventricular fibrillation in 90% of the birds (Gregory, 1992b). Nevertheless, 105 mA per bird should be adequate, provided neck cutting is performed promptly and properly.

An important criticism of some waterbath stunners is that they cause pre-stun shocks in the birds. The problem is peculiar to particular plants, rather than being widespread in the industry. There are four ways in which it occurs. Firstly, in waterbaths that do not have an entry or exit ramp, water is continuously fed into the bath and it overflows from the entry or exit lip. There should in fact be no overflow at the entry lip, otherwise the birds will get an electric shock from this water (which will be electrically live). Secondly, in waterbaths that are fitted with an entry ramp, the ramp becomes wet from water splashes out of the bath. If the ramp is not electrically isolated from the rest of the tank (e.g. by an air space), it will be live wherever there is a wet route to the water in the bath. Thus birds will get an electric shock when their heads make contact with the ramp and are drawn up it. The third way is for the wing of the bird to dip into the waterbath before the head. This is only a problem for slow line speeds, but it is a common feature in turkey plants because this species has a large wingspan and the wings hang below the head. It can be avoided by redesigning the entry ramp such that it holds the body of the bird back and allows the head, body and wings to be drawn together over the edge of the ramp into the waterbath. A fourth way in which broilers can get pre-stun shocks is when the rate at which their heads are immersed in the water is too slow and they recoil before being immersed.

Another fault at some killing lines is that some birds miss the stunner altogether, either because they are runts and do not reach the water level, or because they are flapping their wings and raise their bodies as they pass over the bath. These features are, however, less common. The problem of runts missing the waterbath can be avoided by not hanging them on the line with the other birds, but keeping them back and treating them separately.

The duration of unconsciousness provided by electrical stunning is quite short. For example, when waterbath stunning does not induce a ventricular fibrillation (while applying 105 mA per broiler), the time to onset of recovery is as short as 52 seconds, and in hens it can be as low as 22 seconds. The duration of unconsciousness depends on the current that is used and the duration for which the current is applied.

Inducing a cardiac arrest at stunning is helpful from the welfare point of view because when it occurs it is no longer essential to bleed the bird promptly and efficiently in order to kill it. A cardiac arrest also results in a more prompt and punctual loss of brain function than neck cutting and so it decreases even further the likelihood of the bird regaining consciousness.

The physical signs shown by birds that do not develop a cardiac arrest at stunning are sometimes wrongly diagnosed as signs of consciousness. The characteristic signs of the stunned state without cardiac arrest are an arched neck (dorsoflexion), wings held close to the body and tremor in the wings, with the legs rigidly extended. When there is a cardiac arrest at stunning the birds quickly go limp after stunning, the wings and neck drop and the pupils dilate. One of the most useful signs to look for is the resumption of normal rhythmic breathing during bleeding. A conscious bird is not likely to hold its breath for very long, and so the absence of breathing should indicate unconsciousness. Normal rhythmic breathing is not proof of consciousness, but it indicates that further tests are required to establish whether the birds are stunned. Looking for breathing is not a valid test if the spinal cord was severed at neck cutting (Gregory, 1996a).

Neck cutting is usually performed automatically with a machine. The automatic neck cutters usually make a cut at the side or back of the neck. Studies that have examined the time to loss of brain function following a variety of neck-cutting or slaughtering procedures have shown that cutting the back of the neck takes a relatively long time to kill the birds (Gregory and Wotton, 1986). When this approach is used the carotid arteries, which are the main arteries supplying blood to the brain, are not severed. Failure to sever the carotid arteries greatly increases the risk of resumption of consciousness during bleeding if the birds do not develop a cardiac arrest at stunning. Inducing a cardiac arrest is the most effective method of ensuring that consciousness will not return. The next best methods are decapitation and severing both carotid arteries. On this basis, it has been recommended that birds should either be subjected to a cardiac arrest at stunning or have both their carotid arteries severed at neck cutting. In order to cut both carotid arteries it is necessary to cut the whole of the ventral aspect of the neck, including the trachea and oesophagus.

The optimum time between stunning and neck cutting is determined by three factors. Firstly, it should not be so long that it allows the birds to regain consciousness before they die. Secondly, it should be long enough to allow the supervisor to assess whether the birds are stunned when they leave the waterbath. Thirdly, the birds should be given sufficient time to allow their necks to relax and thus feed into the guide bars of the automatic neck cutter. On average the time to neck relaxation after the end of stunning is 9 seconds in broilers, but this may be influenced by whether they experience a cardiac arrest.

It is general practice for a person to stand alongside the bleeding trough or tunnel and manually cut the necks of any birds that were not cut by the automatic neck cutter. These birds are often those that escaped being stunned by the waterbath stunner and so they are fully conscious when they have their necks cut.

Although decapitation and *neck dislocation* without prior stunning are permitted methods, they do not necessarily cause instantaneous impairment of brain function (Gregory and Wotton, 1990). Evoked responses in the chicken brain take time to fail when either of these methods are used, and they do not produce any immediate changes in the amplitude or latency of the evoked responses, unlike concussion. So there is reluctance to commend these methods as being humane. Nevertheless, they are simple and so they are used for immediate euthanasia where there is no better alternative.

In the future more poultry processing plants could change from electrical stunning to gas stunning systems. One of the potential welfare advantages of gas stunning is that the birds can be stunned in their transport crates. This avoids the preslaughter stress of removing them from the crates and hanging them on the shackles of the killing line. In addition, recent research has shown that electrical stunning may not cause an instantaneous stun in all broilers, even when applied in the prescribed manner, and so gas stunning would avoid the problem of some birds experiencing electric shocks before being stunned.

Carbon dioxide is being used because it has narcotic properties, it is a dense gas and so it is reasonably easy to contain, and it is a naturally occurring gas leaving no undesirable residues in the meat. However, CO_2 is aversive to poultry, and it has been recommended that it should not be used at high concentrations. An acceptable system is to use a low concentration of CO_2 in combination with anoxia (less than 2% O_2) (Mohan Raj *et al.*, 1992). This combination is less aversive.

Chapter 14

Stunning and Meat Quality

REDMEAT SPECIES

The methods used for killing cattle, sheep and pigs can affect the following conditions in their carcasses:

- physical convulsions;
- bruising;
- blood splash;
- blood speckle;
- pelt burn;
- broken bones;
- bleeding efficiency;
- rate of pH fall in muscle.

Three physiological events contribute to these conditions: muscle contractions, elevated blood pressure and variation in the rate of bleeding. The physiological control of convulsive activity and blood pressure was described in Chapter 4.

When an animal is electrically stunned the nervous system is activated, causing contraction of the muscles in the body and constriction of the blood vessels in the capillary bed within the muscles. If the spasm at the onset of stunning is particularly severe, the muscles can tear parts of the capillary bed. In the forequarter this is often at the points where the muscles are attached to the tendons and bones. When the electrical stunning current flows through the animal, the vagus nerve is activated along with other nerves, and this causes a pronounced decrease in heart rate. Once the current is switched off, heart rate and arterial blood pressure rise rapidly and continue to rise well above normal levels. The elevated blood pressure, coupled with capillary tearing, produces haemorrhages in the muscles (Leet *et al.*, 1977). If, on the other hand, a cardiac arrest is induced at stunning or if the carcass is immediately stuck, arterial pressure collapses and there is limited leakage of blood through any capillaries that were torn at the onset of current flow.

The *convulsions* that occur after the animal has been stunned usually last for 0.5–1 minute. Most convulsions are controlled by the nervous system. They are mediated through the spinal cord and some of the activity originates in the brain. Severing the spinal cord in the neck interrupts and stops the activity that originates in the brain. Some of the activity is also provoked through spinal reflexes. For example, if a carcass is bumped and jolted as it is conveyed by the hoist between stunning and sticking, this sets up delayed exaggerated kicking activity. Destroying the spinal cord with a pithing cane stops that spinal reflex activity as well as the convulsions that are initiated in the brain. It is also common to see localized muscle twitching or *fasciculations* in a carcass, especially in beef. Unlike convulsions, fasciculations are not prevented by curare, and so they are not due to nerve activity (McLoughlin, 1970).

The convulsions following electrical stunning come in two phases: a tonic (rigid) phase lasting for about 10 seconds and a clonic (kicking) phase which may last about half a minute. The activities are important because they affect the presence of muscle haemorrhages (e.g. blood splash) and also because they can increase the initial rate of post-mortem muscle metabolism, cause broken bones, endanger safety of the operators and reduce the throughput of the slaughterline (Gregory, 1987). Ways of controlling the clonic activity in the stunned animal include:

- pithing;
- severing the spinal cord;
- inducing a cardiac arrest at stunning;
- spinal discharge;
- electroimmobilization;
- prompt sticking;
- sticking before shackling.

Pithing with a cane is only done in cattle that have been shot with a captive bolt or free bullet. The cane is introduced into the head through the hole created by the bolt or bullet and is passed along the upper part of the spinal column. It is then oscillated up and down the column to macerate the spinal cord. During this action the hindlegs kick but thereafter, once the cord is destroyed, kicking ceases altogether and the carcass is safe to handle. Cattle that have been properly stunned and are due to be pithed are sometimes shot a second time in a position that allows easier entry of the cane into the spinal column. This should not be mistaken for repeat stunning where, in the judgement of the slaughterman, the animal was not effectively stunned. Where attempts have been made to pith an improperly stunned animal, it has been impossible to introduce the cane because of the animal's physical reaction. The kicking that occurs during pithing does not affect muscle metabolism in the longissimus dorsi muscle but it does accelerate ATP utilization in the psoas major. Pithing is regarded as an unhygienic practice and is likely to be phased out for this reason. As the heart is still beating, blood washes bacteria from the pithing cane to the muscles of the carcass (Mackey and Derrick, 1979).

Severing the spinal cord is sometimes done in sheep after they have been gash stuck. The operator first dislocates the vertebrae in the neck by pushing an arm against to the back of the neck whilst holding the jaw with the other hand. The spinal cord is then severed by introducing a knife ventrally through the gap that was created by the dislocation. There is sometimes a misconception that the first procedure (neck dislocation) will ensure that the animal is 'brain dead'. The only real benefit is in severing the spinal cord to reduce carcass kicking.

Cardiac arrest stunning can be highly effective in reducing clonic activity. Tonic activity is not affected, but carcass kicking is greatly reduced when there is a cardiac arrest with head-to-back, head-to-brisket, head-to-foreleg or head-to-hindleg stunning. In lambs, head-to-foreleg stunning causes slightly more carcass activity than the other cardiac arrest stunning methods, but the difference is small. There could be two reasons for the reduction in carcass kicking. Firstly, when there is a cardiac arrest, peripheral nerve hypoxia quickly sets in and this will reduce the duration of the kicking phase. Secondly, when current passes through the body to the heart, some current flows through the spinal cord. This creates a *spinal discharge* and if sufficient current is used, subsequent transmission along the cord is disrupted and kicking fails to occur. In some situations spinal discharge is applied between stunning and sticking, and it is particularly helpful in controlling carcass kicking in cattle. There is a risk in cattle and pigs that spinal discharge currents will cause broken bones (especially vertebrae) but this damage should be reduced by using high frequency currents.

Electroimmobilization is different from spinal discharge in the way the current is applied. In spinal discharge, a short pulse of a high current is used to disrupt subsequent neurotransmission. Electroimmobilization uses low currents, often at low frequencies, which are applied continuously throughout the period that carcass kicking has to be controlled. In some countries, electroimmobilization is the preferred method of controlling kicking in halal beef animals that have been electrically stunned. In other countries, applying an immobilizing current between stunning and sticking is disallowed because it is no longer possible to judge whether the animal is unconscious when movement is controlled by the current. Some pig and sheep slaughtermen try to control kicking when using head-only stunning by applying the current for a long period. This probably works in a similar manner to spinal discharge.

Prompt sticking (e.g. sticking the animal while it is lying horizontally and before it is shackled) is the most common way of avoiding the problems created by carcass kicking. If the carcass is stuck whilst it is in the tonic phase, it does not need to be handled again until after the clonic phase has ended. This minimizes the risk of injury to staff from spontaneous and reflex kicking activity.

When pigs are stuck whilst suspended vertically, the carcass tends to swing if the forelegs start kicking. The swinging is controlled by the operator, who holds a foreleg with one hand and performs a chest stick with the other. If the pig kicks at the wrong moment, there is a risk that the knife is off-centre and goes into the shoulder. This is known as *shoulder sticking* and it causes a haemorrhage in the shoulder joint. It has been known for the operator to cut his own wrist in this situation, and one way of minimizing this risk is to use short-chained shackles, which help reduce the swing of the carcass.

When carcass convulsions are excessive, they use up energy and accelerate the early stages of post-mortem muscle glycolysis. This is particularly pronounced in the case of pigs that have been shot. The convulsions can lead to an initial pH of less than 6.1. In addition the meat is likely to be blood splashed, and the carcass is dangerous to handle. For these reasons shooting pigs with a captive bolt is rarely used or recommended.

Electrical stunning causes severe clonic activity when high voltages are used and the carcass is not bled promptly. Normally this is controlled by bleeding the animal out whilst it is still tonic, and in this situation the rate of post-mortem muscle glycolysis is not markedly different from that observed with low stunning voltages. High voltage electrical stunning, however, can accelerate the rate of *post-mortem muscle glycolysis* if the carcass is allowed to kick violently, or if the current is applied for excessively long periods (more than 12 seconds). The current is not normally applied for periods as long as this and so it is not a real issue. High frequency electrical stunning can induce milder tonic activity but more erratic clonic activity. This would not be expected to have much effect on muscle glycolysis, but the weaker tonic spasm leads to less blood splash in the meat. Head-to-back stunning in lambs has been shown to cause a marginally lower initial pH (by 0.2 of a unit) in the longissimus dorsi muscle, but the effect is so small that it is of no commercial significance. Similarly, suspending a carcass by a hindleg from a shackle adds to the tension in the leg and loin muscles, and this has a small accelerating effect on their rate of post-mortem glycolysis.

In some situations the muscle contractions that occur during electrical stunning cause *broken bones*. Haemorrhages form at the fractures, provided the heart is still beating. Three types of fracture are worth noting. In pigs, which are stunned whilst free-standing on the floor, the sudden extension of the forelegs causes an impact against the floor which is directed upwards against the scapula (shoulderblade). This can cause the end of the scapula to shatter (van der Wal, 1976). The best way of avoiding this condition is to remove the pigs from the floor, and stun them in a restraining conveyor instead. Another condition is broken backs. When head-to-back stunning is used in pigs, the vertebrae are prone to breaking. For this reason, head-to-back stunning is inappropriate for pigs even though it has animal welfare advantages. Slipped discs also occur with head-to-back stunning in pigs, and the discs can be heard popping out of the vertebrae as the current is applied. Unlike broken backs, they are not associated with significant haemorrhaging. Broken sacrums have occurred when spinal discharge currents have been used in cattle.

Carcass *bruising* can occur at the time of stunning and sticking. Typically, this happens when:

- cattle are struck on the back by guillotine gates in the race and stunning pen;
- stock strike gateways and raceway fittings when moving to the restraining conveyor or stunning pen;
- the initial spasm at stunning causes broken bones;
- stunned cattle fall heavily as they roll out of the stunning pen;
- stunned pigs fall from shackles because of excessive carcass kicking;
- the neck is cut; the edges of the sticking wound can appear as bruised tissue when the forequarter is boned out.

If an animal is bruised just before or after sticking, the bruise will be small. If blood is quickly voided through the sticking wound, there will be limited time for blood to leak from the ruptured vessels at the bruised site (Gregory and Wilkins, 1984). Once the carcass has lost half the blood that is due to leave the sticking wound, it can no longer be bruised. The only possible exception to this is where poorly bled heavyweight pigs sometimes acquire post-mortem bruising on the ham as they are tumbled in the dehairing machine.

If the knife is inserted deeply during chest sticking, the heart may be cut in pigs and the pleura may be punctured in cattle. *Back bleeding* occurs if blood adheres to the pleura or infiltrates between the pleura. This may prompt the staff working on the carcasses to strip the pleura from the carcass before it has been inspected by the official meat inspector. The meat inspector needs to examine the pleura for any adhesions.

In forensic science, one of the signs of death from electrocution is the presence of *blood splash* (petechial haemorrhaging). In livestock, electrical stunning is a common cause of blood splash in meat. Its occurrence depends on two factors: the initial spasm at stunning, which tears the muscle capillaries, and an elevated blood pressure following stunning. It occurs in a range of muscles, including the high value muscles in the hindquarter. In pigs it is often present in the shoulder and it can occur in the quadriceps and gracilis muscles. In veal, it is more likely to be seen in the shoulder and the fascia of the loin. Its presence in a whole carcass can be determined from an inspection of the skirt (diaphragm) and, in some situations, the thin flank. These can be useful indicator muscles. It appears as small bleps and streaks of blood, often aligned with the direction of the muscle fibres, and they are dark red in colour. Blood splash gives fresh meat an abnormal appearance and it is likely to be rejected by meat buyers. When it is grilled or fried, the bleps of blood turn brown and take on the appearance of the normal burn or charred marks that are seen in cooked meat.

The following are ways of reducing blood splash and bruising that occur at stunning.

- Keep the interval between stunning and sticking to a minimum. This will not stop the formation of the blood splash, but it will reduce the period during which blood can leak through the ruptured blood vessels.
- In lambs, calves and cattle, use a captive bolt instead of electrical stunning. The muscle spasms are less severe with the captive bolt in these classes of stock.
- In lambs, use an electrical stunning method which simultaneously induces a cardiac arrest (Kirton *et al.*, 1980/81). This reduces the blood pressure.
- Ensure that there is an uninterrupted, continuous flow of current during stunning (Kirton and Frazerhurst, 1983)
- Ensure that the restraining conveyor does not grip the animal too tightly. If necessary, change to a straddle conveyor, or stun pigs while they are free-standing on the floor.
- In pigs, use high frequency electrical stunning or gas stunning. Alternatively, high voltage automatic electrical stunning (700 V) causes less blood splash in pigs than 300 V, presumably because it induces a cardiac arrest (Table 14.1) (Larsen, 1982).
- In venison, reduce preslaughter stress.

Not all blood splash is caused by stunning. It has occurred, for example, in beef slaughtered by shechita where there was no stunning. In that situation, the blood splash was controlled (but not eliminated) by minimizing preslaughter stress. High blood pressure coupled with struggling were the likely causes.

Blood speckle is a fiery rash which occurs in the connective tissue and muscle fascia on the backs and hindlegs of lamb carcasses (Gilbert, 1980).

Table 14.1. Meat quality in pigs stunned by three methods.

	300 V Manual	700 V Automatic	CO_2
Shoulder haemorrhages (g)	145	59	8
Bone fractures (%)	1.2	1.0	0
PSE (%)	19	15	4
DFD (%)	6	8	6

It is associated with head-to-back stunning and often occurs at the site of the back electrode. Reducing the stunning current (from 1.4 to 0.7 A) and applying the current for shorter periods (2 instead of 10 seconds) has reduced blood speckle in the hindleg (Devine *et al.*, 1983). It does not occur with head-to-leg stunning, which also induces a cardiac arrest, and so it is not directly linked to heart function. Instead, it is due to the direct effect of the current on the blood capillaries. Reducing the amount of blood held in the capillaries, by applying an α-adrenergic blocking drug, has been shown to reduce the severity of the condition. Blood speckle often looks worse in young lambs because of their high capillary density in their subcutaneous tissues.

Head-to-back stunning is also linked with *pelt burn*. This is caused by heating of the skin by the electric current at the back electrode. The burn marks are only noticed when the pelt is cured. It can be controlled by increasing the area of contact between the electrodes and the skin, and this is achieved by using a metal plate instead of pins and by thoroughly wetting the back before applying the plate electrode.

Bleeding efficiency is influenced by the stunning method that is used, the way the skin and blood vessels are cut during sticking, the interval between stunning and sticking and the position of the carcass during bleeding. The weight of blood in an animal is usually about 8% of its liveweight. Normally only about half that blood is voided during slaughter. However, very little is retained in the meat; for example, beef only holds about 2–9 ml kg^{-1} of muscle. Most of the remaining blood is in the offal and major blood vessels, and it is removed during evisceration and dressing.

A stunned animal does not need to have a beating heart in order to bleed out properly. The initial rate of blood flow from a carcass with a cardiac arrest may be reduced but in most species, provided it is left long enough, the carcass will drain by gravity and yield the same amount of blood as a carcass which had a beating heart when it was stuck (Warriss and Wotton, 1981; Gregory and Wilkins, 1989). Carcasses that have a cardiac arrest will usually drain more rapidly if they are suspended by a hindleg, in comparison with the horizontal bleeding position. In practice, this has been an issue in lamb slaughterhouses where a protracted bleeding has resulted in excessively bloody floors under the slaughterline. With horizontal bleeding more blood tends to be held back in the viscera (Kirton *et al.*, 1980/81), but this has been overcome by tilting the carcass slightly with the head downwards. Gash sticking gives a more rapid bleed out than spear sticking but, once again, the total amount of blood that is released is not affected provided the carcass is given long enough to drain. Bleeding efficiency can be slightly impaired when pigs are stunned with CO_2 instead of electrically, and if the sticking wound is too small.

In the past it was thought that it is important to bleed an animal out completely, otherwise the meat will not keep. The argument has been that blood is a good incubation medium for bacteria, and it can promote autolysis and oxidation of fats. When ground meat has been mixed with blood and then inoculated with bacteria, the rate of proliferation of the bacteria has been no greater than in mince which had no added blood. Meat is just as good an incubation medium for bacteria as blood. A more important consideration is if blood is left in the veins and it produces an unsightly smear across the surface when it is cut. Blood-enriched meat is more likely to have a salty flavour, because of the high sodium level in blood serum.

The carcass has to be stuck within 3 minutes of heart failure in order to bleed out satisfactorily. If an animal dies and it is not bled promptly, the blood in the larger vessels will start to clot. Clotting does not occur inside the small blood vessels and capillaries. This is because the smaller vessels are thin-walled and they take up low-molecular-weight clotting factors along with some fluid once the circulation stops. The larger blood vessels are thick-walled and less permeable, and so long gels of clotted blood form in the jugular veins, vena cava, aorta and heart if they do not empty out. These gels block the release of unclotted blood in the smaller vessels, should an attempt be made to bleed a dead animal out. Some of the unclotted blood will, however, gravitate within the dead animal if it is not dressed immediately, and this will affect the appearance of the meat. The exact appearance of a poorly bled carcass or one produced by *cold slaughter* (bleeding out a dead animal) depends on the animal's position after it died. If, for example, it was suspended by a hindleg, blood would gravitate to the fore-end, and the lungs, thymus and medial surface of the subcutaneous fat at the split brisket will be noticeably engorged with blood (Gregory *et al.*, 1988).

The early methods used for stunning pigs with *carbon dioxide* had a reputation for causing PSE meat. In recent times the design of CO_2 units has improved and they are now considered to produce less handling stress and less PSE meat than electrical stunning systems (von Zweigbergk *et al.*, 1989). Over the years there have been four types of CO_2 stunning systems: oval tunnel, dip lift, compact stunner and the combi stunner. The oval tunnel was the first system to be developed (see Fig. 13.9). Sybesma and Groen (1970) did an important experiment which demonstrated the effect of handling stress at stunning in causing PSE meat. They had four treatments. In the first treatment, pigs were put through an oval tunnel filled with CO_2, at a normal pace (180 pigs/hour). They measured the proportion of pigs that developed PSE meat, and it was 9%. In the second treatment, they put pigs through the CO_2-filled oval tunnel at a slower pace (90 pigs/hour) but the proportion of pigs with PSE meat was the same (9%). In the third treatment, the pigs were put through the oval tunnel but this time it was filled with air, and the pigs were electrically stunned when they came out the other end. The prevalence of PSE meat was still the same (9%). In the fourth treatment, the pigs were driven along the race up to the oval tunnel in the normal way, but they were redirected across the entrance and electrically stunned at the exit. By preventing them passing through the oval tunnel, the level of PSE meat was reduced to 1%. The conclusion, therefore, was that the stress involved in putting pigs into the oval tunnel unit was sufficient in itself to induce the higher incidence of PSE meat.

The compact stunner operates along the lines of a ferris wheel, and the handling is thought to be less stressful for the pigs. The concentration of CO_2 that is used in stunning the pigs, however, may also influence the development of PSE meat. Pigs subjected to high concentrations (85–90%) show less vigorous physical activity before they collapse and their muscle has a slower rate of pH fall post-mortem (Troeger and Woltersdorf, 1991).

Any stunning or slaughter method that involves penetration of the skin of the animal is liable to raise hygiene risks. It has been found that when bacteria were inoculated on to either the bolt of the captive-bolt gun or on to the blade of the sticking knife, the same bacteria could be recovered from the edible meat in the carcass. In the case of the captive bolt, bacteria are transferred to the brain, which is still irrigated with blood after the animal is shot, and so the microorganisms can be distributed throughout the carcass. The same applies to the pithing cane. For this reason it is appropriate to sterilize the knife and pithing cane between each animal. Sterilizing the bolt of the captive-bolt gun is not a practical proposition with existing gun designs.

Carcass contamination can also occur from oesophageal efflux of rumen contents. This is a particular nuisance where the oesophagus is cut during sticking; the edible meat in the neck is visibly contaminated with digesta and it can acquire a green stain. Three methods can be used for controlling this. The first is to insert a plastic plug into the oesophagus via the mouth after the animal has been shot. The second is to tie off the oesophagus by knotting it or by using a weasand clip. The third is to stimulate the carcass electrically at the time when efflux is likely to occur. Passing a current through the carcass causes closure of the sphincter, but this only works for as long as the current is applied and the muscle of the sphincter is not exhausted. Where blood is collected as an edible food product, a tubular bleeding knife with a hose leading to a tank is used for sticking the animal. This is potentially more hygienic than collecting blood in a trough or gutter, as it is less likely to be contaminated with urine and gut contents.

WHITEMEAT SPECIES

The methods used for killing poultry can affect the following conditions in their carcasses:

- physical convulsions;
- wing and shoulder haemorrhages;
- breast skin colour and haemorrhages;
- breast meat haemorrhages;
- bleeding efficiency;

- breast meat pH fall;
- breast meat texture;
- ease of feather removal;
- removal of inedible offal;
- hygiene of the body cavity.

Other procedures can affect these conditions and so it is important not to blame the stunner arbitrarily whenever a problem arises (Gregory, 1991b).

If birds are slaughtered by neck cutting without any stunning, they beat their wings very violently during the convulsive phase. It has been shown experimentally that denervation of the breast muscle will prevent these convulsions and it also slows the rate of post-mortem muscle glycolysis (Papinaho *et al.*, 1995). Electrical stunning before neck cutting helps to control the convulsions and so it slows the rate of post-mortem glycolysis. This can lead to more tender breast meat by reducing the extent of heat shortening (Thomson *et al.*, 1986). In practice, most birds are electrically stunned before they have their necks cut, but in some processing plants which export frozen broilers, stunning has been stopped because it can cause breast meat haemorrhages. By not stunning the birds, breast meat haemorrhages can be reduced but there is a greater risk of breast meat toughness.

Table 14.2 summarizes the causes of *downgrading* for the haemorrhagic conditions. Research experience indicates that breast meat haemorrhages are inevitably linked with the use of electrical stunning with a low frequency waveform. The stunning currents that cause an increase in the prevalence of *breast meat haemorrhages* are higher than those recommended for producing an effective stun in broilers, turkeys and ducks, and so it should be possible to exert some control over this quality problem

Table 14.2. Causes of haemorrhaging in broiler carcasses.

Downgrading problem	Cause
Red wingtips	Excessive flapping of the wings before death Stunning currents in the range of 110–150 mA per bird* Poor bleeding in combination with harsh plucking
Wing and shoulder haemorrhages	Stunning currents in the range of 110–150 mA per bird Poor bleeding in combination with harsh plucking
Red feather tracts and neck skin	Largely due to poor bleeding
Breast muscle haemorrhages	Usually due to high stunning currents (130–190 mA per bird*). Not influenced by efficiency of bleeding or severity of plucking

* When using a 50 Hz AC, and when compared with currents within the range of 45–220 mA per bird.

whilst achieving an adequate stun. This may not be the case for wing haemorrhages in broilers, but the situation is complicated by the fact that wing haemorrhages can also be due to inadequate bleeding and unduly harsh plucking when removing the feathers. This was demonstrated in the following experiment, which had four treatments (Gregory and Wilkins, 1990). In each treatment the broilers were electrically stunned with 120 mA per bird and all of them had a cardiac arrest at stunning. The birds in the first treatment were bled by severing both carotid arteries and both jugular veins, and they were machine plucked in a normal manner. In the three remaining treatments the birds were not bled, and this was meant to exaggerate the effect of inadequate bleeding. In one of these treatments the birds were hand plucked (mild pluck), in another treatment they were machine plucked (normal pluck) and in the last treatment they were put through the machine plucker twice (severe pluck). Comparing the normal-bleeding–normal-pluck treatment with the not-bled–normal-pluck treatment gives an indication of the effect that very bad bleeding has on downgrading (Table 14.3). *Red wingtips, wing haemorrhages and red feather tracts* were worse in the badly bled carcasses. As the severity of plucking increased, so also did the prevalence of red wingtips, wing haemorrhages, red feather tracts and broken wishbones. Breast meat haemorrhages within the meat were not affected by either the efficiency of bleeding or the severity of plucking.

The reason for the effects on the wings was as follows. When a shackled bird is stunned and bled, its wings go limp as the bird dies and they hang down from the shoulder joint. If this occurs before blood emptied from the wing veins, the veins will contain blood when the carcass enters the pluckers. The rotating plucker fingers can rupture the veins through the skin, causing a post-mortem bruise; the more severe the plucking, the more likely it is that a bruise will form. Poor bleeding from the neck-cut wound increases the likelihood of the wing veins being engorged with blood, and

Table 14.3. Percentages of carcasses downgraded according to bleeding and plucking procedure. (From Gregory and Wilkins, 1990.)

Carcasses downgraded for	Normal bleeding, normal plucking	Not bled		
		Hand pluck	Normal machine pluck	Double machine pluck
Red wingtips	22	0	54	87
Wing haemorrhages	22	0	35	87
Red feather tracts	11	48	85	98
Breast meat haemorrhages	24	31	26	25
Broken wishbones	28	15	25	40

severe plucking increases the likelihood of wing vein rupture. Although this experiment was somewhat synthetic compared with commercial practice, it helped to establish the importance of bleeding efficiency and plucking severity in causing downgrading.

High frequency electrical stunning can reduce the prevalence of *breast muscle haemorrhages* (by as much as 70%) in comparison with 50 or 60 Hz. It is important, however, to bleed the birds correctly to achieve a humane kill as high frequency currents do not cause a cardiac arrest and so there is a greater risk of recovery of consciousness. Gas stunning using a combination of 30% CO_2 and less than 2% O_2 also reduces the amount of breast muscle haemorrhaging in broilers and turkeys.

Consumers often look upon *broken bones* in poultry portions as 'foreign bodies' and the bone fragments can inflict mouth damage if they have sharp edges. If the wishbone (furculum) breaks, a section of the bone may be left attached to the breast meat when it is filleted. Wishbones usually break during the initial body spasm at stunning and during plucking. Increasing the stunning current can increase the prevalence of broken wishbones. Electrical stunning also results in broken coracoid and scapula bones, but this does not occur with gas stunning (Raj *et al.*, 1997).

Automatic neck cutters bleed the birds out by making a cut at the back of the neck. The welfare implications of this method are discussed in Chapter 13. In birds that do not develop a cardiac arrest at stunning, the carotid arteries should be cut by the neck cutter, and this would normally involve making a cut at the front of the neck. In the past, the reason that the cut has been made at the back of the neck was that a frontal cut would have involved severing the trachea, weakening the neck and thus allowing heads to become detached in the pluckers. In both situations a section of trachea would be left attached to the neck flap and would have to be removed by hand further down the line. By cutting the back of the neck the need for this additional procedure was avoided. More recently, new designs of cropping (final inspection) machines have been introduced which remove *residual trachea* from the neck flap automatically. So, the reason for back-of-the-neck cutting no longer applies, and in the future we could see ventral neck cutting instead.

Automatic neck cutters are sometimes set to sever the spinal cord. This makes it difficult to judge whether the bird is conscious or unconscious, but the way to test for this has been described in some detail (Gregory, 1996a). By severing the spinal cord, the nervous activity passing from the brain to the body is interrupted. This helps to reduce carcass convulsions and it quickly arrests the smooth muscle activity that is responsible for vasoconstriction and for gripping the feather shafts in the skin. In birds which are not scalded, *feather removal* is easier if the spinal cord is severed at neck cutting (Levinger and Angel, 1977). There could also be a poorer bleed-out if the spinal cord is cut, because it would result in a prompt vasodilation before the blood has been lost.

The way birds are stunned and slaughtered affects the way in which they convulse as they die, and the convulsions affect muscle metabolism and meat quality. The general principle is that increased muscle activity results in a faster *rate of pH fall.* If this occurs whilst the muscle is hot, there is a greater risk of toughness due to heat shortening. The following serve as examples of situations when this can occur. If birds are bled without being electrically stunned, they convulse violently during bleeding and this causes an accelerated rate of breast muscle pH fall. At high stunning currents the carcass quickly relaxes after it leaves the stunner, and so the rate of breast muscle pH fall is slower. If the carcass is cut into portions and filleted within 4 hours of slaughter, the freshly filleted breast will contain more ATP and so it will be more prone to toughness caused by rigor shortening (Papinaho and Fletcher, 1996). If, on the other hand, the carcass is left whole or the breast is filleted after the muscle has been allowed to metabolize its ATP (i.e. more than 4 h after slaughter), texture is either unaffected or slightly more tender in the birds which received a high stunning current. However, if the stunning current is applied for long periods (e.g. 10 seconds in comparison with 4 seconds), the longer forced contraction can accelerate glycolysis and lead to tougher breast meat through heat shortening (Young *et al.*, 1996). One way of accelerating post-mortem glycolysis whilst minimizing heat shortening is to stun with 30% CO_2 and 60% argon (Raj *et al.*, 1997).

During electrical stunning, some of the birds defaecate and urinate. This is particularly noticeable at high stunning currents, and it causes bacterial *contamination* of the water in the stunner. About one-third of the birds inhale water during the initial tonic spasm that occurs during stunning, and this allows bacterial contamination of the body cavity with dirty stunner water when the respiratory tract is removed during evisceration.

Chapter 15

Caring for Animals and for Quality

In 1996 the Humane Society of the United States released a video which showed a team of men catching broilers at a chicken farm. They were gathering the birds for slaughter. The video was not pleasant viewing, as they were hurling the birds into the modules with no concern about injuring them. The video also showed one catcher kicking a bird that got separated from the flock, as if it was a football, up the shed towards the other birds. Day-old chicks were unloaded from their delivery boxes by throwing them en masse on to the floor. At about the same time, Compassion in World Farming (UK) produced another appalling video. There were live cattle being hoisted from railway wagons by crane with a chain tied around their heads. One of the animals slipped from the chain whilst it was suspended in mid-air, fell to ground on to its rump and broke its spine. It was left overnight with a broken back before it was shot. Both of these videos showed acts of unquestionable cruelty.

This leads to the question: how do people react to cases of blatant cruelty such as these? Your reaction would probably be influenced by your emotions, so let's rephrase the question. What would you feel if you came across a case of blatant cruelty? Would it be anger, shame, horror or distress? I was working in a pig abattoir once when a woman burst into the slaughterhall without any gumboots or overalls. She started haranguing one of the staff, tried to hit him, burst into tears and eventually was led outside. Her outburst came from having to listen to the screams of the pigs in the lairage when she passed by in the street. More recently, I have been showing people a particularly unpleasant video of cases of animal cruelty in Europe. Different groups or individuals have reacted in quite different ways. Some of the students became distressed; they left the room or wept. When managerial staff of a marketing board saw it, they became wide-eyed, thoughtful and I suspect a little alarmed. When veterinarians saw it they wagged their heads, and then took a professional interest by discussing the consequences of the brutality or actions. Finally, when a group of farmers saw it there was complete silence. Not a stir or whisper. Their emotions were private ones, but I suspect there was a mixture of horror, anger and shame for the people in the video. Distress about animal suffering, and shame towards people who are cruel, are two key emotions that influence our attitudes about animal welfare.

Cases of animal cruelty are very harmful to the image of the meat and livestock industry. They cause revulsion amongst the public and they reinforce the move against meat-eating. They create an image of indifference and profit-chasing at the animals' expense.

Non-caring images are also being attributed in a more general way to some of the large corporate companies that are linked to the livestock, meat and food industries. In response to this, there is a growing feeling of anti-corporatism in a sector of the community. Some supermarket companies have recognized this and are trying to reverse the trend. Individual companies are using animal welfare as a way of persuading the public that they are in fact a 'caring' company. They want to create the image that they care about food safety, about the environment and in particular they care for their customers. An ostentatious way of putting this caring image over is through their attitude towards animals. They are showing that they care about animals by marketing welfare-friendly products. The overall aim is to link the company name with a sense of friendliness, security and comfort, all of which are increasingly valued in a society that has to tolerate the seemingly uncaring attitude of competitive accountability that exists in the workplace.

The caring attitude of the retailer has to be translated into real terms. There are three ways in which they can do this:

- by not selling products that are considered welfare-unfriendly (e.g. battery eggs);
- by promoting welfare-friendly products (e.g. free-range chicken);
- by imposing welfare standards on suppliers as part of their contractual relationship (e.g. imposing adoption of recognised Codes of Practice).

Examples of some food labelling schemes that promote animal welfare are shown in Table 15.1. Schemes such as these require credibility, otherwise the whole basis of marketing welfare-improved products is liable to collapse. The retail sector is prone to over-imaginative use of nonsense words such as the following example of labelling:

> This *succulent* pork was produced from *happy* pigs on *selected family-run farms* in the heart of *beautiful Iowa*. The *specially* formulated diet contains *natural* maize and soyabean given to the pigs under *exacting* conditions which were regularly *checked*.

It is important that welfare-improved products are dissociated from this type of jargon. Instead, welfare-friendly products have to be labelled accurately and the labelling must be based on standards that have been developed by a respected independent organization. The systems of production and slaughter need to be audited regularly to ensure that there is compliance with those standards.

Another approach to improving animal welfare is to change the law. The days when the law on animal cruelty and animal welfare only gave general principles are coming to an end. Instead, the official regulations and recommendations on how animals can be treated are becoming more detailed. Enforcement of the law can be made more effective in various ways. One approach that is being considered in New Zealand is to have instant fines for infringement offences involving animal welfare, in much the same way as a traffic officers can issue fines against motorists for parking or speeding offences.

What areas of animal welfare need particular attention? In the public's view, the least acceptable practices are probably those involving:

- prolonged confinement
- mutilations
- slaughter

In terms of animal suffering, there are many other issues in additon to these. Some of the more important ones are listed in Table 15.2: 75% of the problems in this list are strongly influenced by standards of stockmanship (e.g. disease control) and about 50% are innate problems in particular production systems and have an element of inevitability which makes them difficult to control or avoid (e.g. weaning stress). About 25% of the problems (e.g. handling stress) have an impact on the quality and acceptability of the

Table 15.1. Food labelling schemes with animal welfare criteria.

Country	Scheme
France	Label Range
Germany	Neuland
Ireland	Organic Trust Ltd
	10FGA Symbol Scheme
Netherlands	Controlebureau Pluimvee Eieren
	International Scharrelvlees Controle
	Skal Eko Standards
Sweden	KRAV
Switzerland	Agri-Natura
United Kingdom	Freedom foods
	Real Meat Company
	Soil Association

Table 15.2. Some of the main welfare problems in farmed animals.

Dairy cows	Suckler cows	Calves	Beef cattle	Pigs	Sheep	Deer	Hens	Broilers	Farmed fish
Lameness	Handling problems	Loss of maternal care	Transport and handling	Handling in abattoirs	Lameness	Handling	Behavioural deprivations	Leg weakness	Mortality
Mastitis	Disease from neglect	Castration	Disease from neglect	Stunning and slaughter	Transport stress	Trauma	Barren environment	Stocking density	Ineffective treatment of disease
Dystocia	Parasitism	Transport and handling	Parasitism	Confinement in sow stalls	Cold stress at shearing	Antler harvesting	Stocking density	Dehydration in runts	Handling
Over-production disorders	Under/ malnutrition	Disbudding	Trauma	Piglet mortality	Adverse weather	Calf mortality	Broken bones	Catching damage	Slaughter
Flies	Exposure to bad weather			Aggression	Undernutrition	Underfeeding	Cannibalism	Light intensity	Cannibalism
Stray voltages	Flies			Pneumonia and pleurisy	Shearing and worming	Dystocia	Inspection and culling	Heat stress	Overstocking
Heat stress				Tail biting	Mulesing	Osteochondrosis	Beak trimming	Inspection and culling	Cage noise
Calf removal				Osteochondrosis	Parasitism	Heat stress	Light intensity	Poor litter	
Physical discomfort				Barren environments	Untreated disease	Fence pacing	Heat stress		
Downer cow management				Weaning	Washing at abattoirs				
Introducing heifers to the herd					Handling problems				
					Lambing problems				
					Weaning				

carcass or meat and cause downgrading, rejection or dissatisfaction of the product. All of the welfare problems that lead to poor product quality are strongly influenced by the standard of stockmanship. Good stockhandling is a key issue.

Many people decide to work in the livestock industry because they enjoy working with animals. The attractions include an interest in their behaviour, enjoyment from directly interacting with animals, satisfaction in performing work with animals skilfully and pride in owning and controlling animals. Over-exposure and excessive familiarity can change those outlooks. Some farmers, by the time they reach retirement, are glad not to have to milk the cows twice daily or feed and muck out the pigs every morning. The novelty and interest in working with animals can wear off with time, especially if the job is too demanding.

The abattoir industry deals with large numbers of livestock every day. Its outlook towards animals is inevitably different from farmers' attitudes. Whilst a dairy farmer would appraise a cow from its posture, the way it moved, its general health, size and udder conformation, the livestock supervisor at an abattoir thinks in terms of the flow of livestock, their likely temperament and ease of handling. It is wrongly stated that the animals are regarded as machines. More correctly, the animals are considered in terms of their group behaviour and for the reactions of any individuals which indicate that they could cause trouble. When stockhandling is done skilfully it creates a sense of pride and satisfaction. Many of us admire the way a good stockhandler can control and coordinate a Border collie bringing in a flock of sheep. The same applies to animal handling in saleyards and meatworks.

In abattoirs, the job of moving stock is very repetitive and so satisfaction from performing the work skilfully may not persist. Unlike farming, there is no pride in ownership, but there is opportunity for enjoyment from physically handling and interacting with stock in redmeat abattoirs. I well remember one pig abattoir where the stockhandlers and the design of the facilities knitted together perfectly. There was virtually no squealing from the pigs, no use of electric goads, and very little squabbling or pushing as the pigs were herded to the stunning point at over 200 pigs per hour. There was complete satisfaction in doing the job well.

Stockmanship and positive attitudes to stockhandling can be upheld and improved in abattoirs in a number of ways:

- greater interest, encouragement or control from the staff supervisors (a caring attitude from the supervisor will help to promote a similar attitude amongst staff);
- better facilities and transport equipment which allow stockhandlers to do a better job with less stress to themselves and to the stock;
- greater self-control and positive attitudes amongst stockhandlers.

Good stockmanship develops from an understanding of the way that animals behave, their preferences and from learning about the consequences of mishandling. This experience is reinforced by the knowledge that poor welfare can lead to poor meat quality. To summarize some of the key points in this book, poor preslaughter treatment leads to inferior product quality and reduced yield in the following ways:

- greater risk of stress-induced heart failure in poultry and pigs;
- mortality due to heat stress;
- risk of death from smothering in poultry and sheep;
- broken and dislocated bones leading to bruising and bone fragments in the final product;
- ruptured livers;
- torn skin and entry of bacteria;
- burst bellies and autolysis in fish;
- prolapses in benthic fish, leading to downgrading;
- bruising, leading to unsightly collections of blood;
- dog bites and bruising in sheep;
- sale through auction markets and bruising;
- increased risk of oxidative rancidity and warmed-over flavours (WOFs) in processed meat products prepared from bruised tissue;
- preslaughter fasting and loss of carcass weight;
- prolonged preslaughter fasting and poor quality liver;
- fasting with intermittent feeding, leading to a greater risk of *Salmonella* contamination;
- dehydration, leading to dark, dry, sticky meat;
- long-distance transport and high pH_{ult} meat;
- heat stress and PSE-like condition in turkeys;
- heat stress and drip in broiler meat;
- exercise and/or heat stress leading to exaggerated risk of PSE meat in pigs;
- excessive exercise and burnt tuna;
- exercise-induced heat shortening in poultry;
- exercise-induced glycogen depletion in muscle leading to DCB, DFD pork and high pH_{ult} lamb;
- swimwashing and high pH_{ult} meat;
- insufficient rest period in the lairage and PSE meat;
- emotional stress and increased excretion of faeces and *Salmonellas*, leading to greater risk of carcass contamination;
- handling stress and bacterial contamination in crabs;
- handling stress and melanosis in prawns;
- no preslaughter stunning and breast meat toughness in chickens;
- CO_2 stunning and skin damage in salmon;
- delayed sticking and greater expression of blood splash.

High pH_{ult} meat has many effects on subsequent meat quality. Theoretically, one would expect meat from glycogen-depleted non-acidotic animals to:

- develop rigor earlier, because of insufficient ATP to pump the Ca^{2+} re-uptake mechanism;
- be less responsive physically during electrical stimulation;
- have a high water-holding capacity;
- lose less weight during further processing and cooking because of its higher water-holding capacity;
- form less drip in packaged products;
- lose less weight during curing because of its high water-holding capacity;
- lose less weight on thawing;
- be firm (but not tough) because of its high water-holding capacity;
- be more tender and more responsive to tenderization during hot conditioning;
- be less prone to cold shortening and rigor shortening induced by hot deboning;
- be darker in colour;
- be more likely to retain its redness in beef during cooking;
- be more likely to produce heat-stable pinkness in cooked poultry meats;
- be less likely to form Maillard reaction products during cooking, and hence have a more bland flavour and less browning;
- greater likelihood of developing rancid flavours or WOFs;
- be more prone to spoilage by proteolytic bacteria;
- be more prone to turning green when stored in vacuum packs;
- produce re-formed meats with stronger myosin gels which are not prone to falling apart;
- produce ground meat products with enhanced fat retention.

There are other ways, besides poor handling, in which compromised welfare leads to poor product quality. These include:

- lack of familiarity with being handled and high pH_{ult} meat;
- fighting and skin damage plus bruising;
- mixing stress and high pH_{ult} meat;
- overcrowding in lairage and DFD pork;
- overcrowding and fin erosion in farmed fish;
- injection site infections, leading to meat rejection;
- shearing scars and poor quality leather;
- mulesing scars and poor leather quality/scar tissue in meat;
- branding scars and poor leather quality;

- cannibalism in farmed fish and carcass rejection;
- predation and scarring in fish;
- lameness and hockburn in broilers;
- lameness and breast blisters in broilers;
- poor farm sanitation and boar taint;
- poor farm sanitation and increased risk of *Salmonella* contamination in pigs;
- endoparasite diarrhoea and risk of carcass contamination with faeces in sheep;
- facial eczema and tough, bitter-tasting meat;
- *Phalaris* staggers and off-flavours in meat;
- emaciation and high pH_{ult} meat.

There are some situations where poor welfare can be linked with superior carcass and meat quality. These include:

- anaemia/confinement and white colour in veal;
- cramming and high quality foie gras production;
- live de-sliming of eels and improved meat flavour/skin colour;
- castration and absence of boar taint;
- castration in pigs and less fat separation in cut meat;
- tail docking pigs and less risk of abscesses in the carcass from tail biting;
- claw/toe amputation in poultry and less back scratching;
- dystocia and double muscling in cattle;
- stress susceptibility in pigs and superior ham conformation;
- prolonged preslaughter fasting and less PSE meat;
- exercise-induced high pH_{ult} meat and tenderness;
- exercise stress and less muscle gaping in fish;
- preslaughter exercise stress and less fatty mouth-feel to trout;
- absence of thaw shortening in exercise-stressed rapidly frozen fish;
- low stunning currents and less blood splash and wing haemorrhaging;
- low stunning currents and fewer broken bones in poultry;
- low stunning currents less likely to be associated with rigor shortening of breast meat in broilers;
- low stunning currents less likely to be associated with defaecation and contamination of the waterbath stunner;
- CO_2 stunning and less blood splash.

In *the future*, greater thought will probably be given to lairage design, to providing slaughterhouses with cleaner, better quality stock and to providing animals with better conditions during transport. For example, in the pig industry some changes that could develop in the near future include the following.

- Genetic lines of low-boar-taint pig could be bred which have higher activities of skatole-degrading enzymes in their livers.

- When unfamiliar pigs have to be mixed they will only be mixed as they are loaded on to trucks.
- For hygiene and disease control reasons, pigs will be held at farms in separate dedicated piggeries from the grower sheds, prior to despatch to the meatworks. The truck will collect pigs only from this despatch piggery. Only the farm staff, and not the truck driver, will be allowed to enter the despatch piggery. The truck will be cleaned and disinfected when it leaves the abattoir. Straw may be provided in the truck to ensure that there is less urine burn on the pigs' skin and that the pigs arrive at the meatworks in a cleaner condition. Farmers will be penalized for sending dirty pigs in for slaughter.
- Trucks will have insulated roofs to reduce the risk of over-heating. Transport deaths could also be controlled by introducing mechanical ventilation and air conditioning in the trucks. Recent evidence has shown that this can reduce mortality from 0.46% to 0.24%.
- Trucks will be designed with noise-free fittings and air suspension.
- The upper deck(s) of the trucks will be mobile instead of relying on fixed ramps for loading and unloading
- The recommended stocking density on the trucks will be 0.4 m^2 per 100 kg pig. Presently the general range is 0.35–0.39 m^2 per 100 kg pig. High stocking densities (0.3 m^2 per pig) are associated with rindside damage (Guise and Penny, 1989).
- At most abattoirs there will be a minimum 2-hour holding period before slaughter, and any fighting will be stopped by playing water on to the pigs from a hose.
- Electric goads could be phased out. In many situations a yard broom or pointed stick is just as effective. The approach to moving pigs on to and off the trucks may need to be reconsidered, and instead of forcing them to move the emphasis will need to be on encouraging them to move.
- A new system has been developed for CO_2 stunning of pigs which avoids the need to reduce the flow of pigs to a single file during the lead-up to the stunner (Fig. 15.1). Pigs are driven by operator 1 in groups of about 15 to the stunning area, and they are held in the waiting pens by the sliding door D1, which is operated manually. Gate D2 operates automatically and crowds the pigs towards gate D3, which is opened manually by operator 2. Five pigs are allowed into the loading pen, and they are crowded into the lift of the stunner by gate D4 which operates at 90° to gate D3. Gate D2 is a push-hoist gate, in other words, it crowds the pigs by automatically travelling over the ground at pig height. When it has completed its journey it is hoisted up and passes back to the starting position over the heads of the second batch of pigs, which have been loaded into the pen.

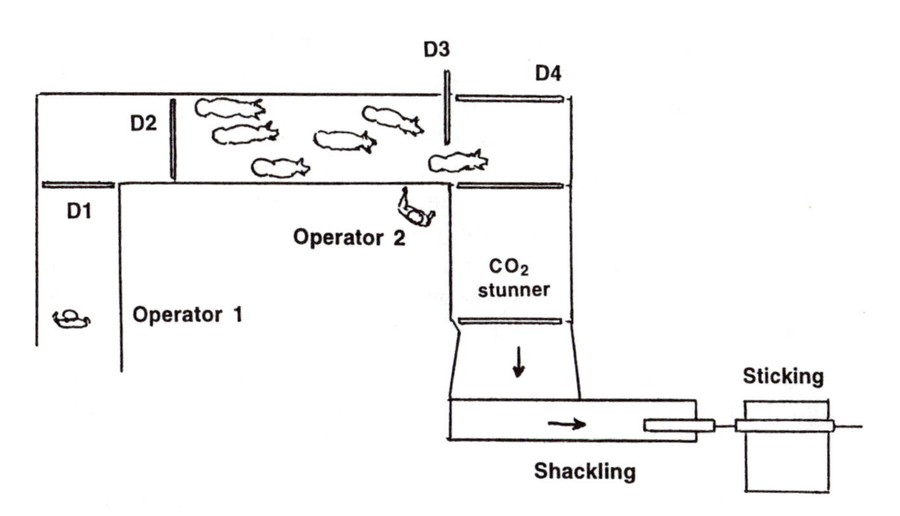

Fig. 15.1. Modern system for handling pigs during CO_2 stunning.

We can look forward to many changes that will benefit animal welfare. However, there will be some developments that will be a hindrance. Some likely changes include the following.

- Stock which are sick and unfit for sending in for slaughter will have to be slaughtered on the farm. The methods used for despatching these animals which are valueless will need to be considered.
- There could be greater emphasis in supplying stock that are suitable for the manufacturing trade. Typically these will be larger animals with a high lean meat yield. Temperament and ease of handling could be affected where this involves changes in breed.
- Feedlot piggeries could develop with an abattoir sited alongside, and large poultry farms will be set up with adjoining processing plants. The public image associated with such large-scale enterprises could be negative, and any welfare problems that arise in these units will help to reinforce this.
- Greater emphasis will be placed in presenting stock for slaughter which are clean and are not shedding *Salmonella*, *Campylobacter*, *Listeria*, *Yersinia* or *Leptospira*. In cattle, the incidence and numbers of *Salmonella* in the intestinal tract, on the hide, and in the areas through which the cattle pass from farm to slaughter is reduced if the time from farm to slaughter is limited (Grau, 1987). Short transport distances will help to promote food safety.
- As farming becomes more competitive, farmers will secure a better income by either scaling up production or cutting costs. Scaling up production means, for example, increasing the number of breeding sows in the herd from 600 to 1000, or putting eight crops of broilers through

the grower sheds in a year, instead of seven. Reducing costs can mean dispensing with a shepherd whilst changing from close management of a flock to running an easy-care system instead. Easy-care inevitably means less care when it comes to treating disease.

- As herd and flock sizes increase, the capital reserve of the small-scale farmer which underpins the farming unit will be stretched. Farmers will either amalgamate or (where there looks to be attractive returns) land, equipment and stock will be capitalized by off-site investors. In this situation, attitudes to livestock care will change as the pressure to service debts and to provide a satisfactory return grows.

Although poor welfare can affect profitability through harming aspects of product quality, we cannot rely on the profit motive as a cure for animal welfare problems. Ultimately the solution to animal welfare problems must rest with our concern for animals. It must be based on a real sense of moral responsibility towards animals. Without a genuine sense of fairness we will end up either paying lip-service to the needs of animals or operating under closely defined rules as to what is acceptable and what is unacceptable. There is a risk that the current interest in animal welfare will create an insincere, if not jaundiced, outlook amongst some people, and in this situation the benefits we give the animals will be imagined rather than real. It must be recognized that many people do care for and about animals and their sense of responsibility should be fostered, encouraged and rewarded – especially when it imposes additional burdens on them as individuals.

References

Aalhus, J.L., Price, M.A., Shand, P.J. and Hawrysh, Z.J. (1991) Endurance-exercised growing sheep. 2. Tenderness increase and change in meat quality. *Meat Science* 29, 57–68.

Aberle, E.D., Thomas, N.W., Howe, J.M. and Arroyo, P.T. (1969) Environmental influence on high energy phosphate and metabolites in porcine muscle. *Journal of Food Science* 34, 600–603.

Abilgaard, C.P. (1775) Tentamina electrica in Animalibus Instituta. In: *Societatis Medicae Haviensis Collectanea* 2, 157.

Alessio, H.M., Goldfarb, A.H. and Cutler, R.G. (1988) MDA content increases in fast- and slow-twitch skeletal muscle with intensity of exercise in a rat. *American Journal of Physiology* 255, C874–C877.

Algers, B. (1984) A note on the response of farm animals to ultrasound. *Applied Animal Behaviour Science* 12, 387–391.

Ames, D.R. (1974) Sound stress in meat animals. Livestock environment proceedings of the livestock symposium. (Publication No. SP–0174). *Transactions of the American Society of Agricultural Engineers*, 324–330.

Anil, M.H. (1991) Studies on the return of physical reflexes in pigs following electrical stunning. *Meat Science* 30, 13–21.

Apple, J.K., Dikeman, M.E., Minton, J.E., McMurphy, R.M., Fedde, M.R., Leith, D.E. and Unruh, J.A. (1995) Effects of restraint and isolation stress and epidural blockade on endocrine and blood metabolite status, muscle glycogen metabolism, and incidence of dark-cutting longissimus muscle of sheep. *Journal of Animal Science* 73, 2295–2307.

Asghar, A., Morita, J.-I., Samejima, K. and Yasui, T. (1984) Biochemical and functional characteristics of myosin from red and white muscles of chicken as influenced by nutritional stress. *Agricultural and Biological Chemistry* 48, 2217–2224.

Azam, K., Mackie, I.M. and Smith, J. (1989) The effect of slaughter method on the quality of rainbow trout (*Salmo gairdneri*) during storage on ice. *International Journal of Food Science and Technology* 24, 69–79.

Badawy, A.M., Campbell, R.M., Cuthbertson, D.P. and Fell, B.F. (1957) Changes in the intestinal mucosa of the sheep following death by humane killer. *Nature* 180, 756–757.

Baile, C.A. and Forbes, J.M. (1974) Control of feed intake and regulation of energy balance in ruminants. *Physiological Reviews* 54, 160–214.

Bailey, M.E. (1992) Meat flavour – the Maillard reaction and meat flavour quality. *Meat Focus International* 1, 192–195.

Barnes, M.A., Carter, R.E., Longnecker, J.V., Riesen, J.W. and Woody, C.O. (1975) Age at transport and calf survival. *Journal of Dairy Science* 58, 1247.

Barton-Gade, P. (1984) Influence of halothane genotype on meat quality in pigs subjected to various pre-slaughter treatments. *30th European Meeting of Meat Research Workers*, Bristol, England, 1:3, pp. 8–9.

Bartos, L., Franc, C., Rehak, D. and Stipkova (1993) A practical method to prevent dark-cutting (DFD) in beef. *Meat Science* 34, 275–282.

Bass, J.J., and Duganzich, D.M. (1980) A note on effect of starvation on the bovine alimentary tract and its contents. *Animal Production* 31, 111–113.

Beardsworth, A. and Keil, T. (1992) The vegetarian option: varieties, conversions, motives and careers. *The Sociological Review* 40, 253–293.

Bendall, J.R. (1966) The effect of pre-treatment of pigs with curare on the post-mortem rate of pH fall and onset of rigor mortis in the musculature. *Journal of the Science of Food and Agriculture* 17, 333–338.

Berends, B.R., Urlings, H.A.P., Snijders, J.M.A. and van Knapen, F. (1996) Identification and quantification of risk factors in animal management and transport regarding *Salmonella* spp. in pigs. *International Journal of Food Microbiology* 30, 37–53.

Bergmann, F., Costin, A. and Gutman, J. (1963) A low threshold convulsive area in the rabbit's mesencephalon. *Electroencephalography and Clinical Neurophysiology* 15, 683–690.

Bianca, W. (1968) Effects of water deprivation on the water content of cattle skin. *International Journal of Biometeorology* 12, 153–157.

Biss, M.E. and Hathaway, S.C. (1994) Wastage due to diseases and defects in very young calves slaughtered in New Zealand. *New Zealand Veterinary Journal* 42, 211–215.

Biss, M.E. and Hathaway, S.C. (1995) Microbiological and visible contamination of lamb carcasses according to preslaughter presentation status: implications for HACCP. *Journal of Food Protection* 58, 776–783.

Biss, M.E. and Hathaway, S.C. (1996) Effect of pre-slaughter washing of lambs on the microbiological and visible contamination of the carcases. *Veterinary Record* 138, 82–86.

Boissy, A. and Bouissou, M.F. (1995) Assessment of individual differences in behavioral reactions of heifers exposed to various fear-eliciting situations. *Applied Animal Behaviour Science* 46, 17–31.

Bolton, W., Dewar, W.A., Morley Jones, R. and Thompson, R. (1972) Effect of stocking density on performance of broiler chicks. *British Poultry Science* 13, 157–162.

Bradshaw, R.H., Parrott, R.F., Forsling, M.L., Goode, J.A., Lloyd, D.M., Rodway, R.G. and Broom, D.M. (1996) Stress and travel sickness in pigs: effects of road transport on plasma concentrations of cortisol, beta-endorphin and lysine vasopressin. *Animal Science* 63, 507–516.

Braggins, J.J. (1996) Effect of stress-related changes in sheepmeat ultimate pH on cooked odor and flavor. *Journal of Agricultural Food Chemistry* 44, 2352–2360.

Bramblett, V.D., Judge, M.D. and Vail, G.E. (1963) Stress during growth. 2. Effects on palatability and cooking characteristics of lamb meat. *Journal of Animal Science* 22, 1064–1067.

Bray, A.R., Graafhuis, A.E. and Chrystall, B.B. (1989) The cumulative effect of nutritional, shearing and preslaughter washing stresses on the quality of lamb meat. *Meat Science* 25, 59–67.

Briskey, E.J. (1964) Pale, soft, exudative porcine musculature. *Advances in Food Research* 13, 89–178.

Broom, D.M., Goode, J.A., Hall, S.J.G., Lloyd, D.M. and Parrott, R.F. (1996) Hormonal and physiological effects of a 15 hour road journey in sheep: comparison with the responses to loading, handling and penning in the absence of transport. *British Veterinary Journal* 152, 593–604.

Brown, A.J., Coates, H.E. and Speight, B.S. (1978) *Muscular and Skeletal Anatomy of the Beef Carcass.* Meat Research Institute, Bristol, UK, 186 pp.

Burrow, H.M. (1997) Measurements of temperament and their relationships with performance traits of beef cattle. *Animal Breeding Abstracts* 65, 477–495.

Cambero, M.I., Seuss, I. and Honikel, K.O. (1992) Flavour compounds of beef broth as affected by cooking temperature. *Journal of Food Science* 57, 1285–1290.

Campbell, J.B. (1988) Arthropod-induced stress in livestock. *Veterinary Clinics of North America: Food Animal Practice* 4(3), 551–555.

Carabelli, R.A. and Kellerman, W.C. (1985) Phantom limb pain: relief by application of TENS to contralateral extremity. *Archives of Physical Medicine and Rehabilitation* 66, 466–467.

Cena, P., Jaime, I., Beltran, J.A. and Roncales, P. (1992) Proteolytic activity of isolated calpains on myofibrils under the conditions of pH, Ca^{2+} concentration and temperature existing in post-mortem muscle. *Zeitschrift für Lebensmittel Untersuchung und Forschung* 194, 248–251.

Chang, S.F. and Pearson, A.M. (1992) Effect of electrical stunning or sticking without stunning on the microstructure of Zousoon, a Chinese semi-dry pork product. *Meat Science* 31, 309–326.

Charpentier, J. (1966) Pigmentation musculaire du veau de boucherie. 1. facteurs de variation. *Annales de Zootechnie* 15, 181–196.

Chrystall, B.B., Devine, C.E., Snodgrass, M. and Ellery, S. (1982) Tenderness of exercise-stressed lambs. *New Zealand Journal of Agricultural Research* 25, 331–336.

Clark, E.G. (1979) Necropsy survey of transport stress deaths in Saskatchewan market weight hogs. In: *22nd Annual Proceedings of the American Association of Veterinary Laboratory Diagnosticians*, pp. 53–60.

Classen, H.L. (1992) Management factors in leg disorders. In: Whitehead C.C. (ed.) *Bone Biology and Skeletal Disorders in Poultry.* Poultry Science Symposium Number 23. Carfax Publishing Company, Abingdon, UK, pp. 195–211.

Cockram, M.S. and Corley, K.T.T. (1991) Effect of pre-slaughter handling on the behaviour and blood composition of beef cattle. *British Veterinary Journal* 147, 444–454.

Cole, N.A., Camp, T.H., Rowe, L.D., Stevens, D.G. and Hutcheson, D.P. (1988) Effect of transport on feeder calves. *American Journal of Veterinary Research* 49, 178–183.

Cook, C.J., Devine, C.E., Tavener, A. and Gilbert, K.V. (1992) Contribution of amino acid transmitters to epileptiform activity and reflex suppression in electrically head stunned sheep. *Research in Veterinary Science* 52, 48–56.

Cook, C.J., Devine, C.E., Gilbert, K.V., Smith, D.D. and Maasland, S.A. (1995) The effect of electrical head-only stun duration on electroencephalographic-measured seizure and brain amino acid neurotransmitter release. *Meat Science* 40, 137–147.

Costill, D.L., Coyle, E., Dalsky, G., Evans, W. and Hoopes, D. (1977) Effects of elevated plasma FFA and insulin on muscle glycogen usage during exercise. *Journal of Applied Physiology* 43, 695–699.

Cramer, J.L., Nakamura, R.M., Dizon, A.E. and Ikehara, W.N. (1981) Burnt tuna: conditions leading to rapid deterioration in the quality of raw tuna. *Marine Fisheries Review* 43(6), 12–16.

Crouse, J.D., Cross, H.R. and Siedeman, S.C. (1984) Effects of a grass or grain diet on the quality of three beef muscles. *Journal of Animal Science* 58, 619–625.

Czochanska, Z., Shorland, F.B., Barton, R.A. and Rae, A.L. (1970) A note on the effect of the length of the resting period before slaughter on the intensity of flavour and odour of lamb. *New Zealand Journal of Agricultural Research* 13, 662–663.

Davie, P.S., Franklin, C.E. and Grigg, G.C. (1993) Blood pressure and heart rate during tonic immobility in the black tipped reef shark, *Carcharhinus melanoptera. Fish Physiology and Biochemistry* 12, 95–100.

Davis, M. (1992) The role of the amygdala in fear and anxiety. *Annual Review of Neuroscience* 15, 353–375.

Dembo, J.A. (1894) *The Jewish Method of Slaughter Compared with Others.* Kegan Paul, Trench, Trubner & Co., London, 105 pp.

de Smet, S.M., Pauwels, H., de Bie, S., Demeyer, D.I., Calleweir, J. and Eeckhout, W. (1996) Effect of halothane genotype, breed, feed withdrawal, and lairage on pork quality of Belgian slaughter pigs. *Journal of Animal Science* 74, 1854–1863.

Devine, C.E. and Chrystall, B.B. (1988) High ultimate pH in sheep. In: Fabiansson S.U., Shorthose, W.R. and Warner, R.D. (eds) *Dark-cutting in Cattle and Sheep, Proceedings of an Australian Workshop.* Australian Meat & Live-stock Research & Development Corporation, Sydney, pp. 55–67.

Devine, C.E., Gilbert, K.V. and Ellery, S. (1983) Electrical stunning of lambs: the effect of stunning parameters and drugs affecting blood flow and behaviour on petechial haemorrhage incidence. *Meat Science* 9, 247–256.

Devine, C.E., Graafhuis, A.E., Muir, P.D. and Chrystall, B.B. (1993) The effect of growth rate and ultimate pH on meat quality in lambs. *Meat Science* 35, 63–67.

Dexter, D.R., Cowman, G.L., Morgan, J.B., Clayton, R.P., Tatum, J.D., Sofos, J.N., Schmidt, G.R., Glock, R.D. and Smith, G.C. (1994) Incidence of injection-site blemishes in beef top sirloin butts. *Journal of Animal Science* 72, 824–827.

Dunn, C.S. (1990) Stress reactions of cattle undergoing ritual slaughter using two methods of restraint. *Veterinary Record* 126, 522–525.

Ehinger, F. and Gschwindt, B., (1981) Der einfluß unterschiedlicher transportzeiten auf die fleischqualitat und auf physiologische merkmale bei broilern vershiedener herkunft. *Archiv für Geflügelkunde* 45, 260–265.

Eldridge, G.A. and Winfield, C.G. (1988) The behaviour and bruising of cattle during transport at different space allowances. *Australian Journal of Experimental Agriculture* 28, 695–698.

Enck, P., Merlin, V., Erckenbrecht, J.F. and Wienbeck, M. (1989) Stress effects on gastrointestinal transit in the rat. *Gut* 30, 455–459.

Enfalt, A.-C., Lundstrom, K., Hansson, I., Lundeheim, N. and Nystrom, P.-E. (1997) Effects of outdoor rearing and sire breed (Duroc or Yorkshire) on carcass composition and sensory and technological meat quality. *Meat Science* 45, 1–15.

Esplin, D.W. and Freston, J.W. (1960) Physiological and pharmacological analysis of spinal cord convulsions. *Journal of Pharmacological and Experimental Therapeutics* 130, 68–80.

Etherington, D.J., Taylor, M.A.J., Wakefield, D.K., Cousins, A. and Dransfield, E. (1990) Proteinase (cathepsin B,D,L and calpains) levels and conditioning rates in normal, electrically stimulated and high ultimate pH chicken muscle. *Meat Science* 28, 99–109.

Evans, D.G. and Pratt, J.H. (1978) A critical analysis of condemnation data for cattle, pigs and sheep 1969 to 1975. *British Veterinary Journal* 134, 476–492.

Everitt, G.C., Jury, K.E., Dalton, D.C. and Ward, J.D.B. (1978) Beef production from the dairy herd. 1. Calving records from Friesian cows mated to Friesian and beef breed bulls. *New Zealand Journal of Agricultural Research* 21, 197–208.

Ewbank, R., Parker, M.J. and Mason, C.W. (1992) Reactions of cattle to head restraint at stunning: a practical dilemma. *Animal Welfare* 1, 55–63.

Farm Animal Welfare Council (1996) *Report on the Welfare of Farmed Fish.* MAFF, FAWC, Surbiton, UK, 52 pp.

Farmer, L.J., Perry, G.C., Lewis, P.D., Nute, G.N., Piggott, J.R. and Patterson, R.L.S. (1997) Responses of two genotypes of chicken to the diets and stocking densities of conventional UK and Label Rouge Production Systems – 2. Sensory attributes. *Meat Science* 47, 77–93.

Fernandez, X., Meunier-Salaun, M.-C., Ecolan, P. and Mormede, P. (1995) Interactive effect of food deprivation and agonistic behavior on blood parameters and muscle glycogen in pigs. *Physiology and Behavior* 58, 337–345.

Fernandez, X., Monin, G., Culioli, J., Legrand, I. and Quilichini, Y. (1996) Effect of duration of feed withdrawal and transportation on muscle characteristics and quality in Friesian-Holstein calves. *Journal of Animal Science* 74, 1576–1583.

Ferris, L.P., King, B.G., Spence, P.W. and Williams, H.B. (1936) Effect of electric shock on the heart. *Electrical Engineering* May 1936, 498–515, 1264, 1265.

Fischer, C. and Hamm, R. (1981) Post-mortem muscle biochemistry and beef quality. In: Hood, D.E. and Tarrant, P.V. (eds) *The Problem of Dark-cutting in Beef.* Martinus Nijhoff Publishers, The Hague, The Netherlands, pp. 387–394.

Flight, W.G.F. and Verheijen, F.J. (1993) The 'neck-cut' (spinal transection): not a humane way to slaughter eel, *Anguilla anguilla* (L.). *Aquaculture and Fisheries Management* 24, 523–528.

Fogd Jørgensen, P. and Hyldgaard-Jensen, J.F. (1975) The effect of physical training on skeletal muscle enzyme composition in pigs. *Acta Veterinaria Scandinavica* 16, 368–378.

Gabr, R.W., Birkle, D.L. and Azzaro, A.J. (1995) Stimulation of the amygdala by glutamate facilitates corticotropin-releasing factor release from the median eminence and activation of the hypothalamic–pituitary–adrenal axis in stressed rats. *Neuroendocrinology* 62, 333–339.

Genigeorgis, C. (1975) Public health importance of *Clostridium perfringens*. *Journal of American Veterinary Medical Association* 167, 821–827.

George, P. and Stratmann, C.J. (1954) The oxidation of myoglobin to metmyoglobin by oxygen. *Biochemical Journal* 57, 568–573.

Geverink, N.A., Bas, E., Lambooij, E. and Wiegant, V.M. (1996) Observations on behaviour and skin damage of slaughter pigs and treatment during lairage. *Applied Animal Behaviour Science* 50, 1–13.

Gilbert, K.V. (1980) Developments in stunning and slaughter. In: *Proceedings of the 21st Meat Industry Research Conference.* MIRINZ, Hamilton, New Zealand, pp. 18–23.

Gill, C.O. and Harrison, J.C.L. (1982) Microbiological and organoleptic qualities of bruised meat. *Journal of Food Protection* 45, 646–649.

Gill, C.O. and Newton, K.G. (1981) Microbiology of DFD beef. In: Hood, D.H. and Tarrant P.V. (eds) *The Problem of Dark-cutting in Beef.* Martinus Nijhoff Publishers, The Hague, The Netherlands, pp. 305–327.

Gill, C.O., Penney, N. and Nottingham, P.M. (1978) Tissue sterility in uneviscerated carcasses. *Applied and Environmental Microbiology* 36, 356–359.

Goldfarb, A.H., McIntosh, M.K., Boyer, B.T. amd Fatouros, J. (1994) Vitamin E effects on indices of lipid peroxidation in muscle from DHEA-treated and exercised rats. *Journal of Applied Physiology* 76, 1630–1635.

Graafhuis, A.E. and Devine, C.E. (1994) Incidence of high pH beef and lamb. 2. Results of an ultimate pH survey of beef and sheep plants in New Zealand. In: *28th Meat Industry Research Conference.* MIRINZ Publication No. 942, Hamilton, New Zealand, pp. 133–141.

Grandin, T. (1982) Pig behavior studies applied to slaughter plant design. *Applied Animal Ethology* 9, 141–151.

Grandin, T. (1984) Race systems in slaughter plants with 1.5 m radius curves. *Applied Animal Behaviour Science* 13, 295–299.

Grandin, T. (1988) Double rail restrainer conveyor for livestock handling. *Journal of Agricultural Engineering Research* 41, 327–338.

Grandin, T. (1990) Design of loading facilities and holding pens. *Applied Animal Behaviour Science* 28, 187–202.

Grandin, T. (1991a) Principles of abattoir design to improve animal welfare. In: Matthews, J. (ed.) *Progress in Agricultural Physics and Engineering.* CAB International, Wallingford, Oxon, UK, pp. 279–303.

Grandin, T. (1991b) *Double Rail Restrainer for Handling Beef Cattle.* Paper No. 91–5004, American Society of Agricultural Engineers, St Joseph, Michigan, USA, 15 pp.

Grandin, T. (1992) Observation of cattle restraint devices for stunning and slaughtering. *Animal Welfare* 1, 85–91.

Grandin, T. (1993) Handling cattle in extensive systems. In: Grandin, T. (ed.) *Livestock Handling and Transport.* CAB International, Wallingford, Oxon, UK, pp. 43–57.

Grandin, T. (1994) Euthanasia and slaughter of livestock. *Journal of the American Veterinary Medical Association* 204, 1354–1360.

Grandin, T. (1995) Restraint of livestock. In: *Proceedings of the Animal Behavior and the Design of Livestock and Poultry Systems International Conference*, Northeast Regional Agricultural Engineering Service, Cornell University, Cooperative Extension, Ithaca, New York, pp. 208–223.

Grandin, T. (1996) Factors that impede animal movement at slaughter plants. *Journal of the American Veterinary Medical Association* 209, 757–759.

Grandin, T. (1997a) Assessment of stress during handling and transport. *Journal of Animal Science* 75, 249–257.

Grandin, T. (1997b) Survey of stunning and handling in Federally inspected beef, veal, pork and sheep slaughter plants. Agricultural Research Service Project Number 3602–32000–002–08G, USDA, Beltsville, Maryland, USA.

Grandin, T. (1998) Genetics and behavior during handling, restraint and herding. In: Grandin, T. (ed.) *Genetics and the Behavior of Domestic Animals*. Academic Press, San Diego, California, USA, pp. 113–144.

Grandin, T., Curtis, S.E., Widowski, T.M. and Thurmon, J.C. (1986) Electroimmobilisation versus mechanical restraint in an avoid–avoid choice test for ewes. *Journal of Animal Science* 62, 1469.

Grau, F.H. (1987) Prevention of microbial contamination in the export beef abattoir. In: Smulders, F.J.M. (ed.) *Elimination of Pathogenic Organisms from Meat and Poultry*. Elsevier Science Publishers, Amsterdam, The Netherlands, pp. 221–233.

Grau, F.H. and Smith, M.G. (1974) Salmonella contamination of sheep and mutton carcasses related to pre-slaughter holding conditions. *Journal of Applied Bacteriology* 37, 111–116.

Grau, F.H., Brownlie, L.E. and Roberts, E.A. (1968) Effect of some preslaughter treatments on the *Salmonella* population in the bovine rumen and faeces. *Journal of Applied Bacteriology* 31, 157–163.

Grau, F.H., Brownlie, L.E. and Smith, M.G. (1969) Effects of food intake on number of *Salmonella* and *Esherichia coli* in rumen and faeces of sheep. *Journal of Applied Bacteriology* 32, 112–117.

Greaser, M.L., Cassens, R.G., Briskey, E.J. and Hoekstra, W.G. (1969) Post-mortem changes of subcellular fractions from normal and pale, soft, exudative porcine muscle. 1. Calcium accumulation and adenosine triphosphatase activities. *Journal of Food Science* 34, 120–124.

Gregory, N.G. (1981) Neurological control of muscle metabolism and growth in stress sensitive pigs. In: Froystein T., Slinde, E. and Standal, N. (eds) *Porcine Stress and Meat Quality*. Agricultural Food Research Society, Ås, Norway, pp. 11–20.

Gregory, N.G. (1985) Stunning and slaughter of pigs. *Pig News and Information* 6, 407–413.

Gregory, N.G. (1987) Effect of stunning on carcass and meat quality. In: Tarrant P.V., Eikelenboom, G. and Monin, G. (eds) *Evaluation and Control of Meat Quality*. Martinus Nijhoff Publishers, Dordrecht, The Netherlands, pp. 265–272.

Gregory, N.G. (1988) Humane slaughter. In: *Proceedings of the 34th International Congress of Meat Science and Technology, Industry Session*, pp. 46–49.

Gregory, N.G. (1991a) Humane slaughter. *Outlook on Agriculture* 20, 95–101.

Gregory, N.G. (1991b) Causes of downgrading during processing in chickens, turkeys and ducks. In: *Welfare, Hygiene and Quality Aspects of Poultry Processing*. Workshop organized by the Meat Technology Service, University of Bristol, UK. Chapter 6.

Gregory, N.G. (1992a) Mobile slaughterlines. *Meat Focus International* 1, 130–131.

Gregory, N.G. (1992b) Stunning in broilers. In: P*roceedings of XIX World's Poultry Congress, Amsterdam*. Vol. 2, pp. 345–349.

Gregory, N.G. (1993) Welfare and product quality: the need to be humane. In: *Safety and Quality of Food from Animals. British Society of Animal Production Occasional Publication* 17, 51–56.

Gregory, N.G. (1995a) Recent developments in gas stunning pigs. In: *Meat '95. Australian Meat Industry Research Conference, Gold Coast.* CSIRO Division of Food Science & Technology, Brisbane, Australia, pp. 9B1–9B4.

Gregory, N.G. (1995b) The role of shelterbelts in protecting livestock: a review. *New Zealand Journal of Agricultural Research* 38, 423–450.

Gregory, N.G. (1995c) Animal trade; welfare regulations. *Meat Focus International* 4, 504–508.

Gregory, N.G. (1996a) Welfare of poultry at slaughter. In: Bremner, A.S. and Johnston, A.M. (eds) *Poultry Meat Hygiene and Inspection.* W.B. Saunders Co. Ltd, London, pp. 53–72.

Gregory, N.G. (1996b) Welfare and hygiene during preslaughter handling. *Meat Science* 43, S35–S46.

Gregory, N.G. (1997) Meat, meat eating and vegetarianism. In: Bass, J. (ed.) *Proceedings of the 43rd International Congress of Meat Science and Technology,* pp. 68–85.

Gregory, N.G. (1998) Physiological mechanisms causing sickness behaviour and suffering in diseased animals. *Animal Welfare* (in press).

Gregory, N.G. and Austin, S.D. (1992) Causes of trauma in broilers arriving dead at poultry processing plants. *Veterinary Record* 131, 501–503.

Gregory, N.G. and Wilkins, L.J. (1984) Effect of cardiac arrest on susceptibility to carcass bruising in sheep. *Journal of the Science of Food and Agriculture* 35, 671–676.

Gregory, N.G. and Wilkins, L.J. (1989) Effect of slaughter method on bleeding efficiency in chickens. *Journal of the Science of Food and Agriculture* 47, 13–20.

Gregory, N.G. and Wilkins, L.J. (1990) The role of electrical stunning, bleeding and plucking efficiency on the downgrading of chicken carcasses. *Veterinary Record* 127, 331–333.

Gregory, N.G. and Wilkins, L.J. (1992) Skeletal damage and bone defects during catching and processing. In: Whitehead, C.C. (ed.) *Bone Biology and Skeletal Disorders in Poultry.* Poultry Science Symposium Number 23. Carfax Publishing Company, Abingdon, UK, pp. 313–328.

Gregory, N.G. and Wotton, S.B. (1981) Autonomic and non-autonomic control of cardiovascular function in stress-sensitive pigs. *Journal of Veterinary Pharmacology and Therapeutics* 4, 183–191.

Gregory, N.G. and Wotton, S.B. (1984a) Sheep slaughtering procedures. 2. Time to loss of brain responsiveness after exsanguination or cardiac arrest. *British Veterinary Journal* 140, 354–360.

Gregory, N.G. and Wotton, S.B. (1984b) Sheep slaughtering procedures. 3. Head to back electrical stunning. *British Veterinary Journal* 140, 570–575.

Gregory, N.G. and Wotton, S.B. (1986) Effect of slaughter on the spontaneous and evoked activity of the brain. *British Poultry Science* 27, 195–205.

Gregory, N.G. and Wotton, S.B. (1988a) Sheep slaughtering procedures. 5. Responsiveness to potentially painful stimuli following electrical stunning. *British Veterinary Journal* 144, 573–580.

Gregory, N.G. and Wotton, S.B. (1988b) Stunning of chickens. *Veterinary Record* 122, 399.

Gregory, N.G. and Wotton, S.B. (1990) Comparison of neck dislocation and percussion of the head on visual evoked responses in the chicken's brain. *Veterinary Record* 127, 285–287.

Gregory, N.G., Wilkins, L.J. and Gregory, A.M.S. (1988) Studies on blood engorgement in beef carcass. *Journal of the Science of Food and Agriculture* 46, 43–51.

Gregory, N.G., Wood, J.D., Enser, M., Smith, W.C. and Ellis, M. (1980) Fat mobilization in Large White pigs selected for low backfat thickness. *Journal of Science in Food and Agriculture* 31, 567–572.

Gregory, N.G., Wilkins, L.J. and Wotton, S.B. (1991) Effect of electrical stunning frequency on ventricular fibrillation, downgrading and broken bones in broilers, hens and quails. *British Veterinary Journal* 141, 71–77.

Grigor, P.N. Goddard, P.J. and Littlewood, C.A. (1997) The movement of farmed deer through raceways. *Applied Animal Behviour Science* 52, 171–178.

Grizzle, J.M., Chen, J., Williams, J.C. and Spano, J.S. (1992) Skin injuries and serum enzyme activities of channel catfish (*Ictalurus punctatus*) harvested by fish pumps. *Aquaculture* 107, 333–346.

Guise, H.J. and Penny, R.H.C. (1989) Factors influencing the welfare and carcass and meat quality of pigs. 1. The effects of stocking density in transport and the use of electric goads. *Animal Production* 49, 511–515.

Hamdy, H.K. and Barton, N.D. (1965) Fate of *Staphylococcus aureus* in bruised tissue. *Applied Microbiology* 12, 464–469.

Hamm, R. (1975) Water-holding capacity of meat. In: Cole, D.J.A. and Lawrie, R.A. (eds) *Meat.* Butterworths, London, pp. 321–338.

Harris, J.A. (1996) Descending antinociceptive mechanisms in the brainstem: their role in the animal's defensive system. *Journal of Physiology (Paris)* 90, 15–25.

Hattula,T., Luoma, T., Kostianen, R., Poutanen, J., Kallio, M. and Suuronen, P. (1995) Effects of catching method on different quality parameters of Baltic herring. *Fisheries Research* 23, 209–221.

Havenstein, G.B., Ferket, P.R., Scheideler, S.E. and Larson, B.T. 1994. Growth, livability, and feed conversion of 1957 vs 1991 broilers when fed 'typical' 1957 and 1991 broiler diets. *Poultry Science* 73, 1785–1794.

Hawrysh, Z.J., Gifford, S.R. and Price, M.A. (1985) Cooking and eating-quality characteristics of dark-cutting beef from young bulls. *Journal of Animal Science* 60, 682–690.

Heffner, R.S. and Heffner, H.E. (1983) Hearing in large mammals: horse (*Equus caballus*) and cattle (*Bos taurus*). *Behavioral Neuroscience* 97, 299–309.

Heir, S. and Wiig, H. (1988) Subcutaneous interstitial fluid colloid osmotic pressure in dehydrated rats. *Acta Physiologica Scandinavica* 133, 365–371.

Hemphill, R.E. and Grey Walter, W. (1941) The treatment of mental disorders by electrically induced convulsions. *Journal of Mental Sciences* 87, 256–275.

Holmes, J.H.G., Ashmore, C.R. and Robinson, D.W. (1973) Effects of stress on cattle with hereditary muscular hypertrophy. *Journal of Animal Science* 36, 684–694.

Holtz, E., Skjoldebrand, C., Jagerstad, M., Laser Reutersward, A. and Isberg, P.-E. (1985) Effect of recipes on crust formation and mutagenicity in meat products during baking. *Journal of Food Technology* 20, 57–66.

Hosobuchi, Y. (1986) Subcortical electrical stimulation for control of intractable pain in humans. *Journal of Neurosurgery* 64, 543–553.

Jacobs, J.A., Field, R.A., Botkin, M.P. and Riley, M.L. (1973) Effect of dietary stress on lamb carcass composition and quality. *Journal of Animal Science* 36, 507–510.

James, N.T. and Cabric, M. (1981) Quantitative studies on the numerical frequency of myonuclei in the mueckes of exercised rats: evidence against the occurrence of fibre-splitting. *British Journal of Experimental Pathology* 62, 600–605.

Janig, W. (1979) Reciprocal reaction patterns of sympathetic subsystems with respect to various afferent inputs. In: Brooks, C.McC., Koizumi, K. and Sato, A. (eds) *Integrative Functions of the Autonomic Nervous System.* University of Tokyo Press, Japan, pp. 263–274.

Janssens, J.J.G., Helmond, F.A. and Wiegant, V.M. (1994) Increased cortisol response to exogenous adrenocorticotropic hormone in chronically stressed pigs: influence of housing conditions. *Journal of Animal Science* 72, 1771–1777.

Jarrett, I.G., Filsell, O.H. and Ballard, F.J. (1976) Utilization of oxidizable substrates by the sheep hind limb: effects of starvation and exercise. *Metabolism* 25, 523–531.

Jensen, J.F. (1976) The influence of transportation on slaughter quality of broilers. *Proceedings of the 5th European Poultry Conference. World's Poultry Science Association* 2, 698–705.

Jeremiah, L.E., Newman, J.A., Tong, A.K.W. and Gibson, L.L. (1988a) The effects of castration, preslaughter stress and Zeranol implants on beef: Part 1 – The texture of loin steaks from bovine males. Meat Science 22, 83–101.

Jeremiah, L.E., Newman, J.A., Tong, A.K.W. and Gibson, L.L. (1988b) The effects of castration, preslaughter stress and Zeranol implants on beef: Part 2 – Cooking properties and flavor of loin steaks from bovine males. *Meat Science* 22, 103–121.

Johansson, G., Olsson, K., Haggendal, J. and Thoren-Tolling, K. (1982) Effect of stress on myocardial cells and blood levels of catecholamines in normal and amygdalectomized pigs. *Canadian Journal of Comparative Medicine* 46, 176–182.

Jones, S.D.M., Schaefer, A.L., Robertson, W.M. and Vincent, B.C. (1990) The effects of withholding feed and water on carcass shrinkage and meat quality in beef cattle. *Meat Science* 28, 131–139.

Jones, S.D.M., Greer, G.G., Jeremiah, L.E., Murray, A.C. and Robertson, W.M. (1991) Cryogenic chilling of pork carcasses: effects on muscle quality, bacterial populations and palatability. *Meat Science* 29, 1–16.

Joseph, K.J., Awosanya, B. and Adebua, B.A. (1994) The effects of preslaughter withholding of feed and water from rabbits on their carcass yield and meat quality. *Nigerian Journal of Animal Production* 21, 164–169.

Joubert, J.P.J., Marais, P.G. and Smith, F.J.C. (1985) Ovine wet carcass syndrome induced by water deprivation and subsequent overhydration. *Journal of the South African Veterinary Association* 56, 17–19.

Kellert, S.R. (1988) Human–animal interactions: a review of American attitudes to wild and domestic animals in the twentieth century. In: Rowan A.N. (ed.) *Animals and People Sharing the World.* University Press of New England, Hanover, New Hampshire, USA, pp. 137–175.

Kellert, S.R. (1993) Attitudes, knowledge and behaviour towards wildlife among the Industrial Superpowers: United States, Japan and Germany. *Journal of Social Issues*, 49, 53–69.

Kenny, F.J. and Tarrant, P.V. (1988) The effect of oestrus behaviour on muscle glycogen concentration and dark-cutting in beef heifers. *Meat Science* 22, 21–31.

Kent, J.E. and Ewbank, R. (1983) The effect of road transportation on the blood constituents and behaviour of calves. 1. Six months old. *British Veterinary Journal* 139, 228–235.

Kestin, S.C., Knowles, T.G., Tinch, A.E. and Gregory, N.G. (1992) Prevalence of leg weakness in broiler chickens and its relationship with genotype. *Veterinary Record* 131, 190–194.

Kettlewell, P., Mitchell, M. and Meehan, A. (1993) The distribution of thermal loads within poultry transport vehicles. *Agricultural Engineer* 48(1), 26–30.

Khan, A.W. and Nakamura, R. (1970) Effects of pre- and post-mortem glycolysis on poultry tenderness. *Journal of Food Science* 35, 266–267.

Kilgour, R. and Dalton, D.C. (1984) *Livestock Behaviour.* University of New South Wales Press, Sydney, Australia. 320pp.

Kirton, A.H. and Frazerhurst, L.F. (1983) Effects of normal, light/normal or double stunning on the incidence and severity of blood splash in lambs. *Meat Science* 8, 1–6.

Kirton, A.H., Moss, R.A. and Taylor, A.G. (1971) Weight losses from milk and weaned lamb in mid Canterbury resulting from different lengths of starvation before slaughter. *New Zealand Journal of Agricultural Research* 14, 149–160.

Kirton, A.H., Woods, E.G. and Smith, B.L. (1976) Facial eczema and the palatability of meat from yearling sheep. *New Zealand Journal of Agricultural Research* 19, 193–196.

Kirton, A.H., Frazerhurst, L.F., Woods, E.G. and Chrystall, B.B. (1980/81) Effect of electrical stunning method and cardiac arrest on bleeding efficiency, residual blood and blood splash in lambs. *Meat Science* 5, 347–353.

Knapp, B.G. and Newell, G.W. (1961) Effect of selected factors on feather removal in chickens. *Poultry Science* 40, 510–517.

Knowles, T.G. and Broom, D.M. (1990) The handling and transport of broilers and spent hens. *Applied Animal Behaviour Science* 28, 75–91.

Knowles, T.G., Warriss, P.D., Brown, S.N., Kestin, S.C., Rhind, S.M., Edwards, J.E., Anil, M.H. and Dolan, S.K. (1993) Long distance transport of lambs and the time needed for subsequent recovery. *Veterinary Record* 133, 286–293.

Knowles, T.G., Warriss, P.D., Brown, S.N. and Kestin, S.C. (1994) Long distance transport of export lambs. *Veterinary Record* 134, 107–110.

Knowles, T.G., Brown, S.N., Warriss, P.D., Phillips, A.J., Dolan, S.K., Hunt, P., Ford, J.E., Edwards, J.E. and Watkins, P.E. (1995) Effects on sheep of transport by road for up to 24 hours. *Veterinary Record* 136, 431–438.

Koohmaraie, M., Wheeler, T.L. and Shackelford, S.D. (1995) Beef tenderness: regulation and prediction. In: *Meat '95. Australian Meat Industry Research Conference, Gold Coast.* CSIRO Division of Food Science & Technology, Brisbane, Australia, pp. 4A1–4A10.

Lambooy, E. (1985) Electro-anesthesia or electroimmobilization of calves, sheep and pigs by Feenix Stockstill. *Veterinary Quarterly* 7, 120–126.

Larsen, H.K. (1982) Comparison of 300 volt manual stunning, 700 volt automatic stunning and CO_2 Compact stunning, with respect to quality parameters, blood splashing, fractures and meat quality. In: G. Eikelenboom (ed.) *Stunning of Animals for Slaughter.* Martinus Nijhoff, The Hague, The Netherlands, pp. 73–81.

Lay, D.C., Friend, T.H. and Randel, R.D. (1991) Behavioral and physiological effects of freeze and hot branding on cross-bred cattle. *Journal of Animal Science* 70, 330–336.

Lay, D.C., Friend, T.H., Randel, R.D., Jenkins, O.C., Neuendorff, D.A., Kapp, G.M. and Bushong, D.M. (1996) Adrenocorticotropic hormone dose response and some physiological effects of transportation on pregnant Brahman cattle. *Journal of Animal Science* 74, 1806–1811.

Lee, G.T. (1986) Growth and carcass characteristics of ram cryptorchid and wether Border Leicester × Merino lambs: effects of increasing carcass weight. *Australian Journal of Experimental Agriculture* 26, 153–157.

Lee, Y.B., Hargus, G.L., Hagberg, E.C. and Forsythe, R.H. (1976) Effect of ante-mortem environmental temperature on post-mortem glycolysis and tenderness in excised broiler breast muscle. *Journal of Food Science* 41, 1466–1469.

Leet, N.G., Devine, C.E. and Gavey, A.B. (1977) The histology of blood splash in lambs. *Meat Science* 1, 229–234.

Leigh, P. and Delany, M. (1987) Use of 'thoracic stick' in halal slaughter of bobby calves *New Zealand Veterinary Journal* 35, 124–125.

Le Neindre, P., Boivin, X. and Boissy, A. (1996) Handling of extensively kept animals. *Applied Animal Behaviour Science* 49, 73–81.

Lester, S.J., Mellor, D.J., Holmes, R.J., Ward, R.N. and Stafford, K.J. (1996) Behavioural and cortisol responses of lambs to castration and tailing using different methods. *New Zealand Veterinary Journal* 44, 45–54.

Levinger, I.M. and Angel, S. (1977) Effect of spinal cord transection on feather release in the slaughtered broiler. *British Poultry Science* 18, 169–172.

Lewis, P.K., Heck, M.C. and Brown, C.J. (1961) Effect of stress from electrical stimulation and sugar on the chemical composition of swine carcasses. *Journal of Animal Science* 20, 727–733.

Lewis, P.K., Brown, C.J. and Heck, M.C. (1962) Effect of stress on certain pork carcass characteristics and eating quality. *Journal of Animal Science* 21, 196–199.

Lewis, P.K., Brown, C.J. and Heck, M.C. (1967) Effect of ante-mortem stress and freezing immediately after slaughter on certain organoleptic and chemical characteristics of pork. *Journal of Animal Science* 26, 1276–1282.

Lister, D. and Spencer, G.S.G. (1983) Energy substrate provision *in vivo* and the changes in muscle pH post mortem. *Meat Science* 8, 41–51.

Lister, D., Sair, R.A., Will, J.A., Schmidt, G.R., Casens, R.G., Hoekstra, W.G. and Briskey, E.J. (1970) Metabolism of striated muscle of stress-susceptible pigs breathing oxygen or nitrogen. *American Journal of Physiology* 218, 102–107.

Lister, D., Gregory, N.G. and Warriss, P.D. (1982) Stress in meat animals. In: Lawrie, R.A. (ed.) *Developments in Meat Science* 2, Applied Science Publishers, London, pp. 62–92.

Long, V.P. and Tarrant, P.V. (1990) The effect of pre-slaughter showering and post-slaughter rapid chilling on meat quality in intact pork sides. *Meat Science* 27, 181–195.

Love, R.M. (1988) *The Food Fishes.* Farrand Press, London, 276 pp.

Love, R.M., Robertson, I., Smith, G.L. and Whittle, K.J. (1974) The texture of cod muscle. *Journal of Texture Studies* 5, 201–212.

Lowe, T.E. and Wells, R.M.G. (1996) Primary and secondary stress responses to line capture in the blue mao mao. *Journal of Fish Biology* 49, 287–300.

Loye, P. (1887) Recherches expérimentales sur la mort par la décapitation. PhD thesis, Laboratoire de physiologie de la Sorbonne, Faculté de Médicine de Paris, 105 pp.

Lyon, B.G. and Lyon, C.E. (1986) Surface dark spotting and bone discoloration in fried chicken. *Poultry Science* 65, 1915–1918.

Mackey, B.M. and Derrick, C.M. (1979) Contamination of the deep tissues of carcasses by bacteria present on the slaughter instruments or in the gut. *Journal of Applied Bacteriology* 46, 355–366.

Martrenchar, A., Morisse, J.P., Huonnic, D. and Cotte, J.P. (1997) Influence of stocking density on some behavioural, physiological and productivity traits of broilers. *Veterinary Research* 28, 473–480.

Marx, H., Brunner, B., Weinzierl, W., Hoffmann, R. and Stolle, A. (1997) Methods of stunning freshwater fish: impact on meat quality and aspects of animal welfare. *Zeitschrift fur Lebensmittel Untersuchung und Forschung* 204, 282–286.

Mayer, D.J. and Liebeskind, J.C. (1974) Pain reduction by focal electrical stimulation of the brain: an anatomical and behavioral analysis. *Brain Research* 68, 73–93.

McDaniel, A.H. and Roark, C.B. (1956) Performance and grazing habits of Hereford and Aberdeen Angus cows and calves on improved pastures as related to types of shade. *Journal of Animal Science* 15, 59–63.

McLoughlin, J.V. (1970) Muscle contraction and post-mortem pH changes in pig skeletal muscle. *Journal of Food Science* 35, 717–719.

McLoughlin, J.V. (1974) Curare and post-mortem changes in skeletal muscle of Piétrain pigs. *Proceedings of the Royal Irish Academy* 74B, 305–312.

McLoughlin, J.V., Tarrant, P.V. and Harrington, M.G. (1973) The effects of contraction and ischaemia on creatine phosphate and adenosine triphosphate in *m. semitendinosus* of the pig. *Proceedings of the Royal Irish Academy* 73B, 95–108.

McNally, P.W. and Warriss, P.D. (1996) Recent bruising in cattle at abattoirs. *Veterinary Record* 138, 126–128.

McVeigh, J.M. and Tarrant, P.V. (1981) The breakdown of muscle glycogen during behavioural stress in normal and beta-adrenoreceptor blocked young bulls. In: Hood, D.E. and Tarrant, P.V. (eds) *The Problem of Dark-cutting in Beef.* Martinus Nijhoff Publishers, The Hague, The Netherlands, pp. 430–453.

Melton, S.L., Black, J.M., Davis, G.W. and Backus, W.R. (1982) Flavor and selected chemical components of ground beef from steers backgrounded on pasture and fed corn up to 140 days. *Journal of Food Science* 47, 699–704.

Merkel, R.A. (1971) Processing and organoleptic properties of normal and PSE porcine muscle. In: Hessel-de Heer, J.C.M., Schmidt, G.R., Sybesma, W. and van der Wal, P.G. (eds) *Proceedings of the 2nd International Symposium on Condition and Meat Quality of Pigs.* Centre for Agricultural Publishing and Documentation, Wageningen, The Netherlands, pp. 261–270.

Mitchell, G., Hattingh, J. and Ganhao, M. (1988) Stress in cattle after handling, transport and slaughter. *Veterinary Record* 123, 201–205.

Mohan Raj, Gregory, N.G. and Wilkins, L.J. (1992) Survival rate and carcass downgrading after the stunning of broilers with carbon dioxide–argon mixtures. *Veterinary Record* 130, 325–328.

Monin, G. (1981) Muscle metabolic type and the DFD condition. In: Hood, D.E. and Tarrant, P.V. (eds) *The Problem of Dark-cutting in Beef.* Martinus Nijhoff Publishers, The Hague, The Netherlands, pp. 63–85.

Moran, E.T. and Bilgili, S.F. (1990) Influence of feeding and fasting broilers prior to marketing on cecal access of orally administered *Salmonella. Journal of Food Protection* 53, 205–207.

Murray, A.C. and Jones, S.D.M. (1994) The effect of mixing, feed restriction and genotype with respect to stress susceptibility on pork carcass and meat quality. *Canadian Journal of Animal Science* 74, 587–594.

Newhook, J.C. and Blackmore, D.K. (1982) Electroencephalographic studies of stunning and slaughter of sheep and calves – Part 2: The onset of permanent insensibility in calves during slaughter. *Meat Science* 6, 295–300.

Newton, K.G. and Gill, C.O. (1978) Storage quality of dark, firm, dry meat. *Applied and Environmental Microbiology* 36, 375–376.

Newton, K.G. and Gill, C.O. (1980) Control of spoilage in vacuum packaged dark, firm, dry (DFD) meat. *Journal of Food Technology* 15, 227–234.

Nicol, D.J., Shaw, M.K. and Ledward, D.A. (1970) Hydrogen sulfide production by bacteria and sulfmyoglobin formation in prepacked chilled beef. *Applied Microbiology* 19, 937–939.

Nielsen, N.J. (1977) The influence of pre-slaughter treatment on meat quality in pigs. *Slagteriernes Forskningsinstitut Svin Kodvalitet MS. Nr. 561E*, Danish Meat Research Institute, Roskilde, Denmark, 14 pp.

Nielsen N.J. (1981) The effect of environmental factors on meat quality and on deaths during transportation and lairage before slaughter. In: Frøystein, T., Slinde, E. and Standal, N. (eds) *Porcine Stress and Meat Quality*. Agricultural Food Research Society, Ås, Norway, pp. 287–297.

Northcutt, J.K., Foegeding, E.A. and Edens, F.W. (1994) Water-holding properties of thermally preconditioned chicken breast and leg meat. *Poultry Science* 73, 308–316.

Olsson, U., Wahlgren, N.M. and Tornberg, E. (1995) The influence of preslaughter stress on muscle shortening, isometric tension and meat tenderness of beef. *Proceedings of the 41st International Congress of Meat Science and Technology*, San Antonio, USA. E–36, 614–615.

Ørtenblad, N., Madsen, K. and Djurhuus, M.S. (1977) Antioxidant status and lipid peroxidation after short-term maximal exercise in trained and untrained humans. *American Journal of Physiology* 272, R1258–R1263.

Oude Ophuis, P.A.M. (1994) Sensory evaluation of 'free range' and regular pork meat under different conditions of experience and awareness. *Food Quality and Preference* 5, 173–178.

Papa, C.M. (1991) Lower gut contents of broiler chickens withdrawn from feed and held in cages. *Poultry Science* 70, 375–380.

Papinaho, P.A. and Fletcher, D.L. (1996) The effect of stunning and deboning time on early rigor development and breast meat quality of broilers. *Poultry Science* 75,672–676.

Papinaho, P.A., Fletcher, D.L. and Buhr, R.J. (1995) Effect of electrical stunning amperage and peri-mortem struggle on broiler breast rigor development and meat quality. *Poultry Science* 74, 1533–1539.

Park, R.J., Corbett, J.L. and Furnival, E.P. (1972) Flavour differences in meat from lambs grazed on lucerne (*Medicago sativa*) or phalaris (*Phalaris tuberosa*) pastures. *Journal of Agricultural Science* 78, 47–52.

Parrott, R.F., Misson, B.H. and Delariva, C.F. (1994) Differential stressor effects on the concentration of cortisol, prolactin and catecholamines in the blood of sheep. *Research in Veterinary Science* 56, 234–239.

Pascoe, P.J. (1986) Humaneness of an electroimmobilization unit for cattle. *American Journal of Veterinary Research* 10, 2252–2256.

Petersen, G.V. (1978) Factors associated with wounds and bruises in lambs. *New Zealand Veterinary Journal* 26, 6–9.

Petersen, G.V. (1983) Preslaughter and slaughter factors affecting meat quality in lambs. PhD thesis, Massey University, Palmerston North, New Zealand, 219 pp.

Petersen, G.V. (1984) Cross-sectional studies of ultimate pH in lambs. *New Zealand Veterinary Journal* 32, 51–57.

Petersen, G.V., Carr, D.H., Davies, A.S. and Pickett, B.T. (1986) The effect of different methods of electrical stunning of lambs on blood pressure and muscular activity. *Meat Science* 16, 1–15.

Pethick, D.W. and Rowe, J.B. (1996) The effect of nutrition and exercise on carcass parameters and the level of glycogen in skeletal muscle of Merino sheep. *Australian Journal of Agricultural Research* 47, 525–537.

Petrie, N.J., Mellor, D.J., Stafford, K.J., Bruce, R.A. and Ward, R.N. (1995) Cortisol responses of calves to two methods of disbudding used with or without local anaesthetic. *New Zealand Veterinary Journal* 44, 9–14.

Puolanne, E. and Aalto, H. (1981) The incidence of dark-cutting beef in young bulls in Finland. In: Hood, D.E. and Tarrant, P.V. (eds) *The Problem of Dark-cutting in Beef.* Martinus Nijhoff Publishers, The Hague, The Netherlands, pp. 462–475.

Purchas, R.W. (1990) An assessment of the role of pH differences in determining the relative tenderness of meat from bulls and steers. *Meat Science* 27, 129–140.

Purchas, R.W. and Aungsupakorn, R. (1993) Further investigations into the relationship between ultimate pH and tenderness for beef samples from bulls and steers. *Meat Science* 34, 163–178.

Purchas, R.W. and Grant, D.A. (1995) Liveweight gain and carcass characterstics of bulls and steers farmed on hill country. *New Zealand Journal of Agricultural Research* 38, 131–142.

Puron, D., Santamaria, R., Segura, J.C. and Alamilla, J.L. (1995) Broiler performance at different stocking densities. *Journal of Applied Poultry Research* 4, 55–60.

Quass, D.W. and Briskey, E.J. (1968) A study of certain properties of myosin from skeletal muscle. *Journal of Food Science* 33, 180–187.

Radak, Z., Asano, K., Inoue, M., Kizaki, T., Oh-Ishi, S., Suzuki, K., Taniguchi, N. and Ohno, H. (1995) Superoxide dismutase derivative reduces oxidative damage in skeletal muscle of rats during exhaustive exercise. *Journal of Applied Physiology* 79, 129–135.

Raj, A.B.M., Wilkins, L.J., Richardson, R.I.R., Johnson, S.P. and Wotton, S.B. (1997) Carcase and meat quality in broilers either killed with a gas mixture or stunned with an electric current under commercial conditions. *British Poultry Science* 38, 169–174.

Ramsgaard Jensen, L. and Oksama, M. (1996) Influence of different housing systems on carcass and meat quality in young bulls. In: Hildrum, K.I. (ed.) *Proceedings 42nd International Congress of Meat Science and Technology*, Norway, pp. 436–437.

Randall, J.M., Stiles, M.A., Geers, R., Schutte, A., Christensen, L. and Bradshaw, R.H. (1996) Vibration on pig transporters: implications for reducing stress. In: Schutte, A. (ed.) *Proceedings of EU Seminar New Information on Welfare and Meat Quality of Pigs as Related to Handling, Transport and Lairage Conditions.* Landbauforschung Volkenrode, 166, 143–160.

Reiland, S. (1975) *Osteochondrosis in the Pig.* Akademisk Avhandling, Stockholm, Sweden, 118 pp.

Richards, R.B., Hyder, M.W., Fry, J., Norris, R.T. and Higgs, A.R.B. (1991) Seasonal metabolic factors may be responsible for deaths in sheep exported by sea. *Australian Journal of Agricultural Research* 42, 215–226.

Richardson, N.J., Shepherd, R. and Elliman, N.A. (1993) Current attitudes and future influences on meat consumption in the United Kingdom. *Appetite* 21, 41–51.

Riches, H., Guise, J. and Penny, R. (1996) Preliminary investigation of frequency of vomiting by pigs in transport. *Veterinary Record* 139, 428.

Roberts, T.A. (1980) The effects of slaughter practices on the bacteriology of the red meat carcass. *Royal Society of Health Journal* 100, 3–10.

Rollin, B.E. (1997) Animal ethics, social change, and the meat industry. In: Bass, J. (ed.) *Proceedings of the 43rd International Congress of Meat Science and Technology*, pp. 140–142.

Rossen, R., Kabat, H. and Anderson, J.P. (1943) Acute arrest of cerebral circulation in man. *Archives of Neurology and Psychiatry* 50, 510–528.

Roy, O.Z., Trollope, B.J. and Scott, J.R. (1987) Measurement of regional cardiac fibrillation thresholds. *Medical and Biological Engineering and Computing* 25, 165–166.

Rushen, J. (1986) Aversion of sheep to electro-immobilization and physical restraint. *Applied Animal Behaviour Science* 15, 315.

Sainsbury, J.C. (1971) *Commercial Fishing methods: an Introduction to Vessels and Gears.* Fishing News Books, West Byfleet, UK, 119 pp.

Sair, R.A., Lister, D., Moody, W.G., Cassens, R.G., Hoekstra, W.G. and Briskey, E.J. (1970) Action of curare and magnesium sulphate on striated muscle of stress-susceptible pigs. *American Journal of Physiology* 218, 108–114.

Saito, M., Mano, T. and Iwase, S. (1989) Sympathetic nerve activity related to local fatigue sensation during static contraction. *Journal of Applied Physiology* 67, 980–984.

Salminen, A., Hongisto, K. and Vihto, V. (1984) Lysosomal changes related to exercise injuries and training-induced protection in mouse skeletal muscle. *Acta Physiologica Scandinavica* 120, 15–19.

Sayre, R.N. (1963) Effect of excitement, fasting and sucrose feeding on porcine muscle phosphorylase and post-mortem glycolysis. *Journal of Food Science* 28, 472–477.

Sayre, R.N., Briskey, E.J., Hoekstra, W.G. and Bray, R.W. (1961) Effect of preslaughter change to a cold environment on characteristics of pork muscle. *Journal of Animal Science* 20, 487–492.

Sayre, R.N., Kiernat, B. and Briskey, E.J. (1964) Processing characteristics of porcine muscle related to pH and temperature during rigor mortis development and to gross morphology 24 hr post-mortem. *Journal of Food Science* 29, 175–181.

Scholtyssek, S., Ehinger, F. and Loman, F. (1977) Einfluß von transport und nuchterung auf die schlachtkorperqualitet von broilern. *Archiv für Geflügelkunde* 41, 27–30.

Schoonderwoerd, M., Doige, C.E., Wobeser, G.A. and Naylor, J.M. (1986) Protein energy malnutrition and fat mobilization in neonatal calves. *Canadian Veterinary Journal* 27, 365–371.

Schuppel, H., Salchert, F. and Schuppel, K.-F. (1996) Investigations into the influence of mastitis and other organ changes on microbial contamination of the meat of slaughter cows. *Fleischwirtschaft* 76, 61–64.

Selwyn, P. and Hathaway, S. (1990) A study of the prevalence and economic significance of diseases and defects of slaughtered farmed deer. *New Zealand Veterinary Journal* 38, 94–97.

Sensky, P.L., Parr, T., Bardsley, R.G. and Buttery, P.J. (1996) The relationship between plasma epinephrine concentration and the activity of the calpain enzyme system in porcine longissimus muscle. *Journal of Animal Science* 74, 380–387.

Shanawany, M.M. (1988) Broiler performance under high stocking densities. *British Poultry Science* 29, 43–52.

Sheally, C.N., Mortimer, J.T. and Hagfors, N.R. (1970) Dorsal column electroanalgesia. *Journal of Neurosurgery* 32, 560–564.

Sigholt, T., Erikson, V., Rustad, T., Johansen, S., Nordtvedt, T.S. and Seland, A. (1997) Handling stress and storage temperature affect quality of farm-raised Atlantic Salmon (*Salmo salar*). *Journal of Food Science* 62, 898–905.

Smith, W.C. and Lesser, D. (1982) An economic assessment of pale, soft, exudative musculature in the fresh and cured pig carcass. *Animal Production* 34, 291–299.

Stafford, K.J. and Mellor, D.J. (1993) Castration, tail docking and dehorning – What are the constraints? *Proceedings of the New Zealand Society of Animal Production* 53, 189–194.

Stawicki, S., Niewiarowicz, A. and Trojan, M. (1976) Effect of pH_1 value on the microflora of chicken meat. In: *Proceedings of the 5th European Poultry Conference. World's Poultry Science Association* 2, 832–839.

Stermer, R., Cramp, T.H. and Stevens, D.D. (1981) *Feeder Cattle Stress during Transportation.* Paper No. 81–6001. American Society of Agricultural Engineers, St Josephs, Missouri, USA, 5 pp.

Stevens, D.A. and Gerzog-Thomas, D.A. (1977) Fright reactions in rats to conspecific tissue. *Physiological Behavior* 18, 47.

Summers, J.D. and Leeson, S. (1979) Comparison of feed withdrawal time and passage of gut contents in broiler chickens held in crates or litter pens. *Canadian Journal of Animal Science* 59, 63–66.

Suuronen, P., Erickson, D.L. and Orrensalo, A. (1996) Mortality of herring escaping from pelagic trawl codends. *Fisheries Research* 25, 305–321.

Sybesma, W. and Groen, W. (1970) Stunning procedures and meat quality. *Proceedings of the 16th European Meeting of the Meat Research Workers*, pp. 341–350.

Tanida, H., Miura, A., Tanaka, T. and Yoshimoto, T. (1995) Behavioural response to humans in individually handled weanling pigs. *Applied Animal Behaviour Science* 42, 249–259.

Tarr, H.L.A. (1966) Post-mortem changes in glycogen, nucleotides, sugar phosphates, and sugars in fish muscles – a review. *Journal of Food Science* 31, 846–854.

Tarrant, P.V. (1989a) The effects of handling, transport, slaughter and chilling on meat quality and yield in pigs – a review. *Irish Journal of Food Science and Technology* 13, 79–107.

Tarrant, P.V. (1989b) Animal behaviour and environment in the dark-cutting condition. In: Fabiansson, S.U., Shorthose, W.R. and Warner, R.D. (eds) *Dark-cutting in Cattle and Sheep, Proceedings of an Australian Workshop.* Australian Meat & Livestock Research & Development Corporation, Sydney, pp. 8–18.

Tarrant, P.V. and Grandin, T. (1993) Cattle transport. In: Grandin T. (ed.) *Livestock Handling and Transport.* CAB International, Wallingford, UK, pp. 109–126.

Tarrant, P.V., McLoughlin, J.V. and Harrington, M.G. (1972) Anaerobic glycolysis in biopsy and post-mortem porcine *longissimus dorsi* muscle. *Proceedings of the Royal Irish Academy* 72B, 55–73.

Thomson, J.E., Lyon, C.E., Hamm, D., Dickens, J.A., Fletcher, D.L. and Shackelford, A.D. (1986) Effects of electrical stunning and hot deboning on broiler breast meat quality. *Poultry Science* 65, 1715–1719.

Thornton, R.N. (1983) The aging of bruises in lambs. PhD thesis, Massey University, Palmerston North, New Zealand, 229 pp.

Troeger, K. and Woltersdorf, W. (1991) Gas anaesthesia of slaughter pigs. *Fleischwirtschaft* 71, 1063–1068.

Trout, G.R. (1989) Variation in myoglobin denaturation and color of cooked beef, pork, and turkey meat as influenced by pH, sodium chloride, sodium tripolyphosphate, and cooking temperature. *Journal of Food Science* 54, 536–544.

Trunkfield, H.R., Broom, D.M., Maatje, K., Wierenga, H.K., Lambooy, E. and Kooijman, J. (1991) Effects of housing on responses of veal calves to handling and transport. In: Metz, J.H.M. and Groenestein, C.M. (eds) *New Trends in Veal Calf Production.* Pudoc, Wageningen, The Netherlands, pp. 40–43.

Tume, R.K. and Shaw, F.D. (1992) Beta-endorphin and cortisol concentrations in plasma of blood samples collected during exsanguination of cattle. *Meat Science* 31, 211–217.

Twigg, J. (1979) Food for thought: purity and vegetarianism. *Religion* 9, 13–35.

van der Wal, P.G. (1976) Bone fractures in pigs as a consequence of electrical stunning. *Proceedings of the 22nd European Meeting of the Meat Research Workers,* C3, 1–4.

van Putten, G. and Elshof, W.J. (1978) Observations on the effects of transport on the well being and lean quality of slaughter pigs. *Animal Regulation Studies* 1, 247–271.

Vieville-Thomas, C. and Signoret, J.T. (1992) Pheromonal transmission of an aversive experience in domestic pigs. *Journal of Chemical Endocrinology* 18, 1551.

Voisinet, B.D., Grandin, T., O'Connor, S.F.O., Tatum, J.D. and Deesing, M.J. (1997) *Bos indicus*-cross feedlot cattle with excitable temperaments have tougher meat and a higher incidence of borderline dark cutters. *Meat Science* 46, 367–377.

von Zweigbergk, A.-J., Lundstrom, K. and Hansson, I. (1989) The incidence of high internal reflectance 45 minutes PM with different stunning methods. In: *Proceedings of the 35th International Congress of Meat Science and Technology,* Copenhagen, Denmark, pp. 1145–1148.

Warriss, P.D. (1982) Loss of carcass weight, liver weight and liver glycogen, and the effects on muscle glycogen and ultimate pH in pigs fasted pre-slaughter. *Journal of the Science of Food and Agriculture* 33, 840–846.

Warriss, P.D. (1984) The behaviour and blood profile of bulls which produce dark-cutting meat. *Journal of the Science of Food and Agriculture* 35, 863–868.

Warriss, P.D. (1987) Liver glycogen in slaughtered pigs and estimated time of fasting before slaughter. *British Veterinary Journal* 143, 354–360.

Warriss, P.D. (1989) The relationships between glycogen stores and muscle ultimate pH in commercially slaughtered pigs. *British Veterinary Journal* 145, 378–383.

Warriss, P.D. (1994) Animal handling. *Meat Focus International* 3, 167–172.

Warriss, P.D. and Bevis, E.A. (1987) Liver glycogen in slaughtered pigs and estimated time of fasting before slaughter. *British Veterinary Journal* 143, 354–360.

Warriss, P.D. and Lister, D.L. (1982) Improvement of meat quality in pigs by β-adrenergic blockade. *Meat Science* 7, 183–187.

Warriss, P.D. and Wotton, S.B. (1981) Effect of cardiac arrest on exsanguination in pigs. *Research in Veterinary Science* 31, 82–86.

Warriss, P.D., Kestin, S.C., Brown, S.N. and Wilkins, L.J. (1984) The time required for recovery from mixing stress in young bulls and the prevention of dark-cutting beef. *Meat Science* 10, 53–68.

Warriss, P.D., Kestin, S.C., Brown, S.N. and Bevis, E.A. (1988) Depletion of glycogen reserves in fasting broiler chickens. *British Poultry Science* 29, 149–154.

Warriss, P.D., Bevis, E.A. and Ekins, P.J. (1989) The relationship between glycogen stores and muscle, ultimate pH in commercially slaughtered pigs. *British Veterinary Journal* 154, 375–383.

Warriss, P.D., Bevis, E.A., Edwards, J.E., Brown, S.N. and Knowles, T.G. (1991) Effect of the angle of slope on the ease with which pigs negotiate loading ramps. *Veterinary Record* 128, 419–421.

Warriss, P.D., Kestin, S.C., Brown, S.N., Knowles, T.G., Wilkins, L.J., Edwards, J.E., Austin, S.D. and Nicol, C.J. (1993) The depletion of glycogen stores and indices of dehydration in transported broilers. *British Veterinary Journal* 149, 391–398.

Warriss, P.D., Brown, S.N., Adams, S.M. and Corlett, I.K. (1994) Relationships between subjective objective assessments of stress at slaughter and meat quality in pigs. *Meat Science* 38, 329–340.

Warriss, P.D., Brown, S.N., Nute, G.R., Knowles, T.G., Edwards, J.E., Perry, A.M. and Johnson, S.P. (1995) Potential interactions between the effects of preslaughter stress and post-mortem electrical stimulation of the carcasses on meat quality in pigs. *Meat Science* 41, 55–68.

Watson, C.L., Morrow, H.A. and Brill, R.W. (1992) Proteolysis of skeletal muscle in yellowfin tuna (*Thunnus albacares*): evidence of calpain activation. *Comparative Biochemistry and Physiology* 103B, 881–887.

Weeding, C.M., Hunter, E.J., Guise, H.J. and Penny, H.C. (1993) Effects of abattoir and handling systems on stress indicators in pig blood. *Veterinary Record* 133, 10–13.

Wertheimer, A., Celewycz, A., Jaenicke, H., Mortensen, D. and Orsi, J. (1989) Size-related hooking mortality of incidentally caught Chinook Salmon, *Oncorhynchus tshawytscha*. *Marine Fisheries Review* 51, 28–35.

White, R.G., de Shazer, J.A. and Tressler, C.J. (1995) Vocalization and physiological response of pigs during castration with and without a local anesthetic. *Journal of Animal Science* 73, 381–386.

Wittman, W., Ecolan, P., Levasseur, P. and Fernandez, X. (1994) Fasting-induced glycogen depletion in different fibre types of red and white pig muscles – relationship with ultimate pH. *Journal of Science in Food and Agriculture* 66, 257–266.

Wood, C.M., Turner, J.D. and Graham, M.S. (1983) Why do fish die after severe exercise? *Journal of Fish Biology* 22, 189–201.

Worsley, A. and Skrzypiec, G. (1997) Teenage vegetarianism – prevalence, social and cognitive contexts, *Appetite* 30, 151–170.

Wythes, J.R., Shorthose, W.R., Schmidt, G.R. and Davis, C.B. (1980) Effects of various rehydration procedures after a long journey on liveweight, carcasses and muscle properties of cattle. *Australian Journal of Agricultural Research* 31, 849–855.

Young, J.B., Rosa, R.M. and Landsberg, L. (1984) Dissociation of sympathetic nervous system and adrenal medullary responses. *American Journal of Physiology* 247, E35–E40.

Young, L.L., Northcutt, J.K. and Lyon, C.E. (1996) Effect of stunning time and polyphosphates on quality of cooked chicken breast meat. *Poultry Science* 75, 677–681.

Young, O.A., Cruickshank, G.J., MacLean, K.S. and Muir, P.D. (1994) Quality of meat from lambs grazed on seven pasture species in Hawkes Bay. *New Zealand Journal of Agricultural Research* 37, 177–186.

Young, R.F. and Brechner, T. (1986) Electrical stimulation of the brain for relief of intractable pain due to cancer. *Cancer* 57, 1266–1272.

Zavy, M.T., Juniewicz, P.E., Williams, A.P. and von Tungeln, D.L. (1992) Effects of initial restraint, weaning and transport stress on baseline and ACTH stimulated cortisol responses in beef calves of different genotypes. *American Journal of Veterinary Research* 53, 552–557.

Student Assignments

1. There is a line breakdown at a pig abattoir. Discuss all the effects that this could have on animal welfare and on product quality.
2. A farmer runs two flocks of breeding sheep on separate properties. The genetic background of the flocks is the same, and the rams are interchanged. The lambs are slaughtered at the same time of year and under the same circumstances, often being delivered to the same abattoir in the same truck. One flock consistently produces lambs which have blood splash in their carcasses, whereas the other flock does not. Design a series of trials aimed at identifying the cause of the blood splash.
3. A duck processor has been criticized by a government inspector for unloading ducks from transport crates by pulling them out by their necks. The processor has agreed to participate in some research which aims at determining whether handling the birds by the neck is any more or less stressful than other methods. Design a research programme which could be used in this situation.
4. Review the ways in which preslaughter handling of bulls affects their meat quality.
5. A poultry processing company is considering changing from electrical stunning to gas stunning. You have been called in to advise them on the advantages and disadvantages of making the change. Prepare a written report which summarizes the key welfare and quality issues.
6. A pig abattoir does contract killing for a number of bacon factories, wholesale distributors and smallgoods manufacturers. One bacon factory consistently claims that the carcasses it receives are badly bruised. The pigs are sourced from particular growers. Describe how you would set about solving this problem.
7. An animal welfare pressure group has publicly criticized a beef packer

for inhumane handling and slaughtering practices. The criticisms are general and not specific. You have been asked by the manager of the beef packing plant to do a complete independent welfare audit on the practices at the plant. Describe how you would go about this, emphasizing particular features you would examine in detail.

8. Describe the ways in which the sarcoplasmic Ca^{2+} concentration during post-mortem muscle metabolism is likely to be influenced by pre-slaughter factors that affect meat quality.

9. A poultry processing company has received complaints from one of its main customers that there are hockburn and breast blisters in the carcasses. Discuss how the plant could deal with this problem.

10. Prepare a document which discusses the welfare, hygiene and quality issues connected with slaughtering late pregnant cattle, sheep and pigs. Take into account that some animals may give birth whilst in the holding pens, and that some well developed fetuses could be removed at evisceration. Produce a set of recommendations.

Index